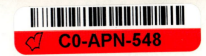

Fundamentals of Monitoring Psychoactive Drug Therapy

Patrick Wong MD

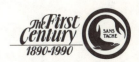

Fundamentals of Monitoring Psychoactive Drug Therapy

C. Lindsay DeVane, Pharm.D., F.C.C.P.

Associate Professor of Pharmacy Practice and Psychiatry
Departments of Pharmacy Practice and Psychiatry
Colleges of Pharmacy and Medicine
University of Florida
Gainesville, Florida

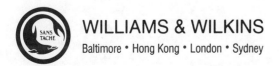

WILLIAMS & WILKINS

Baltimore • Hong Kong • London • Sydney

Editor: John P. Butler
Associate Editor: Linda Napora
Project Editor: Linda Forlifer
Designer: Saturn Graphics
Illustration Planner: Lorraine Wrzosek
Production Coordinator: Barbara J. Felton

Accurate indications, adverse reactions, and dosage schedules for drugs are provided in this book, but it is possible that they may change. The reader is urged to review the package information data of the manufacturers of the medications mentioned.

Printed in the United States of America

Library of Congress Cataloging in Publication Data

DeVane, C. Lindsay.
   Fundamentals of monitoring psychoactive drug therapy / C. Lindsay DeVane.
      p.   cm.
   Includes bibliographies and index.
   ISBN 0-683-02452-3
   1. Mental illness—Chemotherapy.   2. Patient monitoring.   3. Psychopharmacology.   I. Title.
   [DNLM: 1. Mental Disorders—drug therapy.   2. Monitoring, Physiologic.
3. Psychopharmacology.   4. Psychotropic Drugs—therapeutic use.   QV 77 D488f]
RC483.D48 1990
616.89'18—dc20
DNLM/DLC
for Library of Congress   89-14708
                                                                                            CIP

90 91 92 93 94
1   2   3   4   5   6   7   8   9   10

Preface

This book was written for clinicians who monitor patients taking psychoactive drugs, the most widely prescribed medicines in the world. Monitoring means evaluation of the appropriateness of pharmacotherapy for a patient and of the response to therapy, detection of side effects and drug interactions, utilization of plasma concentrations for optimizing therapy with some drugs, and assessment of the appropriate or optimal length of drug therapy. There is a need for all professionals working with the mentally ill (e.g., psychiatrists, family practitioners, clinical pharmacists, nurses, social workers, and psychologists) to have a common knowledge of the factors that influence the selection of pharmacotherapy and the determinants of response. This knowledge should promote appropriate and confident use of psychoactive drugs.

Psychoactive drugs can alter mood, affect psychomotor behavior, and influence thought processes. These effects frequently ameliorate various symptoms of mental illness. The effects of psychoactive drugs are often nonspecific, i.e., they occur regardless of the diagnosis of the patient. For example, sedative-hypnotics may be effective whether the patient has insomnia associated with a mood disorder, an endocrine disorder such as hyperthyroidism, or merely travel-induced sleeplessness. Certain drugs are associated with specific disorders, such as the antidepressants for depressed mood and the antipsychotics for schizophrenia. However, psychoses may be present in a number of mental disorders. Numerous medical disorders are associated with anxiety symptoms. The symptom overlap among various mental illnesses and the broad effects of psychoactive drugs often give the false appearance of an empirical approach to pharmacotherapy in clinical psychopharmacology.

A desirable approach is to identify target symptoms prospectively, select an appropriate psychoactive drug to treat those symptoms, and monitor treatment outcome. By combining an understanding of the time course of drug responses in the body with an appreciation for objective changes in laboratory test results and subjective changes in mental status that drugs can cause, one can objectively monitor psychoactive drug therapy to optimize patient outcome.

The bulk of psychoactive drug prescriptions are written by general medical practitioners. Most clinicians have either received no training in the background areas relevant to clinical psychopharmacology or received instruction in the past when there was little understanding of drug-receptor interactions. Although physicians, and psychiatrists in particular, are most familiar with the presentation of mental illness, their formal training in the principles of pharmacokinetics and pharmacodynamics may be limited. These areas of knowledge are essential for understanding rational dosage regimen design. Similarly, clinical pharmacists and physicians have had training in laboratory test interpretation, but such instruction may not have been included in the training of psychologists and social workers, clinicians who are often in the closest contact with patients and thus in the best position to observe drug-related side effects.

v

The text begins by reviewing some relevant areas of the pharmacological sciences to help in understanding the mechanisms of action and physiological effects of psychoactive drugs. Only fundamental principles are covered, and references are given for the reader who wishes clarification and direction for further study. For clinicians without extensive training in psychiatry, sections on the psychiatric examination and presentation of mental illness have been included. This material is followed by information on the clinical pharmacology of the the major categories of psychoactive drugs. All of the drugs available for use cannot be covered without being encyclopedic. Instead, prototype drug databases are followed by intraclass comparisons to highlight major differences between drugs and refer to alternative pharmacotherapies. This information is derived from observations made in clinical practice and from the psychiatric and psychopharmacology literature. It is hoped that this book will promote the rational use of psychoactive drugs for the benefit of patient care.

Acknowledgments

Numerous individuals influenced my decision to write this book. Michael J. Lynch, M.D., was the first clinician to impress upon me that psychiatry was a scientific discipline. His teaching of the mental status examination led me to pursue an unending path of pharmacy in psychiatry. In various ways, my teachers and colleagues stimulated my interest in clinical science. They include Donald C. McLeod, M.S., William J. Jusko, Ph.D., Ronald B. Stewart, M.S., and Michael A. Schwartz, Ph.D.

The National Fund for Medical Education provided financial support for teaching pharmacokinetic principles in the psychiatric residency program at the University of Florida. I also acknowledge the many psychiatric residents and faculty who brought my attention to interesting cases and participated in our discussions of clinical psychopharmacology.

Finally, several postdoctoral fellows in my laboratory contributed substantially to the atmosphere that motivated the writing of this book. They include Lois J. Birkhimer, Pharm.D., Cynthia S. Dommisse, Pharm.D., and S. Casey Laizure, Pharm.D.

Contents

1

Background of Clinical Psychopharmacology

A

History and Classification of Psychoactive Drugs

Psychoactive drugs have a long and rich history of human use. Evidence of cocaine consumption by Incan civilizations in South America suggest that plants were cultivated for their psychoactive properties as early as 3000 years BC. Extracts of *Rauwolfia*-like plants were used in ancient Hindu medicine in India for a variety of diseases. Cannabis was used in India and China, spreading through Persia to the Arabs, to whom it was known as hashish. It was introduced to Europe and the Americas at about the time of Napoleon. The *U.S. Pharmacopoeia* recognized *Cannabis americana* in a separate monograph in the 1870 edition. Phenobarbital was introduced into therapeutics in 1912. The earliest therapeutic applications of *Rauwolfia*, or reserpine, for psychoses were described in 1931. Until the middle and late 1950s, psychoactive drugs were used essentially for their tranquilizing effects, and then antipsychotics and antidepressants became available for more specific therapeutic use.

Having progressed from the point of using psychoactive drugs primarily for their calming effects on disruptive mental states, modern clinical psychopharmacology is practiced with a better understanding of specific neurochemical changes that drugs evoke. We are still striving to relate these neuropharmacological effects to psychopathology. The mechanisms of psychoactive drug action have been the subject of intense research effort. Unfortunately, none of the psychoactive drugs currently available is curative; their effects are predominantly symptomatic. The symptoms they treat often return when either the medications are discontinued or the episodic nature of the disorders presents as an exacerbation of illness.

The major psychotherapeutic drug classes are listed in Table 1A.1. Within each class there exists one or more prototype drugs with which the other members share common characteristics. Clinicians who monitor psychoactive drug therapy should be familiar with the clinical pharmacology of a prototype drug in each of the major psychotherapeutic categories. Fundamental knowledge about the clinical pharmacology of psychoactive drugs has been divided into 15 topic areas outlined in Table 1A.2. Databases for prototype agents are presented in subsequent chapters. Specialists will find that the scope of these databases is

1

Table 1A.1.
Classification of Psychoactive Drugs

Psychotherapeutic Category	Major Classes	Chemical or Therapeutic Subclass	Prototype Agents
Antidepressants	Cyclic antidepressants	Monocyclics	Bupropion
		Dicyclics	Fluoxetine
		Tricyclics	Amitriptyline, imipramine
		Tetracyclics	Maprotiline
		Heterocyclics	Amoxapine, Trazodone
	Monoamine oxidase inhibitors	Hydrazines	Isocarboxazid, Phenelzine
		Nonhydrazines	Tranylcypromine
	Miscellaneous	Amino acid	L-Tryptophan
Mood stabilizers	Element		Lithium
	Anticonvulsants		Carbamazepine, valproic acid
	Benzodiazepines		Clonazepam
Antipsychotics	Phenothiazines	Aliphatic	Chlorpromazine
		Piperidine	Thioridazine
		Piperazine	Trifluoperazine
	Butyrophenones		Haloperidol
	Thioxanthenes		Thiothixene
	Dihydroindolone		Molindone
	Dibenzoxazepine		Loxapine
Anxiolytics	Benzodiazepines	1,4-substituted	Diazepam
		Triazolo	Alprazolam
	Azaspirode-canediones		Buspirone
Sedative-hypnotics	Benzodiazepines		Flurazepam
	Barbiturates		Secobarbital

narrow, but most clinicians involved in psychoactive drug monitoring should probably have some knowledge about each topic for the major psychoactive drugs routinely encountered in clinical practice. A brief consideration of the history of the major classes of psychoactive drugs (below) illustrates how recent is our pharmacological knowledge of these drugs relative to the length of time psychoactive drugs have been used by humans.

LITHIUM

Lithium was discovered in the early 19th century and was used medicinally for treatment of urinary calculi and gout, as lithium urate was readily water-soluble (1). Mineral water containing lithium was popularly used at health spas. Its use in the United States as a salt substitute for patients with cardiovascular disease in the 1940s abruptly ended with recognition of its toxicity (2). In 1949, the Australian physician John Cade published the first report describing lithium's favorable effects in the treatment of mania (3). Subsequent reports con-

Table 1A.2.
Prototype Database for Psychoactive Drugs

Topic	Discussion
Formulations	Available dosage forms (tablet, capsule, oral solution, etc.), strength, trade names, and manufacturers
Basic pharmacology	Predominant pharmacological actions of the drug, effects on neurotransmitters, relative potency, presumed mechanism of action
Pharmacokinetic properties	A description of the drug's absorption, distribution, metabolism, elimination characteristics, and other relevant data (plasma protein binding, parameters in physically healthy patients or normal volunteers)
Indications	FDA-approved indications; unapproved uses, comparative efficacy data with other drugs in the same category
Dosage regimen design	Initial dosing rate, titration, duration of therapy; maintenance therapy; discontinuation of therapy
Therapeutic drug monitoring	Therapeutic and toxic drug concentration ranges in plasma or serum; blood sampling considerations
Contraindications, warnings, precautions	Conditions or situations that may affect pharmacotherapy
Drug interactions	Information on drug-drug and drug-lab interactions
Adverse reactions	Description, incidence, and management of side effects, clinical laboratory monitoring
Management of overdose	Signs and symptoms, treatment, and the value, if any, of monitoring plasma concentrations
Use in renal and/or hepatic disease	Pharmacokinetic and dynamic considerations pertinent to use when these conditions are present
Use in children and adolescents	Differences that may exist between adults and children in indications, dosing, therapeutic concentration ranges, and pharmacokinetics
Use in the elderly	Special considerations for dosing the drug in the elderly, including pharmacokinetic abnormalities, predisposition to adverse effects
Use in pregnancy	Teratology of the drug and whether the drug is expected to be present in breast milk
Patient information	Information that should be discussed with patients

firmed its benefits in this disorder (4). The Food and Drug Administration approved lithium for use in the treatment of mania in 1970 and for prophylactic use against recurrences in 1974. Several thousand publications have now described experience with lithium in a wide variety of psychiatric and medical disorders. Despite extensive biochemical investigation, lithium's precise mechanism of action remains elusive.

Lithium is rarely used without serum concentration monitoring because of its toxicity at doses just above those producing beneficial effects. In the 1970s, it seemed that lithium could be used with impunity as long as overt toxicity was avoided. However, in 1977, Danish investigators described interstitial fibrosis in renal biopsies obtained from patients who had received chronic lithium therapy

(5). These findings resulted in a crisis of concern that lithium caused irreversible structural kidney damage. Preexisting renal disease or the presence of toxic serum concentrations is currently regarded as a factor that can contribute to lithium's nephrotoxicity, but its propensity to cause progressive renal damage is low when therapy is accompanied by monitoring of renal function.

The efficacy of lithium in the treatment of acute mania has been compared in controlled trials to that of placebo and neuroleptics. Lithium can improve the symptoms of acute mania in as many as 80% of treated patients but requires up to 10 days or longer for expression of its complete benefits. Neuroleptic drugs seem to have some efficacy, but the quality of symptom improvement is superior with lithium. Although lithium has questionable value in the treatment of acute depression, evidence from controlled studies clearly demonstrates that lithium decreases the severity of both manic and depressive episodes in patients with bipolar affective disorder (see Chapters 1F and 2A).

Lithium is not specific for manic-depressive illness, as indicated by reports of its utility for other psychiatric disorders. It has revolutionized the treatment of acute mania, however, and the prophylactic treatment of mood disorders.

ANTIDEPRESSANTS

The tricyclic antidepressants and monoamine oxidase inhibitors were developed during the 1950s. Early observations that a hydrazine derivative, iproniazid, introduced for the treatment of tuberculosis, produced excitement and euphoria in some patients led to its testing as an antidepressant by Nathan Kline (6). However, it was abandoned because of toxicity. Isoniazid became the preferred treatment for tuberculosis but was not an effective antidepressant. Subsequently, it was discovered that iproniazid was a monoamine oxidase inhibitor (MAOI). This led to the testing and introduction of MAOIs that did not share iproniazid's hepatic toxicity. Phenelzine (Chapter 2D) is a widely used hydrazine MAOI and is far less hepatotoxic than iproniazid. Other nonhydrazine MAOIs have been introduced, but all share the need for dietary restrictions to prevent hypertension as a side effect. This has led to unpopularity of the MAOIs in the United States, where the tricyclic antidepressants are favored, but a resurgence of interest occurred in the 1980s as developments in the nosology of depression allowed better classification of subgroups of patients who show favorable response to MAOIs. MAOIs specific for subtypes of monoamine oxidase will be marketed in the future, which should allow further definition of the types of patients most likely to show improvement with this group of drugs.

Imipramine, the prototype tricyclic antidepressant, was tested in depressed patients in 1957 by the Swiss psychiatrist Kuhn (1), who believed that iminodibenzyl compounds, which had been synthesized as potential antihistamine and antipsychotic drugs, might be effective in depression. Imipramine proved to be an effective antidepressant, as did amitriptyline, which was introduced in the early 1960s. These drugs were soon followed by others with slight variations of the tricyclic structure.

All of the tricyclic antidepressants share the same disadvantages of producing troublesome side effects, requiring a lag time of 1 to 4 weeks to produce their full response, and failing to produce adequate benefit in 20 to 30% of treated patients. At about the time of their introduction into clinical practice, the tricyclic antidepressants were found to inhibit the neuronal uptake of catecholamine neurotransmitters, principally norepinephrine and serotonin, in the brains of laboratory animals. This observation led to development of a second generation of antidepressants in the late 1970s, with generally more specificity for one or the other of the major neurotransmitters; however, all of the newer antidepressants retain the disappointing lag time in response. However, their side effect profiles depart in some ways from the traditional tricyclic antidepressants, allowing a basis for clinical selection. Unfortunately, the pathogenesis of depression remains ill-defined, and there is no a priori way to predict reliably which patients will respond to specific antidepressants.

The antidepressants have expanded in number, structure, specificity of neurochemical effects, and diversity of adverse effects with the introduction of several new members. The list now includes bupropion and perhaps soon will include fluvoxamine and citalopram. As a class, these do not have the degree of efficacy expected with optimally effective antidepressants. Overall, the antidepressants require frequent dosage adjustments and occasional intergroup drug changes to find the proper drug and dosage regimen design. When successful, therapy with antidepressants can be a rewarding experience for both patients and clinicians.

ANTIPSYCHOTICS

The modern era in psychopharmacology began with the recognition in 1952 that chlorpromazine had a stabilizing effect on many body processes, including body temperature and excited behavior (1). This drug's development was the result of investigations with antihistamines to characterize their multiple effects. Before this time, the major psychoactive drugs in use included morphine, amphetamine, mescaline, and barbiturates. Haloperidol was developed in the late 1950s during the search for better analgesics. Numerous derivatives of the phenothiazine molecule have been marketed, but none has superceded chlorpromazine (Chapter 3A) in diversity and flexibility of use. The thioxanthenes are similar to the phenothiazines, and all of the available antipsychotic drugs (Table 1A.1) block postsynaptic dopamine receptors as a central action mediating their therapeutic effects.

The phenothiazines, thioxanthenes, and butyrophenones are still the mainstay for treatment of thought disorders such as the schizophrenias and manic psychoses. Unfortunately, little progress has been made in the treatment of tardive dyskinesia, a disabling and sometimes permanent side effect of antipsychotic therapy, but newer drugs (see "Clozapine," Chapter 3C) acting on σ-receptors and dopamine receptor subtypes should produce a lower incidence of neurological side effects.

ANTIANXIETY AGENTS

The benzodiazepines are perhaps the safest class of psychoactive drugs. Compounds in this class were initially synthesized in 1933, and over 2000 different such compounds have been made. Early reports of the taming effects of benzodiazepines in animals led to clinical trials in the 1960s. Chlordiazepoxide was the first to be marketed, followed shortly by diazepam, which has become the most popular sedative in the world. These drugs possess sedative, hypnotic, antianxiety, and anticonvulsant activities and vary mostly in their pharmacokinetic properties. Knowledge of their interactions with a specific benzodiazepine recognition site in the central nervous system has been a great impetus for discovering endogenous substrates that could be responsible for anxiety. Buspirone (Chapter 4B), the first nonbenzodiazepine to be introduced in decades, has a pharmacological profile different from that of the benzodiazepines and has helped further stimulate the field of anxiolytic neuropharmacology.

SEDATIVE-HYPNOTICS

The earliest drugs were sedative-hypnotics. The barbiturates are broad central nervous system depressants and have found therapeutic application in the treatment of various epilepsies. Of over 5000 barbiturate compounds synthesized, about 50 have clinical applications. None of the subsequently introduced drugs for anxiety or sedation, including meprobamate, ethchlorvynol, and methaqualone, has become permanently useful because of high addictive potential and toxicity. Meprobamate was originally synthesized as a muscle relaxant in 1951. It was widely prescribed after its introduction, primarily because of a lack of better agents, and is still used today. Tybamate was a shorter-acting antianxiety agent but was not as popular as meprobamate. However, these agents were widely utilized until the introduction of the benzodiazepines in the 1960s. This latter class of agents dominates the market for sedative-hypnotics and anxiolytics because of its members' superior efficacy and safety, as compared to previously available drugs.

REFERENCES

1. Jacobsen E: The early history of psychotherapeutic drugs. *Psychopharmacology* 89:138–144, 1986.
2. Talbott JH: Use of lithium salts as a substitute for sodium chloride. *Arch Intern Med* 85:1–10, 1950.
3. Cade JEJ: Lithium salts in the treatment of psychic excitement. *Med J Aust* 36:349–352, 1949.
4. Schou M: Lithium in psychiatric therapy. Stock-taking after 10 years. *Psychopharmacology* 1:65–78, 1959.
5. Hestbech J, Hanses HE, Amdisen A, et al: Chronic renal lesions following long-term treatment with lithium. *Kidney Int* 12:205–213, 1977.
6. Kline N: Clinical experience with iproniazid. *J Clin Exp Psychopathol* 19(suppl):72–78, 1958.

▬ B

Mechanisms of Psychoactive Drug Action

Psychoactive drugs exert prominent effects through interactions with specific sites in the brain. Examining the effects of drugs on the brain has been difficult, given the lack of access in vivo and the complex nature of the central nervous system (CNS). Much of our knowledge of how psychoactive drugs act in the CNS is derived from experiments using animal models and from in vitro data. It is assumed that information is transmitted in the brain from cell to cell by

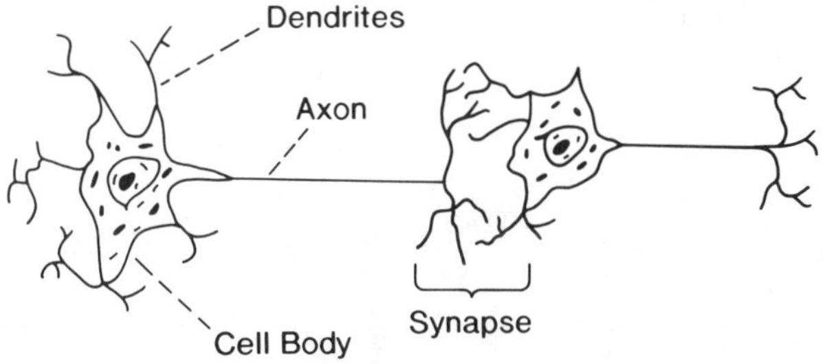

Figure 1B.1.   The neuron.

release of chemicals called neurotransmitters. Inferences on central drug effects have been drawn by examining peripheral measures of CNS drug action, such as changes in neurotransmitter concentrations in plasma, urine, and cerebrospinal fluid (CSF). The strength of conclusions derived from these data relies heavily on the assumption that peripheral changes in neurotransmitter concentrations, or their metabolites, reflect changes occurring in the brain. Through research to define the mechanisms of action of psychoactive drugs, we hope to be better able to determine the pathophysiology of various mental disorders and, therefore, to design better therapy to prevent or treat these illnesses. A brief review of some fundamental concepts of neuropharmacology can greatly aid an appreciation for the actions of psychoactive drugs (1, 2).

NEUROANATOMY

The functional unit of the CNS is the neuron (Fig. 1B.1). An electrical impulse, or action potential, travels away from the body of the cell along a fiber called an axon. At the end of the axon, nerve signals reach the synaptic terminal, a structure containing neurotransmitters that are released in response to the arrival of an action potential. Information is transmitted to other neurons at junctions known as synapses (Fig. 1B.2). Neurotransmitters diffuse across the space between two neurons, called the synaptic cleft, and bind to specific sites, called receptors, located on the membranes of a dendrite, the receiving fiber of another neuron. A neuron that transmits information toward a synapse is a presynaptic neuron, and a neuron that transmits information away from a synapse is a postsynaptic neuron. The neurotransmitter-receptor interaction results in activation of effector mechanisms (see below) that further transmit signals to subsequent neurons. This effect may be either excitatory or inhibitory. A single neuron may have multiple synaptic connections, some inhibitory and some excitatory, from both near and relatively distant nerve sites. A chain of interconnecting neurons is called a pathway. A bundle of pathway neurons is referred to as a tract.

On an organizational basis, the CNS can be anatomically divided into the cerebrum, cerebellum, brainstem, and spinal cord (3) (Fig. 1B.3). Between the brainstem and cerebrum lay the diencephalon and basal ganglia. Each of these major structures can be further subdivided, as outlined in Table 1B.1.

The cerebral cortex is the outer gray matter of the cerebrum. With an arrangement of folds and grooves called gyri and sulci, respectively, it has an enormous surface area. Physiological and anatomical studies have shown that numerous body functions are localized to specific areas of the cortex. Some-

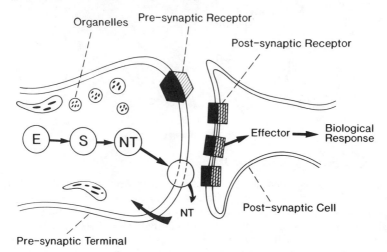

Figure 1B.2. The generalized synapse. Organelles are present in the presynaptic nerve terminal containing enzymes (*E*) for neurotransmitter (*NT*) synthesis (*S*) and storage. After release, NT can undergo an active reuptake, be metabolized in the synaptic cleft, modulate further release through interaction with presynaptic receptors, or interact with postsynaptic receptors. Postsynaptic response can be either excitatory or inhibitory, depending on the nature of the cell, and occurs through an effector mechanism, producing further neurotransmission leading to a biological response.

times in conjunction with other areas of the brain, these include motor and sensory functions, speech, sight, and memory. The prefrontal cortex governs the highest intellectual functions, including judgment, reasoning, and abstract thought. Electrical activity from the cerebral cortex can be recorded with the electroencephalogram, which is used to study sleep patterns (see Chapter 4E) and diagnose various neurological disorders.

The pyramidal tracts are pathways of motor nerves that descend from the cortex into the spinal cord and regulate the activity of skeletal muscles. These neurons are so named because their cell bodies are pyramid-shaped. They are located in an area known as the precentral gyrus. Located nearby are neurons that cause groups of muscles to contract in specific sequences, thereby causing stereotyped movements. For example, this ability is very useful in learning to play musical instruments or in typing. These motor neurons travel in extrapyramidal tracts.

The basal ganglia are groups of nerve cell bodies located deep within each cerebral hemisphere (Table 1B.1). They include the caudate nucleus, amygdala, putamen, and globus pallidus. The latter two structures form the lentiform nucleus. Together the caudate nucleus, the lentiform nucleus, and a band of white matter called the internal capsule are collectively called the corpus striatum because of an appearance like a "striped body." The basal ganglia interconnect with the cortex and other parts of the brain and are involved in controlling skeletal muscle movements. They are considered part of the extrapyramidal system. The extrapyramidal system activates and coordinates

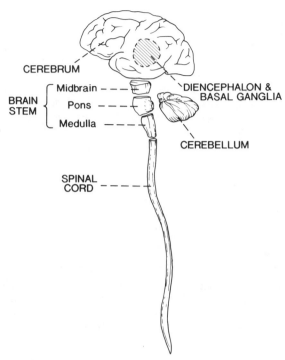

CEREBRUM

BRAIN
STEM { Midbrain — — —
       Pons — — — —
       Medulla — — —

DIENCEPHALON &
BASAL GANGLIA

CEREBELLUM

SPINAL
CORD — — — —

Figure 1B.3.   The central nervous system.

the endless postural adjustments and automatic and stereotyped movements of the body.

Located within the diencephalon are the thalamus and hypothalamus. The thalamus is a major relay and integrating center of the brain. It serves a major sensory role as all sensory fibers on their way to the cortex synapse in the thalamus. The hypothalamus, located beneath the thalamus, comprises several nuclei. Hormones, including oxytocin and antidiuretic hormone, are synthesized here and are released to blood vessels that carry them to the pituitary gland. The hypothalamus is involved in regulating autonomic (peripheral) nervous system activity, body temperature, water balance, appetite, sexual activity, some emotions, and the release of pituitary hormones.

The midbrain, pons, and medulla compose the brainstem. The pons consists of neurons that connect to the cerebellum. Areas in the medulla control vital functions such as heart rate and respiration. Functions that are below the level of consciousness are monitored in the cerebellum.

The CNS can be characterized by structurally distinct nerve pathways such as the nigrostriatal pathway, tuberoinfundibular system, and limbic system. Such systems may have a unique function or may participate in several functions. Many neuronal pathways will have interconnections with other pathways in various parts of the brain.

Intense emotions such as fear or rage are influenced by the hypothalamus, but the limbic system is considered to be particularly implicated in controlling emotional behavior, pleasure, pain, and memory. The limbic system is a wish-

Table 1B.1.
Major Divisions of the Central Nervous System

Major Division	Subdivisions
Cerebrum	The largest and most prominent part of the brain is divided into left and right hemispheres and further divided into the frontal, parietal, occipital, and temporal lobes. The cerebral cortex is the gray matter that lies on the surface of the cerebrum.
Diencephalon	Thalamus, hypothalamus, epithalamus (containing the pineal gland), subthalamus, and portions of the basal ganglia (substantia nigra and red nucleus)
Basal ganglia	Amygdala, claustrum, caudate nucleus, globus pallidus, and putamen
Brainstem	Midbrain, pons, medulla
Cerebellum	Superior, middle, and inferior peduncle that coordinate impulses necessary for posture and organized motor movements.
Spinal cord	Central gray matter containing cell bodies and synapses and peripheral white matter containing ascending and descending nerve pathways

bone-shaped group of structures and includes the olfactory bulbs, the fornix, the amygdala (part of the basal ganglia), the hippocampus (part of the cerebrum), the mamillary bodies, and various thalamic and hypothalamic nuclei. The benzodiazepines are thought to exert their actions within the limbic system.

RECEPTOR CONCEPT

No one has actually visualized a receptor, but it is hypothesized to exist on the basis of substantial evidence. Historically, the concept arose through work of Langley to account for observations that extremely small amounts of drugs or endogenous compounds produced biological responses in various tissues (4). The receptor recognizes the drug or endogenous compound and transmits a signal to elicit a biological response. The classification of receptors can be made on the basis of specific chemicals stimulating the response; for example, cholinergic receptors respond to acetylcholine, whereas dopamine receptors respond to dopamine. In 1926, Clark described the occupancy theory, which stated that the intensity of a pharmacological effect is proportional to the number of receptors occupied (5).

Macromolecules, either drugs or endogenous neurotransmitters, are generally excluded from entering cells. One mechanism of transporting macromolecules to the cellular interior is pinocytosis, but this is a mechanism that is usually involved in the termination of drug or neurotransmitter action, rather than in the initiation of information transfer. Thus, mechanisms to pass information between cells must exist. In the 1960s, binding techniques became available using radioactively labeled ligands to distinguish between nonspecific binding sites and sites meeting strict criteria as receptors.

The earlier belief of a "lock-and-key" analogy of drug-receptor interactions to account for the actions of agonists and antagonists has been mostly abandoned today. A drug is termed an agonist when it combines with a receptor that initiates a series of events leading to a biological response. Thus, the drug has affinity for the receptor and also produces efficacy, a graded response. A drug is an antagonist if it has affinity for the receptor but is devoid of efficacy. An antagonist interacts with the receptor or with some aspect of the effector mechanisms to inhibit the action of the agonist. The phenothiazines, for example, are postsynaptic dopamine receptor antagonists. This implies that they have affinity for dopamine receptors, yet do not actually interact with these receptors to produce a biological response. Their pharmacological effects are a result of preventing the response that would normally occur if dopamine acted on these receptors in the absence of drugs. Drugs that are receptor antagonists are frequently referred to as receptor blockers.

Drugs may also act by being direct or indirect agonists. Direct agonists have efficacy at the postsynaptic receptor. Indirect agonists produce efficacy by enhancing the effects of the natural neurotransmitter at its receptor. This can occur by increasing the presynaptic release of the neurotransmitter. An example is methylphenidate (Chapter 5A). Alternatively, some drugs may enhance neurotransmission by inhibiting the metabolism or reuptake of the transmitter, thereby increasing its effects. Table 1B.2 classifies major receptors and lists examples of agonists and antagonists.

Although agonists and antagonists were once viewed as competing for the same site, they probably bind to different sites to induce an alteration in the stability of a receptor. A drug must bind with a receptor in some way to produce an effect. Therefore, binding forces must attract and maintain interactions with the receptor long enough for the effect to be produced. Drugs may alter both the affinity of receptors and/or the number of receptors in producing their characteristic effects. When the receptor concentration, or density, is altered, the effect is referred to as "downregulation" or "upregulation." The chronic administration of a receptor agonist can result in receptor downregulation, and treatment with a receptor antagonist can increase receptor density. The Scatchard plot and the Hill plot are widely used methods of analyzing data from studies of drug-receptor interactions (6).

A characteristic of drugs and neurotransmitters is that they may interact with multiple receptor subtypes. The earliest identity of receptor subtypes was the division of receptors activated by acetylcholine into either muscarinic or nicotonic receptors. In 1948, Ahlquist divided adrenergic receptors into α and β subtypes (7). We now recognize that α-receptors are further classed as α_1 or α_2 and that β-receptors are either β_1 or β_2, depending upon their location in various tissues and their reponse to specific agonists (8). At least seven different subtypes of serotonin receptors have been proposed.

The control of neurotransmitter release and function is influenced by presynaptic receptors called autoreceptors. The concentration of neurotransmitters within the synaptic cleft serves as feedback control through presynaptic receptors to direct the release and synthesis of neurotransmitters. Several drugs can be shown to be working through such a mechanism.

EFFECTOR MECHANISMS

The action potential that continues the transmission of communication between neurons must be effected by mechanisms beyond the combination of a neurotransmitter with a postsynaptic receptor. The postsynaptic cell membrane (Fig. 1B.2) is viewed as composed of a lipid bilayer containing various proteins, some of which are free to move within the fluid membrane. The receptor is

Table 1B.2.
Classification of Receptors

Type	Subtype	Agonists	Antagonists
Adrenergic	α_1	Phenylephrine, methoxamine, EPI, NE	Prazosin, phentolamine
	α_2	Clonidine, EPI, NE	Yohimbine, phentolamine
	β_1	Isoproterenol	Atenolol, propranolol
	β_2	Salbutamol	Butoxamine, propranolol, pindolol
Dopaminergic	D-1	Dopamine	Phenothiazines, thioxanthenes, butyrophenones
	D-2	Dopamine, apomorphine	Phenothiazines, thioxanthenes, butyrophenones
Serotonergic	5-HT-1	Buspirone, gepirone, ergotamine, m-CPP[a]	Methiothepin
	5-HT-2	Quipazine	Cyproheptadine, mianserin, ketanserin, methylsergide
Cholinergic	Muscarinic	Pilocarpine, acetylcholine	Atropine, various psychoactive drugs used in therapeutics
	Nicotinic	Carbachol, bethanechol	d-Tubocurarine, succinylcholine
GABAergic	GABA-A	Muscimol, isoguvaline	Bicuculline, securinine
	GABA-B	Baclofen	Phaclofen, gaclofen
Opiate	μ	Morphine, meperidine, methadone	Naloxone
	κ	Ketocyclazocine	Naloxone (low affinity)
	∂	N-Allylnormetazocine	Naloxone (low affinity)

[a]m-CPP, m-chlorophenylpiperazine.

fixed in position and partially protrudes into the synaptic cleft. After a neuro-transmitter-receptor interaction, a cascade of events is initiated involving chemical mediators called "second messengers," which function to propagate the nerve signal.

Second messenger activity seems to involve protein phosphorylation by enzymes called protein kinases. In many cases, these reactions seem to be dependent upon the cyclic neucleotides, 3',5'-adenosine monophosphate (cAMP) or cyclic guanine monophosphate (GMP), or an ion such as calcium. Dopamine and norepinephrine stimulate the formation of cAMP through adenylate cyclase. Receptor-activated intracellular metabolism of phospholipids results in changes in membrane permeability, ion release, or other effects that ultimately lead to a subsequent biological response. Thus, drugs could alter neurotransmission through effects on several effector mechanisms.

Table 1B.3.
Some Pharmacological Effects of Psychoactive Drugs on Neurotransmission

Mimicking the agonist action of the natural neurotransmitter: amphetamine, L-DOPA

Blocking the action of the neurotransmitter by acting as an antagonist: phenothiazines, other antipsychotics

Enhancing or inhibiting the synthesis of neurotransmitter(s): phenelzine, disulfiram, monoamine oxidase inhibitors

Blocking the reuptake of transmitter after synaptic release: tricyclic antidepressants

Depleting neuronal stores of neurotransmitter: reserpine

Stimulating the release of neurotransmitter: cocaine, amantadine

Inhibiting the metabolism of neurotransmitter: monoamine oxidase inhibitors

Enhancing or inhibiting postsynaptic receptor sensitivity: benzodiazepines

Altering postsynaptic membrane ionic permeability

MAJOR NEUROTRANSMITTERS

Most drugs demonstrating effectiveness in treating major mental disorders affect one or more of the major neurotransmitters (serotonin, one of the catecholamines, or a peptide). The effects of psychoactive drugs on various aspects of neurotransmitter homeostasis have been well studied for most psychotherapeutic drugs; however, their precise mechanism of action in alleviating the symptoms of mental illness is imprecisely defined. Through animal studies and *in vitro* preparations, various central effects of psychoactive drugs can be demonstrated. Unfortunately, the pathogenesis of mental disorders is elusive. Table 1B.3 lists some actions of psychoactive drugs on neurotransmission. None of these effects alone is sufficient to explain drug efficacy, but they all serve as puzzle pieces in constructing a mosaic of pathogenesis in psychiatry. Some of these pharmacological effects are further discussed in individual drug databases later in the text.

Acetylcholine

The role of acetylcholine as a peripheral nervous system neurotransmitter has long been recognized. Cholinergic receptors were characterized in the early 1900s as muscarinic or nicotinic according to activation by either muscarine or nicotine. An impairment of cholinergic neurotransmission in the periphery is a recognized cause of myasthenia gravis. Recognition of cholinergic pathways in the brain has been accomplished only in recent years. Acetylcholine is now presumed to play a role in Alzheimer's disease and memory and cognition deficits. Acetylcholine mechanisms may also be operative in the affective disorders (9).

Many of the psychoactive drugs produce anticholinergic side effects in the periphery (e.g., dry mouth and blurred vision) by antagonizing muscarinic receptors. The classical acetylcholine antagonists are atropine and related drugs. Anticholinergic side effects are prominent for most antidepressants and antipsychotic agents. CNS toxicity from these produces delirium and disorientation.

Acetylcholine is degraded by acetylcholinesterase-mediated hydrolysis. A useful drug that facilitates cholinergic neurotransmission is physostigmine,

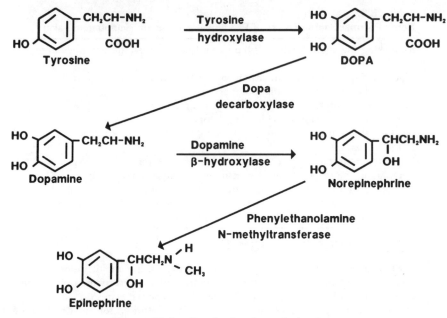

Figure 1B.4.   Synthesis of catecholamines.

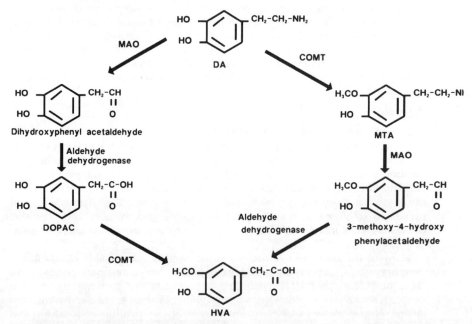

Figure 1B.5.   Degradation of dopamine. *DA*, dopamine; *MAO*, monoamine oxidas *COMT*, catechol-*O*-methyltransferase; *MTA*, 3-methoxytyramine; *DOPAC*, 3,4-dihydro› yphenylacetic acid; *HVA*, homovanillic acid.

which acts by inhibiting the action of acetylcholinesterase. This drug is used topically in the treatment of glaucoma to facilitate a cholinergic-mediated decrease in intraocular pressure, but it has sometimes been used in treating the central anticholinergic delirium produced by antidepressants.

Catecholamines

The term catecholamine commonly refers to three neurotransmitters, dopamine (DA), norepinephrine (NE), and epinephrine (EPI). These neuro-transmitters are synthesized in the brain from tyrosine, their amino acid precursor, through several enzymatic steps (Fig. 1B.4). The enzyme tyrosine hydroxylase catalyzes the formation of 3,4-dihydroxyphenylalanine (DOPA). This reaction seems to be the rate-limiting step in catecholamine synthesis. In areas of the brain where DA is a neurotransmitter, further metabolic steps serve to degrade DA (Fig. 1B.5). In areas in which NE is a neurotransmitter, DA serves only as an intermediate product in its synthesis. EPI seems to have a limited role as a CNS neurotransmitter but is formed outside the CNS from NE in the adrenal glands.

Dopamine exists in high concentrations in three major areas: the nigrostriatal pathway, the basal ganglia, and the limbic system. The nigrostriatal pathway extends from the substantia nigra to the corpus striatum. Degeneration of dopamine neurons in this pathway accounts for many of the symptoms of Parkinson's disease. These symptoms are ameliorated by treatment with L-DOPA, which is converted in the brain to dopamine (Fig. 1B.4). Blockade of dopamine receptors in the corpus striatum by antipsychotic drugs (see Chapter 3) results in extrapyramidal movement side effects, some of which resemble the symptoms of Parkinson's disease. Another result of dopamine receptor blockade by antipsychotic drugs is an elevation of serum prolactin concentration. This can lead to endocrinological side effects such as galactorrhea. The probable cause of this effect is a result of preventing dopamine's physiological role in inhibiting prolactin release. The beneficial effects of antipsychotic drugs are thought to be a result of blocking postsynaptic dopamine receptors in the mesocortical tract, a pathway involving the cortex and limbic systems. There is some evidence that the concentration of dopamine receptors is elevated in the caudate nucleus of untreated schizophrenic patients (10).

NE distribution in the brain occurs in two major tracts. The locus ceruleus in the brainstem is an area of high concentration of NE cell bodies. Its terminals are located in the cerebral cortex, hippocampus, and cerebellum. This NE nucleus has received much attention and is thought to be involved in certain anxiety disorders (11). Other major NE neurons have cell bodies outside the locus ceruleus scattered in the lateral tegmental pathway in the brainstem. No specific behavioral functions have been assigned to these pathways.

The degradation pathways of DA are shown in Figure 1B.5. The end product of dopamine metabolism is homovanillic acid (HVA). HVA has been commonly measured in CSF as an index of CNS dopamine turnover. The degradation of NE and EPI occur along similar pathways (Fig. 1B.6). They have as a final product 3-methoxy-4-hydroxyphenylglycol (MHPG). The monoamine oxidase (MAO) inhibitors (see phenelzine, Chapter 2D) produce effects on these pathways by inhibiting the degradation of monoamines. Numerous studies have investigated the excretion of MHPG in the urine as a reflection of NE activity in the brain and how its excretion is influenced by psychoactive drugs. The

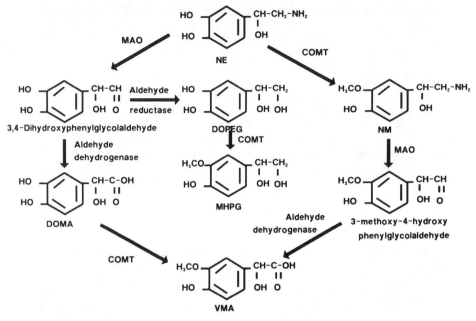

Figure 1B.6. Degradation of norepinephrine. *NE*, norepinephrine; *MAO*, monoamine oxidase; *COMT*, catechol-*O*-methyltransferase; *NM*, normetanephrine; *DOPEG*, 3,4-dihydroxyphenylglycol; *DOMA*, 3,4-dihydroxymandelic acid; *MHPG*, 3-methoxy-4-hydroxyphenylglycol; *VMA*, 3-methoxy-4-hydroxymandelic acid.

monoamine theories of depression relate to deficiencies in one or more of the catecholamines and/or serotonin (12, 13).

Serotonin

Serotonin is a monoamine containing one free nitrogen group, like EPI, NE, and DA, but does not possess the catechol nucleus of these other neurotransmitters. The raphe region of the lower midbrain and upper pons (Fig. 1B.3) contains all of the cell bodies of serotonin-containing neurons. From here, the raphe nuclei send projections to the hypothalamus, cerebral cortex, and cerebellum. Serotonin has been linked to most types of behavioral disorders and to a variety of physiological functions, including sleep, appetite, mood, aggression, blood pressure, sexual activity, and endocrine function.

Serotonin (5-HT) is widely distributed in the body, with only about 1 to 2% found in the brain. Serotonin in the brain must be synthesized there, as 5-HT cannot cross the blood-brain barrier. The synthesis begins by uptake from blood of the amino acid precursor L-tryptophan (Fig. 1B.7). The compound 5-hydroxytryptamine (5-HT or serotonin) is synthesized in the CNS from its amino acid precursor L-tryptophan. L-Tryptophan is hydroxylated to 5-hydroxytryptophan, from which serotonin is synthesized by decarboxylation. Once released into the synaptic cleft, the major route of inactivation of 5-HT is by uptake into the presynaptic terminal (Fig. 1B.2). Many of the tricyclic antidepressants effectively block this reuptake process of 5-HT. Free 5-HT within the presynaptic terminal is degraded by MAO. MAO converts 5-HT into an aldehyde, which in turn is metabolized to 5-hydroxyindoleacetic acid (5-HIAA). Other minor pathways

CH$_2$CH-NH$_2$
COOH
Tryptophan

Tryptophan
hydroxylase

HO
CH$_2$CH-NH$_2$
COOH

5-HTP

5-Hydroxytryptophan

decarboxylase

HO
CH$_2$CH$_2$-NH$_2$

Monoamine
oxidase

HO
CH$_2$CHO

5-Hydroxytryptamine

5-Hydroxyindoleacetaldehyde

Aldehyde
dehydrogenase

HO
CH$_2$COOH

5-Hydroxyindoleacetic acid

Figure 1B.7. Synthesis and degradation of 5-hydroxytryptamine (serotonin).

of metabolism exist, but measurement of 5-HIAA turnover in the CSF has been used as a measurement of the turnover of serotonin in the brain and to assess the effects of various drugs on serotonin metabolism. A drawback to this approach is the need to sample CSF.

A proposed basis for treating some types of depression is to increase brain serotonin by increasing dietary L-tryptophan (Chapter 2). Figure 1B.7 shows the metabolic pathway of tryptophan to serotonin and its metabolites. The first enzyme mediating serotonin degradation is MAO. MAO enzymes have been extensively investigated, and MAO inhibitors have been used as antidepressants (see Chapter 2D). It has recently been determined that MAO has multiple forms, some with preferred substrates. This forms the basis of new drug development for drugs with specific actions on these different types of MAO.

γ-Aminobutyric Acid (GABA)

GABA is one of several amino acids that are candidates for neurotransmitter status within the CNS. They are involved in the bulk of overall neurotransmission, as compared with the catecholamines, which account for neurotransmission in distinct sites. The better-known amino acids that potentially serve this function are glycine, taurine, and glutamic and aspartic acids. A normal constituent of the CNS, GABA is thought to function as a major inhibitory neurotransmitter. GABA is measurable in blood but does not easily cross the blood-brain barrier. The majority of GABA present in the brain is probably formed by the action of glutamic acid decarboxylase on L-glutamate.

GABA is probably metabolized in the postsynaptic cell, where it subsequently enters the Krebs cycle involved with carbohydrate metabolism. GABA receptors have been classified as GABA-A or GABA-B (Table 1B.2). They represent a recognition site on postsynaptic membranes that participates in the regulation of membrane permeability to cations, particularly chloride. Because of their role in inhibitory neurotransmission, GABA receptors are presumed to be involved in a number of mental disorders. As the benzodiazepines facilitate GABAergic neurotransmission, GABA receptors are presumed to be involved in the generation and regulation of anxiety. A number of GABAergic active compounds are known, some with potential therapeutic uses (14).

REFERENCES

1. Cooper JR, Bloom FE, Roth RH: *The Biochemical Basis of Neuropharmacology*, ed 5, Oxford University Press, New York, 1986.
2. Green AR, Costain DW: *Pharmacology and Biochemistry of Psychiatric Disorders*, Wiley-Interscience, New York, 1981.
3. Carpenter MB, Sutin J: *Human Neuroanatomy*, ed 8, Williams & Wilkins, Baltimore, 1983.
4. Langley JN: On nerve endings and on special excitable substances in cells. *Proc R Soc Lond* 78:170–194, 1906.
5. Clark AJ: The reaction between acetyl choline and muscle cells. *J Physiol* 61:530–546, 1926.
6. Marangos PJ, Campbell IC, Cohen RM (eds): *Brain Receptor Methodologies*, Academic Press, Orlando, FL, 1984.
7. Ahlquist RP: A study of the adrenotropic receptors. *Am J Physiol* 153:586–600, 1948.
8. Minniman KP: Alpha-1-adrenergic receptor subtypes, inositol phosphates, and sources of cell Ca. *Pharmacol Rev* 40:87-119, 1988.
9. Janowsky DS, Risch SC: Role of acetylcholine mechanisms in the affective disorders. In: *Psychopharmacology: The Third Generation of Progress*, (Meltzer HY (ed), Raven Press, New York, 1987, pp 527–533.
10. Wong DF, Wagner HN, Tune LE, et al: Positron emission tomography reveals elevated D2 dopamine receptors in drug-naive schizophrenics. *Science* 234:1558–1563, 1986.
11. Gorman JM, Liebowitz MR, Fyer AJ, Stein J: A neuroanatomical hypothesis for panic disorder. *Am J Psychiatry* 146:148–161, 1989.
12. Meltzer HY, Lowy MT: The serotonin hypothesis of depression. In: *Psychopharmacology: The Third Generation of Progress*, Meltzer HY (ed), Raven Press, New York, 1987, pp 513–532.
13. Siever LJ: Role of noradrenergic mechanisms in the etiology of the affective disorders. In: *Psychopharmacology: The Third Generation of Progress*, Meltzer HY (ed), Raven Press, New York, 1987, pp 493–504.
14. Lloyd KG, Morselli PL: Psychopharmacology of GABAergic drugs. In: *Psychopharmacology: The Third Generation of Progress*, Meltzer HY (ed), Raven Press, New York, 1987, pp 183–195.

▬ C ▬▬▬▬▬▬▬▬▬▬▬▬▬

Principles of Pharmacodynamics

Achieving the desired therapeutic effects from administered psychoactive drugs depends upon numerous factors. Pharmacokinetic investigations of the time course of drugs and their metabolites in the body have led to the belief that pharmacological effects are produced when drug concentration reaches some minimal level at the site(s) of action. Thus, pharmacokinetic considerations are important in the dosage regimen design of many drugs (pharmacokinetic prin-

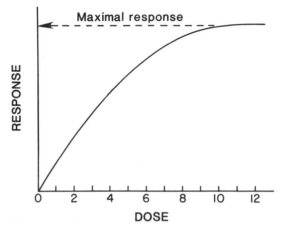

Figure 1C.1.   The graded dose-response curve.

ciples are discussed in Chapter 1D). Patients differ widely in the drug dose or concentration that produces a given effect. This situation reflects individual differences in pharmacodynamic response. Pharmacodynamics is defined as the study of the relationship between drug dosage or concentration in the body and pharmacological response (1). An appreciation of some of the fundamental principles of pharmacodynamics can aid in understanding the response to psychotherapeutic drugs (2).

CONCEPT OF DOSE RESPONSE

The drug effect should have two properties. It should be measurable and should not be present when the drug concentration in the body is zero. From this intuitively obvious principle, a dose-response curve can be plotted in which drug dose or concentration is plotted on the horizontal, or X, axis of an X-Y plot and a measurable drug response is plotted on the vertical, or Y, axis. Thus, the drug dose is the independent variable on which the effect depends. This relationship is illustrated in Figure 1C.1. Ordinarily, as drug dose or concentration increases, the response or effect increases until some maximal response is achieved and a plateau in the response is reached, i.e., a point at which increasing the dose further does not result in a further increase in the response. The height of the plateau is a measure of the drug's *efficacy*. This quality reflects the intrinsic ability of the drug to produce the desired effect. In clinical psychopharmacology, the effect could be an objective measurement (such as the percentage of change in heart rate, reaction time on a psychomotor skill test, or latency time to rapid eye movement sleep) or a subjective measurement (such as a rating of anxiety on a visual analog scale).

When one dose-response curve is compared with another, the left to right position of the curve on the X axis represents drug *potency*. In Figure 1C.2, it can be seen that the two drugs have the same qualitative effect but differ in potency according to dose. At doses above 6.5 dosage units, drug B has greater efficacy; however, below 6.5 dosage units, drug A has greater potency. Drug A produces a greater response at all dosage units below 6.5. Accordingly, one drug may seem to be superior to another at a given dose, but at other dosage levels a different dose-response relationship may exist. In clinical psychopharmacology,

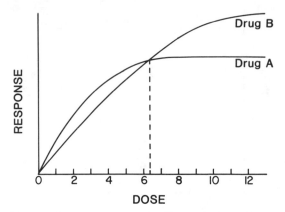

Figure 1C.2.   Potency and efficacy for two drugs.

the antipsychotic drugs are often spoken of as being low potency or high potency, according to the administered dose (see Chapter 3D); however, they often
seem to have equal efficacy if given in equipotent doses. Efficacy, i.e., the
ability to produce a desired pharmacological response, should not be confused
with potency, the dose or the concentration required to elicit the appropriate
effect or response.

In constructing dose-response curves, the X axis is frequently converted to a
logarithmic scale. Also, drug concentration, rather than dose, is sometimes
used as the independent variable. This approach is especially useful when the
measured drug concentration does not relate directly to the dose but relates to
pharmacokinetic factors, such as the degree of absorption and/or the extent of
distribution. Figure 1C.3 shows the typical sigmoid dose-response relationship
that frequently results when drug response is plotted against the logarithm of
the dose. At a low dose or concentration only a marginal effect is produced.
Increasing the dose results in a proportional increase in effect until a plateau is
reached. Above a certain dose, further increases result in little or no additional
response. This relationship often occurs when the drug's response is a consequence of activation of a single type of receptor.

The increase in drug response resulting from an increase in dosage depends
on the steepness of the dose response curve and the starting point on the curve
of the dosage change. Figure 1C.4 illustrates the effect on response of doubling
the dose (arbitrary units). In this example, doubling the dose from 0.25 to 0.5
causes more than a twofold increase in response. At the upper range of doses,
an increase from 3 to 6 dosage units produces only a further 11% increase in
response. Depending on the steepness of an individual's dose-response relationship, these percentage changes will differ. With many patients, when the
dosage of a psychotherapeutic drug is already high, a further increase may not
bring about a significant enhancement in the desired effect.

Drugs rarely have only one pharmacological effect. Most often, they produce
several different actions. For drugs used in clinical psychopharmacology, dose-
response curves for two or more pharmacological effects are usually not super-
imposable because drug effects often differ in intensity for a given plasma concentration. In Fig. 1C.5, this situation is shown for a drug that has both a
desirable therapeutic effect and a toxic effect. Clinical situations reflecting such

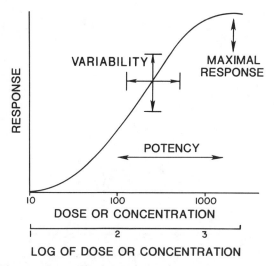

Figure 1C.3.   The logarithmic dose-response curve.

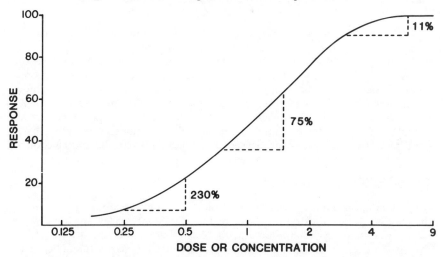

Figure 1C.4.   The effect of increasing dose or concentration on response.

a relationship are encountered frequently with psychoactive drugs. The further the distance between the two dose-response curves, the safer the drug is to administer. This is the same concept embraced in calculating the therapeutic index for a drug (see Chapter 1D). In the example shown in Fig. 1C.5, at 100 ng/ml, nearly 80% of the desired effect is achieved with a relatively low degree of toxicity (25%). However, if 95% of the desired effect is achieved by increasing the dose, and therefore the concentration, to 150 ng/ml, a dramatic increase to 60% occurs in the toxicity, with only a small therapeutic gain. As the drug concentration increases, the increase in toxicity is proportionally greater than the increase in therapeutic response. This is apparent as a steeper slope on the toxicity curve above 100 ng/ml. This situation frequently occurs during anti-

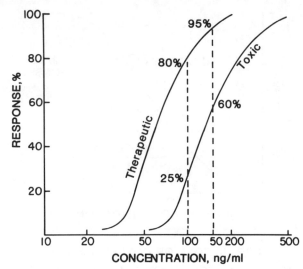

Figure 1C.5.   Dose-response curves for a drug with both a therapeutic and a toxic effect.

psychotic drug therapy as neurological side effects limit the dose that can be safely administered to achieve additional antipsychotic effects.

When a patient seems to be unusually sensitive to a dose-related effect, the situation implies that, for that particular drug and patient, the dose-response curve is steep. When therapeutic effects and toxicity are of similar magnitude, trying other drugs is an accepted practice. Other drugs within the same therapeutic class may have more separation between the dose-response curves for efficacy and toxicity for an individual patient. The relationship between therapeutic and toxic curves of drug classes can be narrow, as for the antipsychotics, or broad, as for the benzodiazepines.

CONCEPT OF LAG TIME

Quite often in clinical psychopharmacology, drug effects do not occur immediately after the administration of a drug dose. Frequently, a lag time, as long as 1 to 4 weeks for cyclic antidepressants, exists before the appearance of full therapeutic benefit. The reasons for such delays may be pharmacokinetic, pharmacodynamic, or both. Pharmacokinetic reasons contributing to lag time are discussed in Chapter 1D.

Pharmacodynamic factors that result in lag-time phenomena may be related to a drug's intrinsic actions. Some drugs are dependent upon alterations of receptor sensitivity to produce desired changes in mood and behavior. The cyclic antidepressants serve as examples. The synaptosomal reuptake inhibition of norepinephrine and serotonin occurs immediately after a single dose. However, during 1 to 2 weeks of continuous therapy, postsynaptic β-adrenergic receptors downregulate, i.e., their density or number decreases (see Chapter 1B). This change in receptor sensitivity seems to correspond more closely to the clinical course of antidepressant effects than do the immediate effects upon neurotransmitter reuptake inhibition caused by these drugs. Thus, lag time can be viewed as an adaptive response to a drug's immediate effects. Other exam-

Table 1C.1.
Lag-Time Phenomena in Clinical Psychopharmacology

Antimanic effects of lithium
Antidepressant effects of cyclic antidepressants
Antipsychotic effects of neuroleptics
Full therapeutic effects of methylphenidate in attention deficit disorder
Antipanic effects of antidepressants in panic disorder
Antianxiety effects of buspirone

ples of lag-time phenomena are given in Table 1C.1. Quite frequently, the existence of a lag time does not necessarily reflect a low plasma drug concentration. Such responses may require periods of adaptation completely unrelated to drug dosage.

Drugs are not instantaneously distributed into the central nervous system and, therefore, concentrations at the site of action may lag behind the concentration in plasma. Such an equilibrium delay results in a plot of the intensity of the pharmacological effect versus the plasma concentration similar to that seen in part **A** of Figure 1C.6. A so-called counterclockwise hysteresis loop can be seen. As concentrations increase, so does response but, as the concentration in plasma begins to decrease, beginning at point a, the intensity of response is still increasing. This situation may occur because of a delay in drug distribution from plasma into the brain. The response continues to increase temporarily, even though the plasma concentration has begun to decline. When performing studies to relate drug concentration to clinical effects, a major reason why plasma drug concentrations should be measured at steady state, when the maximal accumulation for a given dose has occurred, is to allow brain and plasma drug concentrations to reach an equilibrium. Similarly, the lag that can occur in CNS drug concentration also explains why plasma concentrations should be measured at the end of a dosage interval, when equilibrium between plasma and tissues has most likely been completed.

CONCEPT OF TOLERANCE

Tolerance is a fundamental concept in pharmacodynamics. It is frequently used in the drug abuse literature to account for the observation that increasing doses of drugs such as barbiturates must be taken to achieve the same effect as previous doses. This situation represents a change in the intrinsic sensitivity of a receptor or, more properly, a receptor population, to the drug over time. This effect occurs in spite of a constant concentration of drug in blood, in plasma, or at the receptor site. This situation is represented by the clockwise hysteresis loop in Figure 1C.6**B**. Even though drug concentration increases beyond point b, drug response decreases beginning at this time point. An example of this type of relationship is the decline in euphoria ratings after repeated doses, and increasing concentrations, of cocaine.

Tolerance can occur at different rates for different actions of drugs. For example, tolerance to the euphoric effects of cocaine occurs more rapidly than does tolerance to its cardiovascular effects. Another example is the apparent tolerance to gastrointestinal distress produced from caffeine; the cortical stimulation seems to be sustained, thus explaining the popularity of this widely used beverage. Furthermore, tolerance may develop at different rates to drugs within the

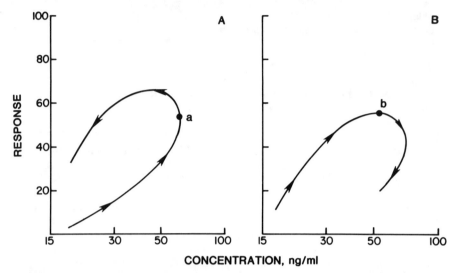

Figure 1C.6.   Hysteresis loops illustrating a delay in effect from rising concentrations (**A**) and tolerance (**B**). At point a, response increases, although concentration begins to decline; at point b, concentration increases, although response begins to decrease.

Table 1C.2.
Examples of Tolerance to Psychoactive Drug Effects

Drug	Effect	Time for Tolerance to Develop
Cyclic antidepressants	Sedation, anticholinergic effects (dry mouth, etc.)	Over first week of chronic therapy
Benzodiazepines	Sedation, ataxia	During acute administration
Morphine	Analgesia, euphoria	Several days
Phenothiazines	Sedation	Days to weeks
Alcohol	Euphoria	Days to weeks
Cocaine	Euphoria	First dose
Amantadine	Decrease in akathisia	After 1–8 weeks of therapy
L-DOPA	Decrease in abnormal movements	Weeks to months

same class. An example is the sedative effects of different benzodiazepines. Table 1C.2 lists other common examples of drug tolerance that occur with psychoactive drugs.

Several mechanisms may be operative in the occurrence of drug tolerance. A pharmacokinetic explanation is increasing metabolism upon chronic dosing. An example is the autoinduction that occurs with carbamazepine. Continued stimulation of receptors by a drug may result in a change in receptor affinity, whereby more drug is required to either occupy or elicit a change in the receptor population over time.

Closely linked to tolerance is the concept of cross-tolerance. This occurs with drugs acting at the same receptor site. For example, methadone will substitute for opiates, preventing the abstinence syndrome in heroin addicts (see Chapter

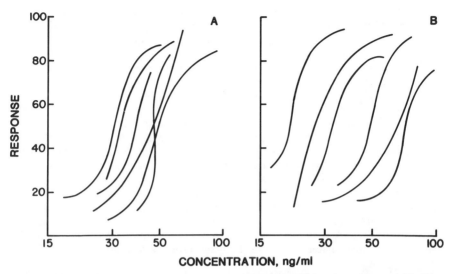

Figure 1C.7.   Concentration versus response relationships for a group of individuals with minimal (**A**) or more pronounced (**B**) variability.

Table 1C.3.
Factors Contributing to Variability in Psychotherapeutic Drug Response

Age
Sex
Race
Genetic phenotype (acetylation, hydroxylation status)
Concurrent drug therapy (drug interactions)
Diet
Disease states
Circadian rhythms
State of fatigue
Smoking status
Ethanol use

6B). The observation that buspirone will not substitute for benzodiazepines in preventing their withdrawal effects suggests that these drugs act at different receptor sites.

VARIABILITY IN DRUG THERAPY

An additional value of understanding dose-response relationships is to realize that each individual has a unique response to a given drug dose (3). A theoretical plot of the response of two groups of patients to the same drug might appear as Figure 1C.7. In one group (Fig. 1C.7A), there is only a small amount of variability among individuals, as compared to the degree of variability present in the other group (Fig. 1C.7B). Such situations can occur because of ageing, the presence of disease, or other variables within a patient group. A frequent situation encountered when monitoring psychoactive drugs is that the same dose or concentration of drug produces a marked effect in one individual and almost no effect in another. Table 1C.3 lists contributing factors causing interindividual differences in drug responses. These factors illustrate the difficulty in dosage regimen design and the need for individualization of therapy when treating patients with psychoactive drugs.

Intrasubject variability in drug pharmacodynamics should also be appreciated. Rarely does an increase in drug dose produce the linear or predictable increase in response depicted in the above figures. As an example, consider the response of a depressed patient to treatment with a cyclic antidepressant. What is important is the overall trend in target symptom changes, not necessarily the day-to-day changes. Target symptom changes in depression are often like the fluctuations of the stock market. What is most important is not the day-to-day variation, but the trend over time. In psychotherapeutic drug monitoring, one should appreciate this type of variability.

Intrasubject variability can be viewed as a reverberating curve, never motionless but in a constant state of flux, changing in terms of intensity and potency for a given drug concentration because of the factors listed in Table 1C.3 and in relation to the dose-response curves for other effects of the drug. Figure 1C.3 summarizes these major aspects of the dose-response relationship.

REFERENCES

1. Tallarida RJ, Jacob LS: *The Dose-Response Relation in Pharmacology*, Springer-Verlag, New York, 1979.
2. Dingemanse J, Danhof M, Breimer DD: Pharmacokinetic-pharmacodynamic modeling of CNS drug effects: an overview. *Pharmacol Ther* 38:1–52, 1988.
3. Rowland M, Sheiner LB, Steimer J-L (eds): *Variability in Drug Therapy: Description, Estimation, and Control*, Raven Press, New York, 1985.

▬ D ▬

Principles of Pharmacokinetics

Pharmacokinetics is the scientific discipline describing the time course and effects of drugs and their metabolites through the body. This discipline overlaps with pharmacodynamics in the study of the relationship of drug concentrations to clinical effects. Mathematical models are frequently used to interpret concentration versus time data obtained in experimental studies. Essentially, pharmacokinetics describes what the body does to the drug, while pharmacodynamics (Chapter 1C) describes what the drug does to the body.

The term pharmacokinetics has existed only since the early 1950s, but in the last two decades there has been an explosion of knowledge in this field (1). Progress has been largely due to advances in analytical chemistry. Methods such as radioimmunoassay, gas chromatography, and high-performance liquid chromatography (see Chapter 1G) have become available to allow very small amounts of drugs and their metabolites (down to the picogram range, 10^{-12} gm), to be quantified in body fluids and tissues. The theoretical pharmacokinetic basis has now been developed for most types of dosage regimens (2), and

Table 1D.1.
Pharmacokinetic Parameters Used to Define a Drug

Animal and Human Pharmacokinetic Parameters	Disease States and Other Conditions Affecting Pharmacokinetics
Clearance	Renal function
Renal excretion	Hepatic function
Metabolic pathways	Blood flow changes
Volume of distribution	Smoking
Half-lives	Posture
Protein binding	Drug interactions
Blood to plasma concentration ratio	Age (young & old)
Placental transfer	
Bioavailability	
Peak time and maximal concentration	
Toxic concentrations	
Effective concentrations (in patients)	

therapeutic plasma concentration ranges have been identified for several drugs that are used routinely to aid dosage regimen design in medical practice (3). There is a general acknowledgment that application of pharmacokinetic principles can help to optimize psychoactive drug therapy (4).

Pharmacokinetic data have no inherent use unless they provide the clinician with a more rational dosage regimen. The need for individualized drug dosage regimens results from recognition of a large intersubject variability in the dose-response relationships for psychoactive drugs (see Chapter 1C, Figs. 1C.3 and 1C.7), interactions occurring with other drugs and the environment that influence the elimination of drugs, and noncompliance of many patients with prescribed therapy. In addition, some dosage forms may cause drug absorption to be erratic and incomplete. Because of these factors, a better correlation frequently exists between plasma drug concentration and pharmacological response than between the prescribed dose and response.

The pharmacokinetic parameters that are usually determined during the development of a new drug from its initial study in animals to its study in human volunteers and ill patients are listed in Table 1D.1. It is most important to evaluate pharamcokinetic parameters in the patient population for which the drug has been devised. The effects of disease states, particularly those diseases that may be related to the action of the drug, are critical in determining how the body will react to a particular drug and thus modify the pharmacodynamic response observed in an individual patient. The need for such studies will become apparent with an appreciation for the basic pharmacokinetic parameters discussed below.

When a clinician prescribes a psychoactive drug and the patient takes it, the main concern is with the effect on the patient's mental status. Ideally, designing dosage regimens should be based on therapeutic response, but this is not always feasible, especially in psychiatry, in which most types of therapeutic response are difficult to evaluate objectively and the onset of response is often delayed (see Table 1C.1). Table 1D.2 lists some factors that make correlations between drug plasma concentration and therapeutic response difficult with psychoactive drugs. Studies that purport to show a concentration-effect rela-

Table 1D.2.

Factors Contributing to Difficulty in Establishing Relationships between Plasma Concentrations and Clinical Effects for Psychoactive Drugs

Drug-related Factors	Patient Factors
Variety of commercially available products	Variable presentation
Multiple active metabolites	Altered pharmacokinetics in different age groups
Low plasma concentrations near the lower limits of assay sensitivity	High and variable protein binding
Multiple drug interactions	Difficulties in objective assessment of clinical response
	Lack of standardized rating scales

tionship must be rigorously designed to avoid pitfalls that can obscure the true relationship between drug concentration and clinical effects. Table 1D.3 lists some of the desirable design features for this type of study. This list may be useful in assessing the value of published data for clinical application.

The study and description of pharmacokinetics are often subdivided into four major processes: absorption, distribution, metabolism, and elimination. These processes are all occurring concurrently from the time a drug dose is administered. Figure 1D.1 shows conceptually the four major pharmacokinetic processes. When drugs are given by any route other than an intravenous one, they undergo an absorption process. The rate at which this happens is partially controlled by formulation factors, for example, administration of chlorpromazine to a psychotic patient as a hard-coated tablet may not provide effective concentrations as rapidly as would administration as a syrup. Once a drug dose is absorbed, a general distribution in the body takes place. In many cases, the initial dose is high enough so that an adequate concentration occurs at the site of action to produce the desired clinical effects. However, both the appearance of drug in the circulation and its presence at the site of action will be modified by how rapidly drug elimination occurs through clearance by renal, hepatic, and/or other processes.

Drugs are eliminated or cleared primarily in two ways—either through renal excretion in an unchanged form (e.g., lithium (Chapter 2A)), or by biotransformation to metabolites. Drug metabolites themselves are either further metabolized or excreted in the urine but may first contribute to pharmacological effects by also being distributed to sites of action (Fig. 1D.1).

A typical pharmacokinetic study consists of monitoring the concentration or amount of drug in blood (or plasma) and/or urine as a function of time after a dose and subsequently plotting the observed data on suitable graph paper. Conceptually, this is what happens after a single drug dose: as drug is absorbed, concentrations increase until a peak concentration occurs in plasma (Cmax). The rate of drug absorption will largely determine the time and magnitude of the Cmax. As drug molecules are being rapidly distributed throughout the body, plasma concentrations decline from a peak. This part of the concentration versus time curve is generally regarded as the drug distribution phase. Eventually, a slower elimination phase becomes apparent, with drug concentration declining over time in a straight line when the data are displayed using semilogarithmic graph paper (plotting the logarithm of the concentration versus time). The ideal time to sample blood when monitoring the plasma concentra-

Table 1D.3.
Desirable Study Conditions for Determining the Relationship between Plasma Concentration and Effect

Plasma concentrations measured at steady state: standardized sample times for all patients
Measurement of parent compounds and all active metabolites with appropriate and sensitive assay
Patients should not be on multiple drugs: homogeneous treatment
Large enough sample for statistical significance
Inclusion of placebo to eliminate placebo responders
Exclusion of nonresponders
Reasonably florid symptoms
Controlled dosage: equal for all patients
Outcome criteria specified as quantitative measures
Blinded raters as to dose, plasma concentration, and active or placebo treatment
Established interrater reliability
Adequate duration of therapy

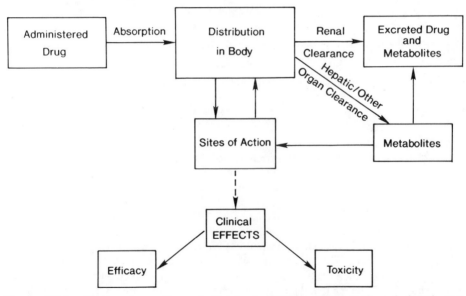

Figure 1D.1. Drug sojourn through the body. During absorption and distribution, elimination begins by means of renal, hepatic, or other clearance processes. Some active metabolites may also be distributed to sites of action to produce clinical effects.

tion of most psychoactive drugs is sometime after the elimination phase commences, usually 8 to 12 hours after a dose.

The concentration versus time course of desipramine and its major metabolite after a single dose is shown in Figure 1D.2, which illustrates the absorption, distribution, and elimination phases commonly observed in single-dose pharmacokinetic studies (5). The above description of the observed plasma concentra-

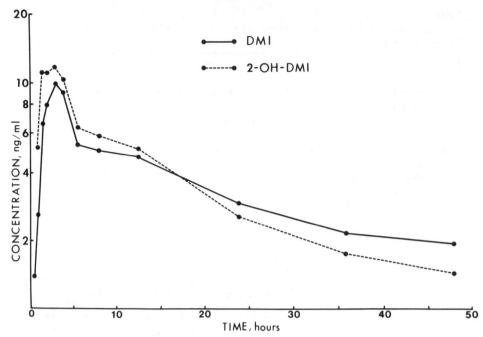

Figure 1D.2.   Concentration versus time profile of desipramine (*DMI*) and its major metabolite, 2-hydroxydesipramine (*2-OH-DMI*) in a healthy volunteer after a single 50-mg oral dose. Drug concentration increases steeply during the initial absorption phase and then falls during a rapid distribution phase until the slower elimination phase predominates.

tion changes is a simplification of reality, as the absorption, distribution, and elimination processes all occur simultaneously. As soon as drug absorption begins, some drug molecules undergo both distribution and elimination. Similarly, some drug continues to be absorbed after the occurrence of the peak concentration, even though the plasma concentration is declining.

What is the use of predicting the rates of drug absorption, distribution, and elimination? When pharmacological effects are related to some drug concentration in blood, we can control the intensity and duration of effects by manipulating the concentration. When an understanding of how a given patient will absorb and eliminate a drug is coupled with knowledge of the pharmacological effect of a given plasma concentration, then drug dosing that will result in clinical efficacy with minimal toxicity can be selected. This can be visualized conceptually in Figure 1D.3. If a drug dose produces a concentration that exceeds the therapeutic range, then toxicity can result.

The ratio of the lowest concentration that produces toxicity to the lowest concentration that produces desired therapeutic effects is called the *therapeutic index* of a drug, a frequently used measurement of the relative safety of a drug. Of course, minimally effective and toxic concentrations are not usually as precise as Figure 1D.3 would suggest. The same concept of a therapeutic range is apparent in Chapter 1C (Fig. 1C.5), which shows the risk of toxicity increasing to an unacceptable degree as plasma concentration increases.

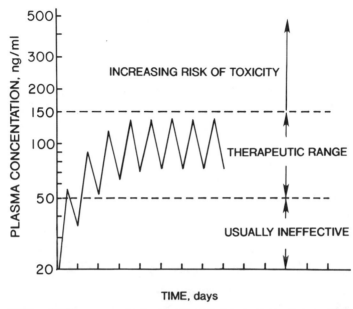

Figure 1D.3.   Time course of plasma drug concentration after multiple doses for a drug with a defined therapeutic concentration range. Below 50 ng/ml, there is a greater possibility of therapeutic failure and greater risk of toxicity for dosage regimens producing concentrations above 150 ng/ml. The sawtooth pattern of drug concentrations occurs with multiple doses.

The application of pharmacokinetics in the clinical setting is not as difficult as it might appear. However, an understanding of three fundamental pharmacokinetic concepts—volume of distribution, half-life, and clearance—is necessary. These are most clearly understood with the aid of a few equations, but complicated mathematics is rarely necessary to appreciate the interrelationships among these parameters or to derive benefit from knowledge of their values for different drugs in individual patients. Excellent nonmathematically oriented textbooks of pharmacokinetics explain these concepts (6, 7).

CONCEPT OF VOLUME OF DISTRIBUTION

Using the most simple pharmacokinetic model, the body can be viewed, as in Figure 1D.4, as a single compartment. Two assumptions are made for this model: (a) input of a drug dose is instantaneous, i.e., we can ignore the absorption process; and (b) distribution of a drug is homogeneous within the compartment. X_D is used to represent the drug dose, X_B is the amount of drug in the body, X_E is the amount of drug eliminated, and K is a first-order elimination constant. The elimination of most drugs in humans and animals after therapeutic or nontoxic doses can be characterized as an apparent first order process, i.e., the rate of elimination of drug from the body at any time is proportional to the amount of drug in the body at that time. The elimination rate constant, K, reflects this fact. It is a proportionality constant relating the rate of elimination to the amount of drug in the body. Its units are reciprocal time. For example, a

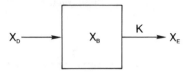

Figure 1D.4. Single-compartment pharmacokinetic model. See text for abbreviations.

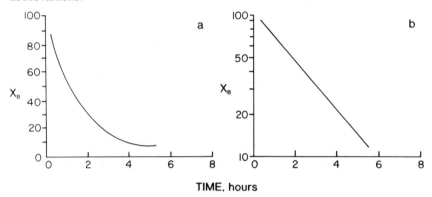

TIME, hours

Figure 1D.5. Predicted time course of drug in the body (X_B) described by a single-compartment pharmacokinetic model. Drug declines over time as shown in **a** proportional to the amount of drug left in the body or in a linear manner when X_B is plotted with a semilogarithmic axis (**b**).

rate constant equal to 0.2 hr^{-1} means that 20% of the drug remaining in the body is eliminated in 1 hour.

A differential equation can be written and solved to describe the behavior of this single-compartment model. For simplicity, it suits our purpose to observe the predicted behavior of this model. The single-compartment model predicts that, after instantaneous input, drug in the body (X_B) declines over time, as shown in Figure 1D.5. However, we can assay only for the concentration of drug in the blood or plasma, not for the entire amount of drug in the body. The concept of volume of distribution allows us to compensate for this inability.

Consider the following general relationship:

$$\frac{X}{V} = C \qquad \text{(Equation 1)}$$

where X equals the amount of any substance, V equals the volume in which the substance is dissolved, and C equals the concentration of X. Because of this equality, a proportionality factor, called the *volume of distribution* (V_D), has been invented to relate the measured plasma concentration of a drug to the amount of drug in the body. This is done by rearranging Equation 1 as follows:

$$X \text{ (amount)} = C \text{ (concentration)} \times V \text{ (volume)} \qquad \text{(Equation 2)}$$

or:

$$V \text{ (volume)} = \frac{X \text{ (amount)}}{C \text{ (concentration)}} \qquad \text{(Equation 3)}$$

It should be intuited that the concentration of drug in the plasma or blood depends on how the drug distributes in the body and the total amount of drug in the body.

V_D is frequently calculated using the above relationship in the following form:

$$V_D = \frac{\text{Dose}}{Cp^0} \qquad \text{(Equation 4)}$$

where Cp^0 is the concentration that occurs immediately after the drug dose is administered, i.e., at time zero before any elimination has occurred. Therefore, at this point in time, the drug dose approximates the amount of drug in the body. The volume of distribution can be thought of as that conceptual volume that would be necessary to contain all of the drug in the body if it were at the same concentration throughout the body as measured in the plasma. V_D has units of volume or volume/mass when related to body weight.

An example from general medicine may help to clarify the V_D concept. The volume of distribution of theophylline in adults has been found to average 0.45 liter/kg. Assume that a patient who requires theophylline treatment weighs 70 kg. Using these data, calculate what bolus intravenous dose of theophylline (administered as aminophylline) would give an initial plasma concentration of 15 µg/ml, a concentration associated with therapeutic effects in the treatment of asthma. To solve this problem, Equation 3 or 4 is rearranged to give

$$\text{Dose} = (V_D) \text{ (desired } Cp^0) \qquad \text{(Equation 5)}$$

By making the appropriate substitutions

$$\text{Dose} = (0.45 \text{ liter/kg}) \text{ (70 kg) (15 µg/ml)}$$

and solving gives

$$\text{Dose} = 472.5 \text{ mg}$$

If this patient has an average volume of distribution for theophylline, then a dose of 472.5 mg will yield a maximal plasma concentration of 15 µg/ml. Of course, the drug will not be administered instantaneously, as in our one-compartment model, and some drug will begin to be eliminated immediately, causing the plasma concentration to fall. In practice, a maintenance infusion is often started to replace the drug that is eliminated in order to maintain a therapeutic plasma concentration. Nevertheless, this example serves to illustrate how V_D is used to relate amount of drug and concentration.

Consider another example of a V_D calculation using a psychoactive drug. Suppose we administer a single oral lithium carbonate dose of 900 mg, or approximately 24 mEq, to a patient. Further, assume that the dose will be completely absorbed 18 hours after administration. Urine collections are made over this time interval to quantify the amount of lithium that has been excreted. A measurement is then made of the plasma lithium concentration, which is found to be 0.3 mEq/liter. A total of 6 mEq is found in the total urine collections. What is the V_D? By recalling that V_D is equal to the proportionality factor that relates the amount of drug in the body to the plasma concentration (Cp), we can write

$$V_D = \frac{\text{Amount of drug in the body}}{\text{Plasma concentration}} = \frac{X}{Cp} \qquad \text{(Equation 6)}$$

Because lithium is completely excreted in the urine, the amount in the body is the difference between the absorbed dose and that collected in the urine. Thus, we can substitute and solve the equation:

$$V_D = \frac{24 \text{ mEq} - 6 \text{ mEq}}{0.3 \text{ mEq/liter}} = \frac{18}{0.3 \text{ liter}} = 60 \text{ liters} \qquad \text{(Equation 7)}$$

There is no relationship between the apparent (calculated) and actual volume of distribution of a drug. The actual distribution volume is related to body water and cannot exceed total body water, which is about 60% of body weight. Body water can be divided into at least three distinct compartments: plasma or blood, extracellular fluid, and intracellular fluid. Some high-molecular-weight substances like indocyanine green are essentially confined to the circulating plasma and have been used to estimate plasma volume. For highly plasma-protein bound drugs, the V_D is less than body water. When body tissue binding of drugs is high, the amount of drug outside the plasma is great, and the calculated V_D is typically far greater than that of body water.

In the last example, the apparent volume of distribution of lithium more closely approximates its true V_D because lithium's binding to plasma proteins and tissues is negligible (see Chapter 2A). For most other psychoactive drugs, this is not the case. Most psychoactive drugs are significantly bound in either the vascular or the extravascular space, or both. Drugs that are predominantly bound to extravascular tissues have large apparent volumes of distribution.

What are the implications of knowing a drug's V_D? The larger a drug's V_D, the more likely that the tissue binding is greater than plasma protein binding and the more likely that most of the drug in the body exists outside the vascular space. An example is imipramine, which has a typical V_D of approximately 20 liters/kg (Chapter 2B). This large V_D reflects extensive tissue distribution and helps explain why hemodialysis is of limited value in the treatment of imipramine overdosage (8). As hemodialysis removes drug from the plasma compartment and most of the drug is outside the circulation, it follows that hemodialysis will have limited effectiveness in removing the body burden of drug.

CONCEPT OF DRUG HALF-LIFE

Consider again the one-compartment model depicted in Figure 1D.4. There are various ways of mathematically representing the decline in concentration over time. The most common way is to use an equation written in logarithmic (base 10) form:

$$\log X_B = \log X_B^0 - \frac{K \times t}{2.303} \qquad \text{(Equation 8)}$$

This equation describes the linear decline of drug amount or concentration over time seen in Figure 1D.5 when amount of drug is plotted on a semilogarithmic scale. Log X_B is the logarithm of the amount of drug in the body, X_B^0 is the initial amount of drug in the body at time zero, and $-K/2.303$ is the slope, with t representing time. Equation 8 has the familiar look of the algebraic expression, $y = mx + b$, which is a general equation for a straight line. Equation 8 can be rewritten using plasma concentrations (Cp) instead of amount of drug in the form of natural logarithms (ln) as

$$\ln Cp = \ln Cp^0 - K \times t \qquad \text{(Equation 9)}$$

Solving for time in Equation 9 gives

$$t = \ln \frac{(Cp/Cp^0)}{-K} \qquad \text{(Equation 10)}$$

Thus, the time for any proportional change in drug concentration to occur can be calculated by substituting in the quotient Cp/Cp^0. To solve for the time required for plasma drug concentration to decrease by one-half (half-life, $t_{1/2}$), a substitution is made in Equation 10:

$$t_{1/2} = \frac{\ln (1/2)}{-K} \qquad \text{(Equation 11)}$$

or

$$t_{1/2} = 0.693/K \qquad \text{(Equation 12)}$$

Half-life is defined as the time required for amount of drug in the body or drug concentration to fall by one-half, or 50%. Thus, it takes the same amount of time for the drug in the body to decline from 50 to 25 mg as it does to decline from 100 to 50 mg. This concept is identical to the concept of radioactive decay. Equation 12 shows that half-life is a simple function of the elimination rate constant. This equation will be seen to be useful below.

Half-life is easily determined by graphical means or by inspection, as long as data are used from the terminal, log-linear portion of the elimination curve (Figs. 1D.2 and 1D.5b). Data obtained before the terminal elimination phase commences may result in an underestimation of the true drug half-life. In Figure 1D.6, the basic pharmacokinetic concepts are summarized. Elimination half-life can be seen through inspection to be 4 hours. Therefore, when drug concentration is decreasing in its terminal elimination phase, in one half-life 50% will be eliminated. In another half-life, half of the remaining drug will be eliminated; thus, a total of 75% will be gone. This increases to 87.5% by three half-lives and ultimately to over 95% between four and five half-lives. Thus, knowing a drug's half-life will predict what length of time is necessary for a drug to be totally washed out of the body. This is useful information, for example, when waiting

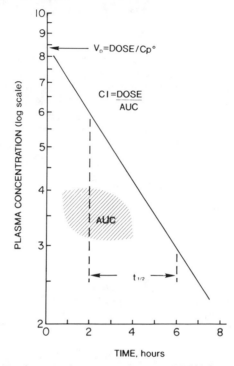

Figure 1D.6. Basic pharmacokinetic parameters. Half-life ($t_{1/2}$) can be observed by inspection to be 4 hours. The equations for volume of distribution (V_D) and clearance (Cl) are explained in the text.

for an antidepressant to be eliminated from the body before starting a monoamine oxidase inhibitor (see Chapter 2D).

Part of the value of knowing a drug's half-life is that this parameter also predicts certain characteristics about drug accumulation during multiple dosing situations. It is intuitively obvious that if a second drug dose is administered to a patient before the first drug dose has been completely eliminated from the body, which takes an elapsed time of four to five half-lives, some drug accumulation will occur. If drug doses are continually administered on a regular schedule, eventually a steady-state situation will exist. With a constant dosage interval, 75% of the ultimate steady state will occur by the end of two elapsed half-lives, 87.5% by the end of the third half-life, and so on, increasing to a plateau. Steady state occurs when the amount eliminated is equal to the amount administered. It takes four to five half-lives to achieve steady state at a constant dosing rate or to achieve a new steady state when the dosing rate is changed. This relationship applies regardless of the route of drug administration or the number of drug doses per day. These implications of half-life are shown in Figure 1D.7.

CONCEPT OF CLEARANCE

Although half-life determines the time to achieve steady state, it does not determine the magnitude of the steady-state concentration. This is determined

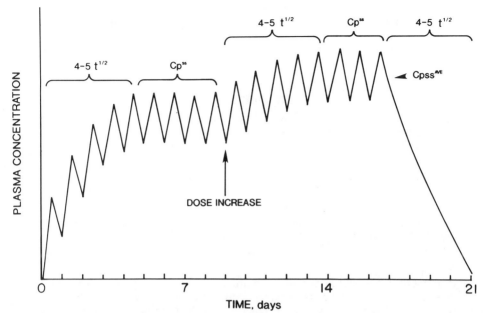

Figure 1D.7. Accumulation of drug during multiple dosing. It takes four to five half-lives (4–5 $t_{1/2}$) to achieve initial steady state (Cp^{ss}) on a constant dosage regimen, to achieve a new steady state upon an increase in dosage, or for drug to wash out from the body upon discontinuing dosing. The average steady-state concentration ($Cpss^{AVE}$) lies somewhere between the peaks and troughs of drug concentration during a dosage interval.

only by the clearance of the drug from the body. Clearance is defined as the volume of blood or other fluid from which drug is irreversibly removed per unit time. Thus, clearance has units of volume/time. Drug clearance is completely analogous to creatinine clearance by the kidney (see Chapter 1G).

To understand drug clearance, one can picture a drug entering and leaving an organ, as shown in Figure 1D.8. Assume that this organ does not accumulate drug, so that all drug that enters either exits the organ on the right side or is eliminated through the bottom by some irreversible process. This process could be hepatic metabolism, renal excretion, pulmonary exhalation, or another route of elimination. The amount of drug that is removed by the organ is simply that which is extracted over time. The extraction ratio, E, is simply the amount entering (the product of blood flow, Q, and arterial concentration, Ca) less the amount leaving (the product of Q and venous concentration, Cv) as a proportion of the entering amount. Thus,

$$\text{Clearance (Cl)} = Q\,(Ca - Cv)\,/\,Ca \qquad \text{(Equation 13)}$$

or

$$Cl = Q \times E \qquad \text{(Equation 14)}$$

Equation 14 states that the clearance of drug by any organ or tissue is equal to the blood flow to that eliminating organ times the extraction ratio of the organ.

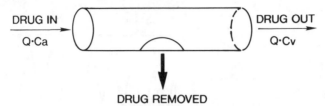

DRUG REMOVED

Figure 1D.8.   Organ clearance model for drug elimination. Drug entering the organ is the product of blood flow (Q) and arterial drug concentration (Ca), and the amount leaving is the product of blood flow (Q) and venous concentration (Cv).

Therefore, the maximal clearance of any drug by the liver is equal to 1500 ml/min, the average hepatic blood blow. An exception to this generalization, explained below, exists for drugs undergoing first-pass elimination.

Although Equation 14 is conceptually correct to represent organ clearance, in practice, body clearance is often calculated as

$$Cl = Dose/AUC \qquad \text{(Equation 15)}$$

where AUC is the area under the concentration versus time curve of drug in the plasma after a single dose. The *shaded area* in Figure 1D.6 reflects the AUC. AUC represents the extent of systemic exposure of the body to the drug. Thus, if the AUC is small after a drug dose, clearance must be high, according to Equation 15. How small or how large the AUC is, as well as its shape, is dependent upon how rapidly the body can eliminate or clear the drug.

Clearance is also frequently calculated as

$$Cl = V_D \times K \qquad \text{(Equation 16)}$$

Equation 16 is a mathematically correct way to calculate a drug's clearance and can frequently be found in pharmacokinetic literature, but it is a gross misrepresentation of the clearance concept. One should keep in mind that clearance and volume of distribution of a drug are independent parameters and that neither depends upon the other nor upon half-life. Rather, half-life is determined by the relative values of clearance and volume of distribution.

Recalling Equation 12, rearranging it to solve for K and substituting the result into Equation 16 gives

$$t_{1/2} = \frac{0.693 \times V_D}{Cl} \qquad \text{(Equation 17)}$$

Equation 17 is an extremely useful relationship in pharmacokinetics. It shows that half-life is a function of both how extensively a drug is distributed in the body (V_D) and how efficiently it is eliminated (Cl). It should be obvious that, as clearance increases, then $t_{1/2}$ will be shorter. Conversely, if body clearance is decreased due to ageing, drug interactions, organ dysfunction, or other causes, then half-life will show a proportional increase when volume of distribution remains constant.

As previously stated, drugs can be eliminated by both renal excretion and hepatic metabolism. As each of these processes may contribute to the elimination of a drug, clearance becomes an additive property. Therefore, total body clearance, Cl_{body}, becomes

$$Cl_{body} = Cl_{renal} + Cl_{hepatic} + Cl_{other} \qquad \text{(Equation 18)}$$

Depending on which of these processes predominates in the total clearance of a drug, predictions can be made as to whether a drug dosage adjustment is necessary in a patient with renal or hepatic impairment. One caution is warranted. Many psychoactive drugs are highly metabolized with very low values for renal clearance of parent drug. However, metabolites are generally more water-soluble than their precursors and undergo a higher degree of renal clearance. In animals and humans, renal failure has resulted in accumulation of antidepressant metabolites with minimal effect on parent drug disposition (9, 10). These observations suggest that renal impairment requires cautious dosing of psychoactive drugs with active metabolites, regardless of the proportion of total clearance of the parent drug contributed by renal clearance.

Although half-life determines the time to accumulate drug to steady state, it is clearance, how efficiently a drug is removed, that determines the magnitude of steady-state accumulation. For drugs administered orally or by any intermittent method, there will be peaks and troughs during a dosing interval. This can be seen in Figures 1D.3 and 1D.7. A commonly used equation to express the average steady-state concentration (Cp_{ss}) over a dosage interval is

$$Cp_{ss} = F \times \text{dose}/Cl_{body} \times t^* \qquad \text{(Equation 19)}$$

where F is the bioavailability factor for orally administered drugs and t^* is the dosage interval. This equation reflects the previous discussion that steady state is determined by clearance and not by half-life or volume of distribution alone. These parameters contribute to the magnitude of peaks and troughs during dosage intervals but not to the overall steady-state concentration.

In summary, volume of distribution is the proportionality factor, which relates plasma concentration of a drug to the amount of drug in the body. Knowledge of its value suggests how extensively a drug is distributed beyond the systemic circulation. Clearance is an overall assessment of how efficiently a drug is removed from the body. It is defined as the volume of blood or other fluid from which drug is irreversibly removed per unit of time. By knowing the clearance in an individual or the average value for a group of individuals, we can calculate the dosage regimen to achieve a desired steady-state drug concentration (2). Half-life is a function of both the extent of drug distribution and the magnitude of drug clearance. The utility of knowing $t_{1/2}$ is that, with a constant dosing regimen (i.e., the same amount of drug administered at constant intervals of time), a period of time equal to four to five half-lives is required to reach steady state, to achieve a new steady-state level if the dosage regimen is increased or decreased, or to eliminate a drug completely from the body when dosing is discontinued (Fig. 1D.7).

INTEGRATION OF BASIC CONCEPTS
Combined Pharmacotherapy in the Same Patient

Consider a hypothetical patient receiving 15 mg of diazepam twice daily and 100 mg of imipramine once daily. A computer-simulated plasma concentration accumulation pattern generated from pharmacokinetic parameters chosen from

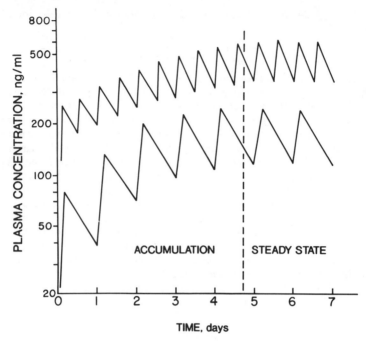

Figure 1D.9. Simulated plasma concentrations of imipramine and diazepam in the same patient using population values for pharmacokinetic parameters. Clearance and volume of distribution were 10 times higher for imipramine than for diazepam, and the half-life was 24 hours for both drugs. The average steady-state concentration achieved between four and five half-lives was 450 ng/ml for diazepam (*upper curve*) and 150 ng/ml for imipramine (*lower curve*).

population ranges (see Chapters 2B and 4A) is shown in Figure 1D.9. Half-life was considered to be 24 hours for each drug, and both volume of distribution and clearance were set at 10-fold higher values for imipramine than for diazepam. Average steady-state plasma concentrations were calculated using Equation 19 by assuming 100% drug absorption.

The predicted average steady-state concentration of diazepam was 450 ng/ml, and the imipramine steady state was 150 ng/ml. Although the antidepressant dose (100 mg/day) is more than threefold higher than the antianxiety drug dose (30 mg/day), the resulting steady-state plasma concentration is only one-third. This difference is predicted because imipramine's clearance was 10-fold greater than that of diazepam. Recall that total body clearance determines steady-state drug concentration, regardless of the values of volume of distribution or half-life. In this example, the V_D of diazepam, like its clearance, is also smaller than the V_D of imipramine, yet the half-lives are identical. This result is predicted from Equation 17 because half-life is a function of both distribution and clearance. When therapy with any two drugs with similar half-lives is initiated in the same patient, the drugs would be expected to accumulate to their respective steady-state concentrations in the same length of time, as is predicted by the concept of half-life. However, the drugs' ultimate steady-state concentrations can differ widely, depending on the relative values of clearance. In this example, imipramine's steady state is lower because of its faster clearance as compared with that of diazepam, although the time to achieve steady state is the same (Fig. 1D.9).

Monotherapy in Different Patients

The clearance of several tricyclic antidepressants has been found to be reduced in the elderly. However, no difference has generally been found in the volume of distribution between young and aged adults. The decreased clearance means that the same dose given to a representative elderly person as to a younger adult will generally produce a higher average steady-state plasma concentration (Equation 19); in addition, the reduced clearance in the elderly results in a prolonged half-life (Equation 17). Therefore, a longer time will be required to achieve steady state in the average elderly patient, the magnitude of steady-state drug concentration will be higher, and a longer time will be required for drug washout once pharmacotherapy is discontinued.

A clinical implication of slower drug clearance in the elderly is that dosage changes should be made at less frequent intervals to allow maximal steady-state accumulation to occur. Drug elimination will also generally take longer to occur in the elderly after discontinuation of dosing. For example, if it is decided to give a monoamine oxidase inhibitor to an elderly person after an unsuccessful trial of a tricyclic antidepressant, it will take longer for the tricyclic antidepressant to clear the body of an average elderly patient than that of a younger person.

CONCEPT OF DRUG ABSORPTION

Once administered, drugs must be absorbed to be effective. Oral administration is the most frequent route for psychotherapeutic drugs. Bioavailability (F) is used to represent the percentage of a drug dose that reaches the systemic circulation intact when referenced to a completely available dose, one usually given intravenously. Bioavailability considers both the completeness of absorption and also the rate of absorption.

The formulation, among other factors, will influence how rapidly a drug is absorbed. This may be an important consideration when rapid relief of symptoms is needed in a psychiatric emergency. Drugs are not absorbed as tablet particles and must first solubilize. This requires a finite time. Capsules must also dissolve to release their contents, which are often solids that must form a solution to be absorbed across the gastrointestinal membranes. These processes frequently result in delays of 30 minutes or more. A general rank order from the most rapid to the slowest bioavailable formulations would be solution, suspension, capsules, tablets, and enteric-coated tablets. A pertinent example of the effect of formulation is that of temazepam; its encapsulation has been blamed for reducing its effectiveness in producing a rapid onset of sleep (see Chapter 4E).

Antacids often decrease the rate of drug absorption and sometimes the extent of absorption. The peak concentration of diazepam after administration with food or antacid is lower and occurs later, as compared to that of drug administration with the patient in the fasting state. However, the completeness of absorption remains the same (see Chapter 4A). This implies that the reinforcing euphoric effects sometimes experienced from oral diazepam could be blunted by administering the drug with antacid. However, the long-term antianxiety

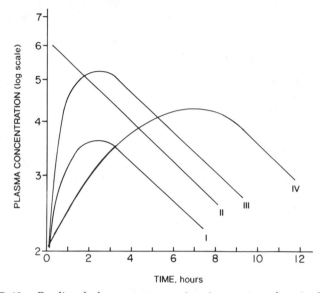

TIME, hours

Figure 1D.10. Predicted plasma concentration time course after single doses of a drug in an intravenous formulation (*II*), a totally absorbed oral formulation (*III*), a more slowly absorbed oral formulation (*IV*), and an incompletely absorbed dose (*I*). As absorption does not alter the elimination rate, the terminal half-lives are similar, as indicated by parallel decline.

effects should be unchanged as the completeness of absorption is expected to be unaltered.

For drugs administered intramuscularly, absorption is usually considered to be faster than from oral forms but may be erratic. An example is that of chlordiazepoxide. Its absorption is less rapid and more erratic after intramuscular (IM) administration than it is after oral administration in the fasting state (11). IM administration cannot be generally depended on to produce the rapid drug absorption that has been attributed to this route of administration. Other disadvantages include pain on administration and local muscular damage.

In Figure 1D.10, concentration versus time profiles are shown for a drug that is administered intravenously (*II*), in a rapidly and completely absorbed oral dosage form (*III*), in an incompletely absorbed formulation (*I*), and in a slowly but completely absorbed oral dosage form (*IV*). As compared to an intravenously administered dose (*II*), there will not be as high a peak concentration for the oral doses, but the total systemic exposure should be the same. This is commonly determined by comparing the area under the curves (AUCs), which should be identical for formulations II, III, and IV. The AUC for formulation *I* is reduced because of incomplete absorption.

CONCEPT OF PRESYSTEMIC ELIMINATION

The concentration versus time profile shown in Figure 1D.11 was observed after an IM and after an oral dose of imipramine on different occasions in the same healthy volunteer. The decreased AUC for the oral dose suggests that absorption of the antidepressant was incomplete. However, urinary recovery studies demonstrated that oral absorption was virtually 100% (12). This profile,

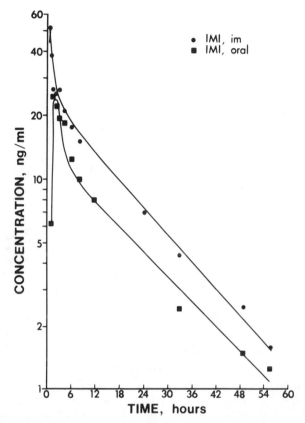

Figure 1D.11.   Plasma concentration versus time course after oral (*IMI, oral*) and intramuscular (*IMI, im*) doses of imipramine in the same volunteer on different occasions.

which seemingly appears to conflict with the comments about AUC above, is a result of the "first-pass" effect, or presystemic elimination (13). This phenomenon results from the loss of drug by metabolism as it passes through the gastrointestional membranes and the liver during the absorption process. Therefore, some administered and absorbed drug never reaches the systemic circulation intact. Presystemic elimination explains why some drugs must be given in much larger oral than intravenous doses to achieve the same pharmacological effects. Many psychoactive drugs, including most cyclic antidepressants and antipsychotics, undergo extensive presystemic elimination (Chapters 2 and 3).

For many psychoactive drugs, the loss of parent drug by oral administration may be partly compensated for by the generation of active metabolites. In Figure 1D.12, the intramuscular and oral plasma concentration profiles for imipramine are shown for another volunteer in whom three of imipramine's active metabolites were also measured (12). The sum of the AUCs for the four active species was nearly identical between doses. The primary effect of first-pass elimination on imipramine disposition is in the rate of metabolite forma-

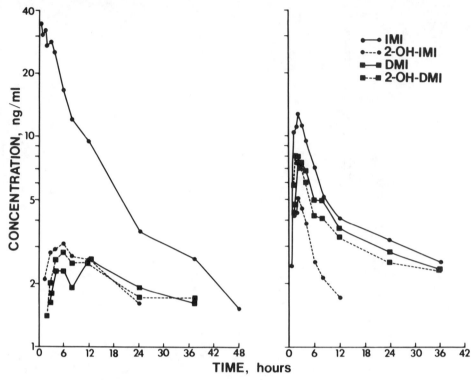

Figure 1D.12.   Plasma concentration time course for imipramine and its major metabolites after intramuscular (**left**) and oral (**right**) doses on different occasions. *IMI*, imipramine; *DMI*, desipramine; *2-OH-IMI*, 2-hydroxyimipramine; *2-OH-DMI*, 2-hydroxydesipramine.

tion with loss of part of the imipramine dose without a marked loss in the yield of pharmacologically active metabolites. First-pass metabolism is an important phenomenon affecting the response to many psychoactive drugs.

IMPORTANCE OF PSYCHOACTIVE DRUG METABOLITES

With the exception of lithium, most of the drugs used in clinical psychopharmacology generate pharmacologically active metabolites. Metabolites arise because of the need for conservation of water. As a general rule, the resulting metabolite displays an increased water solubility, as compared to the parent molecule. This rule has been explained in terms of animal evolution and is linked with the transition from aquatic to terrestrial life. Indeed, water becomes a precious element for nonaquatic beings. As a consequence, natural selection would tend to favor those species that eliminate nonnutritive foreign compounds with maximal water economy and that have acquired enzymatic systems able to increase chemically the water solubility of a large variety of substrates. This explains the ultimate fate of ingested drugs as renally excreted biotransformation products.

Metabolites produce difficulties for psychoactive drug monitoring. The half-life of a drug metabolite will always be equal to or longer than that of its parent drug. This is intuitively obvious because a metabolite cannot be eliminated any faster than it is formed (14). For drugs with major active metabolites, like the cyclic antidepressants, antipsychotics, and some anxiolytics, a longer time may be necessary between dosage adjustments, for both the drug and its metabolites to reach a new steady state than would be predicted by knowing only the half-life of the parent drug. In general, hydroxylated or demethylated metabolites should be considered to be pharmacologically active unless proven otherwise. Another difficulty posed by metabolites is the correlation of plasma concentrations to clinical effects. These issues are discussed later in the text.

Three major factors determine the importance of psychoactive drug metabolites: how much is present (i.e., quantitatively, how much is present in relation to the parent drug); their plasma protein binding, which will reflect how much of the drug is available to diffuse to active receptor sites; and, finally, the intrinsic activity of the metabolite at the receptor site, a function of the affinity of the metabolite for the receptor.

The plasma concentration of m-chlorophenylpiperazine (m-CPP), the major active metabolite of trazodone, can be seen in Figure 1D.13 to be much lower than that of trazodone in plasma after a single dose in rats (CL DeVane, L Faust: Disposition of trazodone and its major metabolite m-chlorophenylpiperazine in rats, unpublished data). On this basis, the metabolite would be predicted to have minimal importance in producing central nervous system (CNS) effects, as compared to trazodone. However, in brain tissue, the m-CPP concentration exceeded that of trazodone. As m-CPP is active as a serotonin receptor agonist, it probably contributes to the overall actions of trazodone. Whether this situation is also present in humans is unknown. Similarly, bupropion, a monocyclic antidepressant, was present in low concentration in the CSF of depressed patients at steady state (15). Although the concentration of its metabolite was also low relative to the metabolite concentration in plasma, the metabolite concentration far exceeded that of bupropion in the CNS. It is likely that the degree of plasma protein binding of hydroxybupropion is far less than that of bupropion, allowing a greater amount of drug to diffuse to the CNS. These two examples point out the difficulty in relating plasma concentrations of psychoactive drugs and their metabolites to clinical effects and the paradox of drawing conclusions about the importance of metabolites without knowing their penetration into the CNS. Whenever possible, active metabolites should be included in psychoactive drug therapy monitoring.

CONCEPT OF NONLINEAR ELIMINATION

The elimination of most drugs in humans after nontoxic doses can be characterized by an apparent first-order process, i.e., the rate of elimination is proportional to how much drug is in the body. With certain drugs, even in the usual dose range, and for any drug in a large enough dose, the kinetics can be described as being nonlinear. For drugs with linear kinetics, a linear relationship exists between dose and plasma concentration. For a few notable examples, this relationship breaks down, causing a disproportionate increase in concentration for a change in dose. Table 1D.4 lists some known examples of nonlinearity in clinical psychopharmacology.

We usually increase doses of psychoactive drugs with the assumption that a proportional increase in plasma concentration will occur at the new steady state. With rigorously designed studies, this relationship can occasionally be

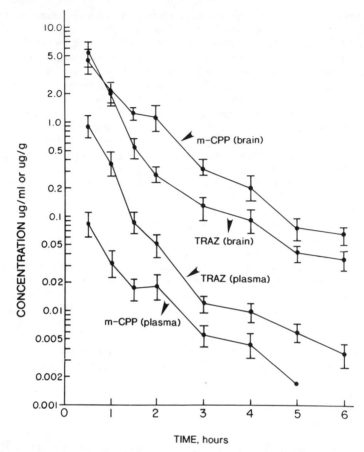

Figure 1D.13.   Time course of trazodone (*TRAZ*) and its major metabolite, *m*-chlorophenylpiperazine (*m-CPP*) in brain tissue and plasma of rats after an intraperitoneal dose of 30 mg/kg. Each *point* represents the mean value of four to five animals.

observed to break down. The examples in Table 1D.4 emphasize the need for caution when increasing drug dosing at the upper range of usually employed doses or in special populations who may be at greater risk for nonlinear disposition because of the presence of medical illness or advanced age.

IMPORTANCE OF DRUG INTERACTIONS

Drug interactions may be either pharmacokinetic or pharmacodynamic. Most often, interacting drugs produce enhancement of the clinical effects of one or both drugs. Examples are given for each of the prototype drugs discussed later in the text. A major cause of drug interactions is disturbance in metabolism by another drug. This may occur by hepatic enzyme induction or inhibition. Table 1D.5 lists some drugs known to cause these effects. Only a few interactions have been thoroughly studied. Impairment of hepatic clearance by a coadministered inhibitor could be expected to decrease total body clearance of a highly metabolized drug (16). As predicted by Equations 17 and 19, half-life would

Table 1D.4.
Evidence for Nonlinear Disposition in Clinical Psychopharmacology

Drug	Effect	Comment
Carbamazepine	Steady-state concentrations decrease with chronic dosing	Due to autoinduction; can influence other coadministered drugs
Lithium	Extended half-life upon dosing for several years	Could be due to renal function decline; emphasizes need for long-term monitoring
Imipramine	Increase in desipramine to imipramine concentration ratio with increasing doses in the elderly	Represents the borderline of capacity-limited disposition in the elderly
Desipramine, nortriptyline	Disproportionate increase in steady state with increase in dose	A rare but apparently real phenomenon
Chlorpromazine	Decreased steady-state concentrations after years of chronic dosing	Mechanism unknown

increase, as would steady-state concentration. Concurrent therapy with any of these drugs or the presence of certain environmental conditions, such as smoking, may require more vigilant monitoring to avoid adverse effects on psychoactive drug therapy.

Another mechanism of drug interactions is interference with the drug absorption process. As explained above, this may involve a decrease in the rate and/or extent of absorption but usually results in a diminution of effects. Drugs that have similar pharmacological effects may cause pharmacodynamic interactions when coadministered. An example would be increased anticholinergic effects when any of the drugs from different classes with muscarinic antagonist activity are coadministered.

ROLE OF PLASMA PROTEIN BINDING

Psychoactive drugs, with the exception of lithium, circulate in the blood bound to some degree to plasma or serum proteins. The major drug-binding proteins are albumin and α_1-acid glycoprotein. For most drugs, the percentage bound is relatively high, in the range of 80 to 95% bound. It is generally accepted that only the free or nonbound portion can diffuse to pharmacologically active sites to interact with receptors. Therefore, drug interactions or other conditions that affect plasma protein binding may alter the free or available drug that produces effects. For the most part, protein binding interactions are of little consequence but should not be ignored. Whenever inflammatory disease states are present or a drug-binding interaction is suspected, more vigilance should be exercised in monitoring therapy. Interested readers are referred elsewhere for explanations of the kinetics of binding interactions (3, 7).

REFERENCES
1. Wagner JG: History of pharmacokinetics. *Pharmacol Ther* 12:537–562, 1981.
2. DeVane CL, Jusko WJ: Dosage regimen design. Pharmacol Ther 17:143–163, 1982.

Table 1D.5.
Known Hepatic Microsomal Enzyme Inducers and Inhibitors

Inducers	Inhibitors
Phenobarbital	Allopurinol
Carbamazepine	Cimetidine
Rifampin	Disulfiram
Ethanol	Ethanol
Phenytoin	Isoniazid
Tobacco smoking	Metronidazol
Brussels sprouts	Valproic acid
Charcoal-broiled beef	Oral contraceptives

3. Evans WE, Schentag JJ, Jusko WJ (eds): *Applied Pharmacokinetic Principles of Therapeutic Drug Monitoring, ed 2*, Applied Therapeutics, San Francisco, 1986.
4. Greenblatt DJ, Shader RI: Introduction: pharmacokinetics in clinical psychiatry and psychopharmacology. In: *Psychopharmacology: The Third Generation of Progress*, Meltzer HY (ed), Raven Press, New York, 1987, p 1339.
5. DeVane CL, Savett M, Jusko WJ: Desipramine and 2-hydroxy desipramine pharmacokinetics in normal volunteers. *Eur J Clin Pharmacol* 19:61–64, 1982.
6. Greenblatt DJ, Shader RI: *Pharmacokinetics in Clinical Practice*, WB Saunders, Philadelphia, 1985.
7. Rowland M, Tozer TN: *Clinical Pharmacokinetics, Concepts and Applications*, Lea & Febiger, Philadelphia, 1980.
8. Pentel PR, Bullock ML, DeVane CL: Hemoperfusion for imipramine overdose: elimination of active metabolites. *J Toxicol Clin Toxicol* 19:239–248, 1982.
9. Dawling S, Lynn K, Rosser R, Braithwaite R: Nortriptyline metabolism in chronic renal failure: metabolite elimination. *Clin Pharmacol Ther* 32:322–329, 1982.
10. DeVane CL, Laizure SC: The effect of experimentally induced renal failure on accumulation of bupropion and its major basic metabolites in plasma and brain of guinea pigs. *Psychopharmacology* 89:404–408, 1986.
11. Greenblatt DJ, Shader RI, Kock-Weser J, Franke J: Slow absorption of intramuscular chlordiazepoxide. *N Engl J Med* 291:1116–1118, 1974.
12. Sutfin TA, DeVane CL, Jusko WJ: The analysis and disposition of imipramine and its active metabolites. *Psychopharmacology* 82:310–317, 1984.
13. George CF, Shand DG, Renwick AG (eds): *Presystemic Drug Elimination*, Butterworth Scientific, London, 1982.
14. Houston JB: Drug metabolite kinetics. *Pharmacol Ther* 15:521–552, 1981.
15. Golden RN, DeVane CL, Laizure SC, Rudorfer MV, Sherer MA, Potter WZ: Bupropion: the role of metabolites in clinical outcome. *Arch Gen Psychiatry* 45:145–149, 1988.
16. Curry SH, DeVane CL, Wolfe MM: Cimetidine interactions with amitriptyline. *Eur J Clin Pharmacol* 29:429–433, 1985.

▬ E ▬

Psychiatric Database

The psychiatric examination consists of patient interviews; a mental status examination; physical, neurological, and laboratory examinations; and, when appropriate, psychological testing and interviews with family or friends. This material is collated into a meaningful diagnosis, prognosis, and treatment plan. The purpose of this chapter is to help readers who do not routinely collect a psychiatric database to understand its general format, to explain why certain questions are asked in the mental status examination, and to suggest where information might be available that will assist in monitoring treatment.

Several mental health professionals usually contribute to the psychiatric database. Psychiatrists are highly skilled at performing mental status examinations and usually direct the overall care of patients; however, all members of a patient care team should be able to make independent assessments about behavior. Clinical pharmacists are often skilled at determining medication histories. Neuropsychological testing is the unique expertise of the psychologist, and social workers are frequently the best professionals to determine social and occupational functioning of patients. Data from several sources will be available in the patient's records; however, answers to some questions relevant to monitoring drug therapy can be obtained only by patient interview. Competent monitoring of psychoactive drug therapy requires the opportunity to obtain information directly from the patient.

All professionals working with psychoactive drugs need to be conversant with the various parts of the psychiatric history and mental status examination. The psychiatric examination is similar to that conducted with other types of patients with the inclusion of a formal mental status examination. A complete psychiatric examination generally covers the areas listed in Table 1E.1. The following outline is meant to serve as a suggested approach for reviewing and organizing patient data for drug therapy monitoring. Standard references should be consulted for further discussion (1–3).

IDENTIFYING DATA

These data include the patient's name, age, sex, occupation, home address, length of current address, and names of other persons living at the same residence.

CHIEF COMPLAINT AND PRESENT ILLNESS

The chief complaint is the problem for which the patient seeks professional help. It may or may not be relevant to the present illness. The patient could be referred by his/her family, by another professional, or by the authorities. A chronology of the problem is determined, beginning with its onset and continu-

Table 1E.1.
The Psychiatric Database

   I. Identifying data
  II. Chief complaint and present illness
 III. Family history
  IV. Personal history
   V. Medical and medication history
  VI. Mental status examination
    A. Attitute toward the examiner
    B. Appearance and grooming
    C. Psychomotor behavior
    D. Affect or mood
    E. Thought
    F. Sensorium
        1. Level of consciousness
        2. Memory
        3. Orientation
        4. Judgment
        5. Insight
        6. Ability to abstract
 VII. Physical evaluation
VIII. Neurological evaluation
  IX. Laboratory examination
   X. Further diagnostic reports
  XI. Diagnosis, prognosis, and treatment plan

---

ing with the course of the problem, the circumstances under which it occurs, and aggravating and alleviating factors.

FAMILY HISTORY

Contributions from the field of genetics demonstrate the importance of hereditary factors in a variety of mental disorders (4). By learning whether relatives have or have not been diagnosed as having major mental disorders, one may make clearer decisions regarding drug maintenance therapy for patients with affective or psychotic disorders. It is useful to know the family's attitude about and insight into the patient's illness. Family members are sometimes the only assurance that prescribed drugs will be taken on schedule.

PERSONAL HISTORY

Included under this heading is information about the patient's past life, from the prenatal period through adulthood. This information can be an important reflection of influences on the current presentation of illness. For example, the history of past school performance can be important in monitoring the response to stimulant therapy in a patient with attention deficit hyperactivity disorder. Patients with panic disorder may relate a history of shyness in school at an early age. This area of inquiry can be extensive and time-consuming, depending on the nature of the present illness. Topics covered include educational, sexual, and occupational functioning, plus other pertinent areas in the patient's past (5).

MEDICAL AND MEDICATION HISTORY

It is necessary to learn of medical illnesses that could be causing or contributing to the patient's problem. Many medical illnesses produce psychological symptoms that disappear when the medical problem is appropriately treated. Hypothyroidism presenting with depressed mood is an example. Records from previous hospitalizations may be available for review. The medical history will suggest the extent of physical and laboratory examinations needed to rule out organic illness.

A complete medication history should be taken (6). A surprisingly high frequency of hospital admissions is due to drug-related problems, including drug abuse, side effects, and noncompliance. Present medications often give indications of problems being treated. The use of an organ system approach is recommended for obtaining these data to determine both prescription and over-the-counter medications that the patient may be taking. Many patients do not consider nonprescription products as drugs. Also included in the medication history should be questions about substance abuse. The inquiry should cover the following classes of substances: opiates, hypnotics and sedatives, stimulants, hallucinogens, volatile substances, cannabinoids, and alcohol. Caffeine and tobacco use should be determined. Smoking directly effects the ability to metabolize most psychoactive drugs, and caffeine should not be overlooked as a source of anxiety.

When patients cannot recall the names of medications that they may be taking, it can be useful to determine the color of the medicine, whether it is a capsule or tablet, or other identifying features about the dosage form. Patients should always be asked if they have any drugs with them. The medication history should also assess the regularity of compliance.

A complete drug history should include questions about drug allergy and side effects. When offending drugs are named by the patient, an attempt should be made to be specific as to the type and intensity of allergic reaction or side effects. Positive responses should be categorized as to definite or questionable, and allergic reactions should be classified as anaphylactic, immediate, or delayed. It is important to keep in mind that patients often report allergy to medication when in fact they mean other reactions such as nausea, vomiting, dizziness, etc.

MENTAL STATUS EXAMINATION

This is a collection of observations about a patient's mood, behavior, and mental operations. This detailed record is a necessary foundation for understanding the patient, for planning further evaluation and treatment, and for providing a baseline against which to measure change. It is analogous in psychiatry to the cardiac examination in cardiology or the neurological examination in neurology.

The mental status examination is performed for the purpose of determining the patient's current mental condition, that is, emotional status, mental capacity, and functioning. When recorded systematically in a meaningful way, it enables the examiner to establish a baseline of current findings with which to compare future changes.

There are many variations of the formal mental status examination (7, 8). Its content and completeness will vary according to the information sought, the time available for interview, the style of the interviewer, whether it is an initial or follow-up assessment, and other factors. The outline below contains many of the topic areas that will be covered in any form of the mental status examination. An understanding of the various parts of this procedure is necessary to assess optimally the response to drug therapy. It is through the mental status examination that most of the target symptoms of illness will be monitored (see Chapter 1F).

Attitude toward the Examiner

This is a statement regarding what seems to be the patient's general view of the examiner. For example, the patient may be withdrawn, open, guarded, suspicious, angry, hostile, friendly, or cooperative. In considering the patient's condition and attitude toward the examiner, one should assess the reliability of the information given by the patient. This also serves as an indication of potential compliance by the patient with prescribed drug therapy.

Appearance and Grooming

One should note what the patient is wearing and whether it is appropriate for his or her age and educational and social background. Questions that should be considered include: Is the patient neat, clean or disheveled? What is the condition of the patient's hair, teeth, and nails? Nonverbal behavior can be informative (9).

Psychomotor Behavior

This consists of a description of the patient's gait, posture, motor activity, facial expression, and speech. Is the patient limp, stiff, sprawled, slouching, unsteady, or poorly coordinated? Is the face expressive, and are facial expressions appropriate to what is being said by the patient? What are the characteristics of the patient's speech? This could include intensity, pitch, productivity, spontaneity, diction, vocabulary, rate, relevance, reaction time, and mannerisms. These observations give indications of the problem and frequently reflect drug-related side effects. For example, a depressed patient may exhibit a prolonged reaction time to questions, speak in a monotone with low intensity, and not speak spontaneously. In contrast to this type of patient, a person with mania may exhibit loud, overly productive speech that rambles. Many neurological side effects of antipsychotic drugs are reflected by a patient's psychomotor behavior.

Affect or Mood

Affect is the feeling tone, pleasurable or unpleasurable, that accompanies an idea. Affect and emotion are often used interchangeably. Affect determines the general attitude, whether of rejection, acceptance, flight, fight, or indifference to an idea. When an affective state is sustained for a considerable period, one speaks of a mood. Thus, mood is a sustained affect. A useful analogy is that affect is to mood as weather is to climate. Most mental status examinations will include a statement about the patient's affect. Affect may be described as shallow or inadequate (emotional flatness), inappropriate (when the emotion does not correspond to the stimulus), or labile (changeable). Other descriptors include optimistic, euphoric, elated, exalted, ecstatic, pessimistic, sad, depressed, melancholic, anxious, fearful, angry, hostile, suspicious, guilty, shameful, prideful, jealous, or humiliated.

Thought

Thought is broken down into the stream of thought and thought content. Stream of thought refers to the rate of thought and associations made. For example, the rate may be slowed or normal, or speech may be pressured, with flight of ideas present. The associations between thoughts may be reduced; there may be blocking; or the patient's thought pattern may be circumstantial, scattered, tangential, or incoherent.

The term "thought content" refers to a constellation of ideas that is emotionally charged for that person. Some examples include trends, complexes, phobias, obsessions, delusions, hallucinations, hypochondriacal ideation, ideas of reference, and paranoid ideation. The assessment of thought content may require specific directed questions, e.g., "Have you ever thought that someone was trying to do you harm?" Hallucinations may be caused by various drugs, including cocaine and amphetamines, or by toxicity from anticholinergic agents or antidepressants.

Delusions are false beliefs that cannot be reconciled to reason and are inappropriate for that person's social and educational background. A complex is a group of associated ideas having a common, strong emotional tone. These are largely unconscious and significantly influence attitudes. A phobia is an obsessive, persistent, unrealistic, intense fear of an object or situation. Ideas of reference refer to the incorrect interpretation of causal incidents and external events as having direct reference to oneself. These may reach sufficient intensity so as to constitute delusions. These and other thought processes, often pathological, are discussed elsewhere in detail (1).

Sensorium

The sensorium relates to the patient's consciousness and ability to concentrate and perform intellectual tasks. Areas of sensorium include the following:

Level of Consciousness   The patient may be alert, hyperalert, confused, stuporous, or in a coma. Drug intoxication is often associated with a disturbance of sensorium. Disorders involving consciousness can cause problems in areas such as memory, judgment, and orientation.

Memory   This is determined for immediate, recent, and remote events and memory deficits in sensory areas. Several conditions can cause memory deficit out of proportion to other cognitive deficits. These include the alcohol amnestic syndrome in alcoholic patients and Alzheimer's dementia in its early stages of progression.

Orientation   This is usually determined for time, place, person, and situation.

Judgment   This area is evaluated for personal matters, whether the patient is logical and practical in handling activities, and for nonpersonal matters, whether the patient can distinguish between different concepts. Gross impairment in judgment may suggest an organic cause or a severe psychosis.

Insight   This is the degree of awareness and understanding on the part of the patient that he is ill. There may be complete denial of illness, a slight awareness of being sick, or an awareness of illness due to something unknown.

Ability to Abstract   The ability to make valid generalizations is most frequently tested with the use of proverbs (10). This is considered by most psychiatrists to be important in evaluating the presence of mental illness. In interpreting this ability, the patient's ethnic, socioeconomic, and educational background must be considered.

PHYSICAL EVALUATION

This is necessary to rule out medical disorders, particularly those that could be responsible for the patient's psychopathology, such as tertiary syphilis, subdural hematoma, and others.

NEUROLOGICAL EVALUATION

Neurological disorders affect many patients with psychiatric problems. Also, many drugs produce neurological symptoms. Distinguishing between psychiatric and neurological problems is a complicated task, but recent technological innovations (e.g., computed axial tomography (CT scan)) are improving the situation.

LABORATORY EXAMINATION

This topic is discussed in Chapter 1G. One should always review available laboratory data as part of the physical examination.

FURTHER DIAGNOSTIC REPORTS

These include the results of psychological testing and reports from social workers and other consultants.

DIAGNOSIS, PROGNOSIS, AND TREATMENT PLAN

When possible, a diagnosis or differential diagnosis should be recorded according to the classification in DSM-III-R (3). The prognosis is an opinion as to the probable future course of the problem. The treatment plan is a summary of recommendations and should include measurable outcomes to assess the patient's progress. The treatment plan would also include the role of medication, including length of therapy and an outline of target symptoms.

Although the depth of inquiry into a particular part of a mental status examination will vary with the patient's presenting complaints, past history, etc., the available data should be reviewed thoroughly at the beginning of drug therapy monitoring. Only by starting at this point can the logic be seen for further diagnostic studies, the development of a treatment plan, and the definition of target symptoms.

REFERENCES

1. Kaplan HI, Saddock BJ (eds): *Comprehensive Textbook of Psychiatry, ed 4*, Williams & Wilkins, Baltimore, 1985, pp 487–499.
2. Taylor MA, Sierles FS, Abrams R: The neuropsychiatric evaluation. In: Hales RE, Yudofsky SC (eds), *Textbook of Neuropsychiatry*, American Psychiatric Press, Washington, DC, 1987.
3. Othmer E, Othmer SC: *The Clinical Interview Using DSM-III-R*, American Psychiatric Press, Washington, DC, 1989.
4. Slater E, Cowie V: *The Genetics of Mental Disorders*, Oxford University Press, London, 1971.
5. Gould RL: The phases of adult life: a study in developmental psychology. *Am J Psychiatry* 129:521–531, 1972.
6. Caranasos GJ, Stewart RB, Cluff LE: Drug induced illness leading to hospitalization. *JAMA* 228:713–717, 1974.
7. Folstein MF, Folstein SE, McHugh PR: Mini-mental state. *J Psychiatr Res* 12:189–198, 1975.

8. Spitzer RL, Skodol AE, Gibbon M, Williams JBS: *DSM-III Case Book*, American Psychiatric Association Press, Washington, DC, 1981.
9. Hill D: Non-verbal behaviour in mental illness. *Br J Psychiatry* 124:221–230, 1974.
10. Carson RC: Proverb interpretation in acutely schizophrenic patients. *J Nerv Ment Dis* 135:556–564, 1962.

▬ F ▬

Target Symptom Monitoring of Mental Illness

This chapter summarizes the major categories of the Diagnostic and Statistical Manual of Mental Disorders, Third Edition-Revised (DSM-III-R), the most widely recognized classification of mental disorders (1). So the reader can appreciate the logic in monitoring pharmacotherapy with psychoactive drugs, briefly reviewed are the disorders of mood, psychosis, and anxiety as they are usually associated with the antidepressant, antipsychotic, and antianxiety drugs. These drugs are used to treat many of the same target symptoms that occur in mental illnesses other than these three major groups of mental disorders.

Table 1F.1 lists categories of major mental disorders. Drugs are listed that have been used for treating disorders from each category, on either an experimental or a routine basis. It should be apparent that various psychoactive drugs may be used in the treatment of many different disorders. The drugs are far less specific in their effects on symptoms of mental illness than are psychiatric diagnoses in classifying symptoms into disorders. In addition, the clinician will encounter some patients with more than one mental illness and other patients who also have coexisting medical problems requiring pharmacotherapy. A lack of objective measurements in rating psychopathological states requires us to make subjective judgments about what symptoms are present and to what severity. This presents a challenge to the clinician to predict the outcome of psychoactive drug therapy.

It should be intuitive that drugs are given for specific reasons but that they frequently produce global effects. An example is the resulting psychomotor blunting from administration of haloperidol to excited or agitated patients, regardless of the cause of the problem. It is the subset of symptoms responsive to drug therapy that reflects the essential features of the illness that the clinician should strive to identify (2, 3). These *target symptoms* frequently show repeating patterns of change. For example, some symptoms of schizophrenia, such as auditory hallucinations and disruptive behavior, frequently disappear sooner than the social isolation and ineffective planning for the future that frequently accompany the chronic psychotic state.

The physician, pharmacist, or other professional monitoring drug therapy should identify at the outset of therapy what changes can be expected in the mental status examination of each monitored patient treated with a specific

Table 1F.1.
Major Mental Disorders and Pharmacotherapy

Major Disorder	Examples: Drugs Used Routinely or Experimentally in Treatment for Either Primary or Associated Symptoms
Disorders evident in infancy, childhood, or adolescence	Mental retardation, conduct disorder, anorexia nervosa, attention-deficit disorder, bulimia nervosa CA, STIM, LI[a], MAOI[b]
Organic mental disorders	Alzheimer's disease, multi-infarct dementia A-PSYCH, BENZO, HYP
Substance use disorders	Alcohol dependence, cocaine dependence, opioid dependence CA, LI, BENZO, clonidine, disulfiram, methadone, propranolol
Psychotic disorders	Brief reactive psychosis, schizoaffective disorder, schizophrenia A-PSYCH, CA, LI, HYP[a], BENZO[a]
Mood disorders	Bipolar disorder (manic), major depression CA, STIM, BENZO, HYP, MAOI, A-CONVUL
Anxiety disorders	Panic disorder, agoraphobia, posttraumatic stress disorder BENZO, HYP, CA, MAOI, A-CONVUL[a]
Dissociative disorders	Multiple personality disorder, psychogenic fugue
Disorders of impulse control	Pathological gambling, intermittent explosive disorder LI, A-CONVUL
Personality disorders	Antisocial, borderline, narcissistic, schizotypal LI, BENZO, A-PSYCH

[a]Drug used experimentally.
[b]CA, cyclic antidepressants; STIM, stimulants; A-PSYCH, antipsychotics; BENZO, benzodiazepines; LI, lithium; A-CONVUL, anticonvulsants used as mood stablizers; HYP, hypnotics; MAOI, monoamine oxidase inhibitors.

drug. Most major psychiatric diagnoses are first made early in the patient's life, and the disorder typically follows a longitudinal course of symptom remissions and recrudescences. However, patient presentations are diverse and variable, sometimes even from one episode of illness to another within the same patient.

Through direct observation and verbal examination of the patient, changes in target symptoms can be assessed. By virtue of integrating individual assessments from a team of people with different health care perspectives, the patient's psychiatric database and mental status examinations are an invaluable source of information. This topic is discussed in the previous chapter. In each of the databases for prototype psychoactive drugs presented later in this book, laboratory tests are identified for monitoring that are expected to show changes or to remain unaffected by typical drug dosage regimens. Thus, psychoactive drug monitoring combines subjective assessment of behavioral changes with expectations about the time course of drug concentrations and effects in the body (Chapters 1C and 1D).

Table 1F.2.
Classification of Mood Disorders

   I. Major depression
      A. Single episode
      B. Recurrent
  II. Dysthymia
 III. Bipolar disorder
      A. Mixed
      B. Manic
      C. Depressed
 IV. Cyclothymia

MOOD DISORDERS

The most widely recognized mood disorders are mania and depression (4, 5). These are severe emotional disturbances that superficially seem to be the opposite of each other. We all experience different moods at times. As mood goes up from normal, we may describe ourselves as happy, optimistic, euphoric, elated, or ecstatic. As our mood goes below normal, we may feel disinterested, sad, pessimistic, depressed, melancholic, or even in a state of desperation. In everyday usage, people state frequently that they are depressed when they mean despondent. However, at the extremes of mood swings, functioning can be impaired. These states frequently require social or medical intervention and may constitute the presence of a mood, or affective, disorder (1). The prevalence is high. As many as 10 to 20 million people in the United States experience a clinically significant depressive episode in any given year.

Until recently, most literature referred to these illnesses as affective disorders. The term affect refers to the emotional feeling that we attach to an object, an idea, or thought, and it includes inner feelings and their external manifestions. Mood is the term used to describe the emotional feeling experienced by a person internally. These two concepts are frequently interchanged but have subtle differences in meaning (6). When an affect is sustained, we speak of mood. Inferences about affect are made from present observations, whereas generalizations about one's mood are made on the basis of present observations and knowledge of past events. The importance of this distinction for monitoring psychoactive drug therapy is that acute drug administration more likely alters affect, whereas chronic therapy is generally needed to elicit sustained changes in mood.

The mood disorders include major depression, bipolar disorder, dysthymia, and cyclothymia. The distinguishing feature between a major depression and bipolar disorder is whether there has ever been a manic episode. When there has been one or more manic episodes, with or without a history of a major depressive episode, the classification bipolar disorder is appropriate. Bipolar disorder is subclassed as mixed (having symptoms of both mania and depression), manic, or depressed, whereas major depression is characterized as single episode (first depression) or recurrent. Table 1F.2 is adapted from the DSM-III-R classification of mood disorders.

A major depression is a serious illness frequently requiring hospitalization. The mortality from suicide associated with depression in the United States may be as great as 70,000 people annually. The illness is recurrent for most people, therefore, careful observation and documentation of symptom presentation and changes during therapy may aid in subsequent therapy.

The biological basis of depression is unknown. The catecholamine and indolamine hypotheses of depression (7, 8) have stimulated productive research into the causes of depression but do not encompass a sufficient number of relevant clinical and biochemical observations to provide a unifying hypothesis. Undoubtedly, the major neurotransmitters, norepinephrine, dopamine, and serotonin, are involved in the pathogenesis of depression and, by inference, their major neuronal pathways in the brain (Chapter 1B). The promise of *in vivo* imaging with positron emission tomography (PET) is that in the future specific physiological abnormalities in mental illnesses will be identified and will provide markers of the progress or remission of mental disease (9). At present, the simplest hypothesis to explain depression is that it involves not a single neurotransmitter but an imbalance between major neurotransmitters.

The symptoms of depression may be present in all of the various subtypes of mood disorders but not to the same degree of severity. These symptoms can be broadly divided into two groups: the emotional or cognitive manifestations of depression and the physical, vegetative, or biological symptoms. It should be emphasized that "depression," along with the symptoms listed below, are normal human emotions. It is only when their collective presence impairs functioning for a sufficient period that a mood disorder is considered to be present. The manifestations of these symptoms are diverse. The essential criteria for diagnosis of a major depressive episode by DSM-III-R criteria are the presence of a dysphoric mood or loss of interest or pleasure in all or almost all usual activities and pasttimes, plus a specified minimal number of symptoms that have been present nearly every day for a period of at least 2 weeks. Many patients who do not meet DSM-III-R criteria for a specific diagnosis frequently benefit from drug therapy. The presence or absence of a precipating event preceding the onset of depression seems to have little correlation with the likelihood of a clinical response to antidepressant therapy.

Major depression is accompanied by both cognitive and physical symptoms. A dysphoric mood is an essential feature. The person often feels profound sadness and a sense of hopelessness about the future. This may be accompanied by suicidal thoughts and attempts. The activities, people, and ideas that usually give the person pleasure become seemingly hollow. Pessimistic thinking is usual, with low self-esteem. There is a lack of motivation to accomplish everyday activities. Physical symptoms are often prominent. Anorexia leading to weight loss is frequent, as are sleep disturbances and loss of libido. Table 1F.3 lists target symptoms potentially useful used for monitoring recovery from depression.

The essential feature of a *manic episode* is a distinct period when the patient's predominant mood is elevated, expansive, or irritable (1). Associated with this mood is the presence of manic syndrome symptoms that may include hyperactivity, pressure of speech, flight of ideas, inflated self-esteem, and involvement in high risk activities. Table 1F.4 lists target symptoms for monitoring response to antimanic therapy. Extensive clinical experience and research results have confirmed the efficacy of lithium in the treatment of acute mania and as prophylaxis of manic-depressive illness (10).

Table 1F.3.
Target Symptoms for Monitoring Response to Antidepressant Therapy

Cognitive Symptoms	Physical Symptoms
Dejected mood	Loss or increase of appetite
Self-blame	Psychomotor agitation or retardation
Low self-esteem	Sleep disturbance
Self-depreciation	Loss of libido
Loss of gratification	Gastrointestinal upset
Loss of attachments	Diurnal fluctuation of mood
Loss of sense of humor	
Negative expectations	
Increasing ambivalence	
Delusions	
Increasing dependence	
Hallucinations	
Suicidal ideation	
Loss of motivation	

Table 1F.4.
Target Symptoms for Monitoring Response to Antimanic Therapy

Affective Symptoms	Psychomotor Symptoms	Cognitive Symptoms
Irritability	Sleep disturbance	Delusions (e.g., sexual
Labile mood	Pressured speech	prowess, persecutory,
Short attention span	Talkative	religious, grandiosity)
Euphoria	Flight of ideas	Racing thoughts
Manipulative behavior	Assaultive behavior	Ideas of reference
Elevated or expansive mood	Increased activity	Hallucinations
		Flight of ideas

In *cyclothymia* there are intermittent symptoms characteristic of both the manic and depressive syndromes, but they are not severe enough to constitute a major depressive or manic episode. In *dysthymia*, the symptoms are not of sufficient severity to meet the criteria for a major depression. Symptoms must be present for at least 2 years to meet the criteria for dysthymia.

PSYCHOTIC DISORDERS

Psychosis is a general term describing a severe behavioral disturbance that is characterized by an impaired sense of reality, impaired ability to communicate, and loss of emotional awareness and control, and/or cognitive abilities. When sustained, this state leads to an inability to maintain personal relations and to compromised daily functioning. Behavior may be of psychotic proportions in several mental disorders, including mania, severe depression, organic brain syndrome, and schizophrenic disorders. The antipsychotic drugs are used to calm disturbed patients, whatever the cause, but their greatest use is in the treatment of schizophrenias.

To be considered schizophrenic, a patient must have certain psychotic features for at least 6 months; must have sufficiently deteriorated in occupational, interpersonal, and self-supportive functioning, with an onset before 45 years of age; and must currently show some signs of illness (1). Many patients show a *prodromal phase* of schizophrenia characterized by social withdrawal, impaired work functioning and self-care, peculiar behavior, a blunted or inappropriate affect, and symptoms of a thought disorder (e.g., circumstantial or metaphorical speech, odd or magical thinking).

An *active phase* may involve a number of characteristic symptoms. A major disturbance in content of thought may appear as delusions or hallucinations. Common delusions are persecutory in nature, e.g., a belief that someone is spying on the patient. In delusions of reference, the patient believes that causal events, everyday objects, or other people hold some particular significance in the patient's life. Hallucinations are most commonly of the auditory type. Frequently, the voices make insulting and derogatory statements about the patient. Command hallucinations, if obeyed, may make the patient dangerous to himself or others. The most common disturbance in the form of thought is a loosening of associations, in which ideas shift from one subject to another, completely unrelated, without the patient showing any awareness that the topics are unconnected. Speech may be incomprehensible ("word salad") when loosening of associations is severe.

The onset of schizophrenia is usually during adolescence or early adulthood, but it may appear later in life. To meet DSM-III-R criteria for schizophrenia, symptoms must be present for at least 6 months during which an active phase, if treatment was given, was present for nearly 1 week. An active phase may last weeks or months. Usually the patient can expect to have recurrences periodically throughout his life, which will be separated by months or years.

For many patients, a *residual phase* of schizophrenia persists after the active phase of the illness has abated. This characteristic of the illness is similar to the prodromal phase, although affective blunting or flattening and impairment in role functioning tend to be more common in the residual phase. At this point, the patient displays psychotic symptoms, but they are no longer accompanied by a strong affect. Schizophrenia is usually a chronic disorder, with a patient gradually becoming more withdrawn and eccentric over a period of years. Some patients experience low-level delusions and hallucinations for many years.

The biology of schizophrenia is still being defined. The most widely accepted hypothesis for its pathological basis is that it involves a relative overactivity of central dopaminergic systems (11). This view has arisen partly from recognition that the effective anti-psychotic drugs (Chapter 3) are dopamine receptor antagonists. Like other mental illnesses, a genetic basis and environmental factors play an important but as yet undefined role in its origin (12).

There have been numerous subclassifications of schizophrenia in the past, most of which were unsatisfactory in describing all presentations of the illness. The DSM-III-R recognizes five subtypes listed in Table 1F.5. In the *disorganized* type, the patient has a blunted, silly, or inappropriate affect, is frequently incoherent, and shows bizarre mannerisms. *Catatonic* patients display bizzare postures and may resist attempts to be moved. In the *paranoid* type, the essential features are prominent persecutory or grandiose delusions or hallucinations with a persecutory or grandiose content. The *undifferentiated* type is a type of schizophrenia in which there are prominent delusions, hallucinations, incoherence, or grossly disorganized behavior that does not seem specific for the preceding three categories. Finally, in the *residual* type, the patient is in remission from active psychosis but displays many of the symptoms of the residual phase

Table 1F.5.
Classification of Psychotic Disorders

I. Schizophrenia
   A. Disorganized
   B. Catatonic
   C. Paranoid
   D. Undifferentiated
   E. Residual
II. Schizophreniform disorder
III. Brief reactive psychosis
IV. Schizoaffective disorder
   A. Bipolar type
   B. Depressive type
V. Induced psychotic disorder
VI. Delusional (paranoid) disorder

(e.g., social withdrawal, inappropriate affect, eccentric behavior, illogical thinking).

A disorder clinically indistinguishable from schizophrenia is *schizophreniform disorder* in which the symptoms of the disturbance last less than 6 months. The patient's symptoms begin and end more abruptly than in the schizophrenias, and there is frequently a higher level of functioning after recovery. A *brief reactive psychosis* is an illness in patients who experience an acute psychotic episode lasting less than 1 month that immediately follows an important life stress. The illness comes as a surprise and is frequently referred to by laymen as a nervous breakdown.

Schizoaffective disorder or, more properly, schizomood disorder, has characteristics in common with both mood disorders and schizophrenia. Depending upon the most prominent clinical features, patients with this disorder may be treated with antipsychotics, antidepressants, or both. Two additional, less common psychotic disorders are *induced psychotic disorder* and *delusional (paranoid) disorder*. In the former, a delusional system develops in a second person as a result of his relationship with another psychotic individual. Persons with paranoid disorders lack the bizarre features of schizophrenia but have elaborate delusions, often of persecution, jealousy, or grandiosity. The psychotic symptoms present in these disorders are amenable to treatment with various antipsychotic drugs.

The antipsychotic drugs, as their name implies, ameliorate various symptoms of schizophrenia and other psychoses. These drugs have been shown to act by interfering with dopaminergic transmission throughout the brain by blocking postsynaptic dopamine receptors. Consequently, neurological side effects are troublesome.

The odds favor that any schizophrenic will improve if given medication. Unfortunately, overall prediction of response to antipsychotic drugs is far less than adequate (13). A few predictors, however, are obvious. Chronic illness is likely to remain chronic; an acute illness usually gets better. If patients have a poor premorbid social adjustment, they are not as likely to attain a high level of adjustment after recovery. Finally, if a patient has been previously treated with

Table 1F.6.
Target Symptoms for Monitoring Response to Antipsychotic Therapy

Positive Symptoms	Negative Symptoms
Delusions	Poor social skills
Hallucinations	Impaired judgment
Bizarre behavior	Inability to prioritize tasks
Grandiosity	Inability to initiate conversation
Paranoid ideation	Loss of punctuality

drugs, the prior response may be a good guide to future therapy. These topics are further discussed in Chapter 3.

Target symptom changes are an effective way to monitor the effectiveness of antipsychotic therapy. Generally, the "positive" symptoms of psychoses (hallucinations, delusions, agitation) show good response as compared to the "negative" symptoms (affective blunting, social withdrawal). A listing of these symptoms is presented in Table 1F.6. A rank order of symptoms from most to least responsive would include combativeness and hostility, tension and hyperactivity, hallucinations, sleep disturbances, peculiar dress, delusions, poor social skills, realistic planning, judgment, and insight.

ANXIETY DISORDERS

Anxiety may be defined as apprehension, tension, or uneasiness that occurs from anticipation of an unpleasant future event. The source of anxiety is largely unknown or unrecognized. This feeling should be distinguished from fear, which is the response from a consciously recognized and externally perceived threat. Anxiety is pathological when it interferes with the person's optimal functioning or achievement of personal goals or satisfactions or compromises emotional well-being.

Anxiety is a universal human experience. It may occur alone as the predominant symptom or in conjunction with other manifestations of emotional disorders. Anxiety is frequently the central feature of many psychiatric illnesses.

The biology of anxiety involves the neurotransmitter γ-aminobutyric acid (GABA) and unknown endogenous anxiety-provoking substrates (14). Catecholamines are also likely to be involved. Altering the activity of the GABA receptor complex in the brain seems partly to be the basis of antianxiety drug action.

The DSM-III-R describes seven specific anxiety disorders listed in Table 1F.7. A *panic disorder*, first delineated by Klein (15), is manifested by a sudden intense feeling of apprehension or fear, frequently accompanied by the perception of impending doom. Physical symptoms may include dyspnea, palpitations, chest pain, choking sensations, dizziness, sweating, and trembling. A *panic attack* usually lasts for minutes, rarely up to an hour. It may be present with or without *agoraphobia*. The essential feature of agoraphobia is a marked fear of being alone or of being in public places from which escape might be difficult. This feeling results in the individual avoiding situations that create the anxiety. The individual may stay at home, decreasing activities to the extent that irrational fears or avoidance behavior dominate the individual's mental life.

A *social phobia* presents with a persistent irrational fear of situations that expose the individual to scrutiny by others and is associated with significant distress. *Simple phobias* frequently focus on an object or a situation other than being

Table 1F.7.
Classification of Anxiety Disorders

I. Panic disorder
   A. Without agoraphobia
   B. With agoraphobia
II. Agoraphobia without history of panic disorder
III. Social phobia
IV. Simple phobia
V. Obsessive-compulsive disorder
VI. Posttraumatic stress disorder
VII. Generalized anxiety disorder

alone or in public places (agoraphobia) or being humiliated or embarrassed in certain social situations (social phobia). Typical simple phobias involve animals or heights.

In *generalized anxiety disorder*, persistent anxiety is present for at least 6 months without the specific features of the disorders described above. The manifestations of generalized anxiety vary widely among individuals.

In an *obsessive-compulsive disorder*, recurrent, persistent ideas, thoughts, images, or impulses that are not voluntarily experienced by the patient become a significant source of distress and interfere with social functioning. A *posttraumatic stress disorder* may occur anytime after the experience of a traumatic event (participation in war, natural disasters, etc). A recognized stressor is usually present, and the traumatic event is relived by the individual in a variety of ways. This includes painful recollections of the event in recurrent dreams or nightmares or in flashbacks during usual daily activities. Often, there is a trigger, some sound or smell, which evokes the memory of the traumatic event. Patients frequently have sleep disturbances, symptoms of hyperalertness, decreased concentration, and survival guilt.

In all of the anxiety disorders, treatment may include psychotherapy and behavioral and supportive therapy. At times, conditioning patients to accept aversive or anxiety-provoking stimuli may be helpful. The support offered by positive family and professional relationships can be expected to have beneficial effects.

Pharmacotherapy is extensively used for the management of anxiety (see Chapter 4). Several chemical classes have been used, but the benzodiazepines are predominant because of both effectiveness and safety. β-Adrenergic blockers, particularly propranolol, and tricyclic antidepressants are sometimes useful in managing anxiety disorders. Imipramine (Chapter 2B) and the monoamine oxidase inhibitor phenelzine (Chapter 2D) have both been proven effective in reducing the frequency of panic attacks.

Regardless of the drug class or classes from which pharmacotherapy is chosen, the target symptoms are similar. The recommended approach to therapy is to identify those symptoms most troublesome to the patient and watch for changes in intensity or resolution. The patient should be questioned frequently, especially after medication changes, regarding his/her subjective impression of anxiety. Table 1F.8 lists various target symptoms that may be useful in drug therapy monitoring.

Table 1F.8.
Target Symptoms for Monitoring Antianxiety Therapy

Motor tension
  Tremor
  Muscle tension
  Startle reactions
  Inability to relax
  Teeth grinding
  Nail or lip picking
  Sleep disturbances
  Sensitivity to noise levels
Autonomic hyperactivity
  Sweating
  Cardiac palpitations
  Cold, clammy hands
  Dry mouth
  Frequent urination and urgency
  Gastrointestinal discomfort, diarrhea
  Paresthesias
  High resting pulse and respiration rate
  Faintness
  Sighing
Cognitive
  Apprehensive expectations
  Excessive worry
  Rumination
  Feelings of unreality
  Avoidance behavior
  Constant vigilance
  Feelings of being "on edge"
  Difficulty in concentration
  Feelings of "pressure"

Anxious patients should be questioned about their acceptance of pharmacotherapy. Side effects may occur with any drug, and the incidence should be specifically sought. When using benzodiazepines, some patients will voluntarily escalate their own dosage in an attempt to further combat their feelings of anxiety. This situation is to be avoided, as it places an undue reliance on drug therapy and may lead to psychological dependence.

It is likely that many patients can be withdrawn from their antianxiety medication for short periods without return of pretreatment levels of distress. Such trials should be encouraged. Nevertheless, some patients' anxiety will not be completely alleviated by drug therapy. It may be necessary for these individuals to accept that a certain degree of anxiety will be present.

CHILDHOOD MENTAL DISORDERS

Mental disorders arising in infancy, childhood, or adolescence are being increasingly recognized. DSM-III-R places many disorders in this category. Pharmacotherapy for some disorders, like the various developmental disorders

Table 1F.9.
Major Child and Adolescent Mental Disorders Having Pharmacotherapy Treatment Options

  I. Disruptive behavior disorders
       A. Attention-deficit hyperactivity disorder
       B. Conduct disorder
 II. Eating disorders
       A. Anorexia nervosa
       B. Bulimia nervosa
III. Tourette's disorder
IV. Elimination disorders
       A. Enuresis
       B. Encopresis
 V. Autistic disorder

Table 1F.10.
Target Symptoms for Monitoring Response to Treatment in Attention-Deficit Hyperactivity Disorder

Decreased attention span
Distractability
Irritability
Poor cooperation with authority figures
Low self-esteem
Lack of motivation
Shouting at siblings, peers, and adults
Low alertness
Social withdrawal
Verbal production

(e.g., mental retardation) and gender identity disorders, is disappointing or unavailable. Table 1F.9 lists those disorders for which drugs have shown some success in therapy or are currently being investigated for their efficacy.

Attention-deficit hyperactivity disorder (ADHD) is the name given to a disorder characterized by inappropriate degrees of inattention, impulsiveness, and hyperactivity evident during childhood development. Its presence can be manifested by difficulty in educational progress, in peer and sibling relationships, and in social and family adjustment. Most children with the disorder display some symptoms before the age of 4, but it may not be recognized until the child matriculates through school. This disorder has been widely discussed in the mass media. Some support groups openly oppose the use of CNS stimulants in children, the principle form of pharmacotherapy. Methylphenidate is the preferred agent (see Chapter 5A). Table 1F.10 outlines target symptoms that may be present and that can be monitored during therapy of ADHD.

Conduct disorder is a form of disruptive behavior arising during childhood or adolescence. Aggression is common, and affected patients commonly deny the rights of others. Pharmacotherapy is not the usual form of treatment unless symptoms of hyperactivity are present. The common eating disorders are *anorexia nervosa* and *bulimia nervosa*. In anorexia, there is a refusal to maintain

Table 1F.11.
Target Symptoms for Monitoring Response to Treatment for Psychoactive Substance Use Disorders

Drug-seeking behavior
Craving
Anxiety
Rumination
Guilt

body weight, an intense fear of gaining weight or becoming fat, and a distorted self-image. Weight loss can continue until death in severe cases. In bulimia, which is characterized by recurrent episodes of binge eating followed by purging, cyclic antidepressants and monoamine oxidase inhibitors have shown some efficacy.

Tourette's disorder is a major tic disorder. Patients typically have multiple motor and one or more vocal tics. Common presentations include frequent eye blinking and repetitive vocal utterances. The most established pharmacotherapy is haloperidol, although clonidine, an α_2-adrenergic agonist, has shown some promise in limited research studies.

The most common elimination disorder is *enuresis*. Children with primary enuresis have never achieved urinary continence; secondary enuresis refers to those children who have subsequently lost it after at least 6 months of continence. This disorder is much more common than incontinence of stool, or encopresis. Enuretic children are frequently seen by pediatricians or urologists. Imipramine has been the standard drug therapy and is superior to the anticholinergic agents. A reduction in bedwetting frequently occurs during the first few days after beginning drug therapy.

Autistic disorder is a severe form of developmental disorder with an onset during infancy or childhood. It has been immortalized in the famous short story "Silent Snow, Secret Snow" by Conrad Aiken. Children display a turning away from the external world of reality to an internal world of fantasy and hallucination. Antipsychotic drugs, notably thioridazine and haloperidol, have received extensive use in the pharmacotherapy of this disorder. More recently, fenfluramine, a drug that reduces blood serotonin concentration, has been tried with some success.

PSYCHOACTIVE SUBSTANCE USE DISORDERS

DSM-III-R recognizes abuse and dependence disorders involving alcohol, amphetamines, or similarly acting sympathomimetics, cannabis, cocaine, hallucinogens, inhalants, nicotine, opioids, phencyclidine, and sedative-hypnotics. Depending on the substance, various organic mental disorders can result from abuse.

The most widely known drugs in treating substance abuse are disulfiram, used as aversive therapy in alcoholics, and methadone, used for detoxification and maintenance of opiate addiction. Databases are included for these drugs in Chapter 6. Target symptoms that may be present in substance abuse disorders are listed in Table 1F.11.

REFERENCES

1. American Psychiatric Association: *Diagnostic and Statistical Manual of Mental Disorders,* ed 3, revised, American Psychiatric Association, Washington, DC, 1987.
2. Gray TK: Endpoints of therapy: a vital concept in surveillance and drug records. *J Clin Pharmacol,* April:221–224, 1975.
3. Stewart RB: Drug Therapy Monitoring. In: *The Practice of Pharmacy: Institutional and Ambulatory Pharmaceutical Services,* ed 1, Miller W, McLeod D (Eds), Harvey Whitney Books, Cincinnati, 1981, pp 70–82.
4. Beigel A, Murphy DL: Unipolar and bipolar affective illness. *Arch Gen Psychiatry* 24:215–220, 1971.
5. Andreasen NJ, Grove WM: The classification of depression: traditional versus mathematical approaches. *Am J Psychiatry* 139:45–52, 1982.
6. Owens H, Maxmen JS: Mood and affect: a semantic confusion. *Am J Psychiatry* 136:97–99, 1979.
7. Siever LJ: Role of noradrenergic mechanisms in the etiology of the affective disorders. In: *Psychopharmacology: The Third Generation of Progress,* Meltzer HY (ed), Raven Press, New York, 1987, pp 493–504.
8. Meltzer HY, Lowy MT: The serotonin hypothesis of depression. In: *Psychopharmacology: The Third Generation of Progress,* Meltzer HY (ed), Raven Press, New York, 1987, pp 513–526.
9. Andreasen NC: Brain imaging: application in psychiatry. *Science* 239:1381–1388, 1988.
10. Goodwin F, Zis A: Lithium in the treatment of mania. *Arch Gen Psychiatry* 36:835–844, 1979.
11. Losonczy MF, Davidson M, Davis KL: The dopamine hypothesis of schizophrenia. In: *Psychopharmacology: The Third Generation of Progress,* Meltzer HY (ed), Raven Press, New York, 1987, pp 715–726.
12. Kendler KS: The genetics of schizophrenia: a current perspective. In: *Psychopharmacology: The Third Generation of Progress,* Meltzer HY (ed), Raven Press, New York, 1987, pp 705–713.
13. Van Putten T, May PRA, Marder SR: Prediction of response to antipsychotic drugs. In: *Drugs in Psychiatry, Vol. 3, Antipsychotics,* Burrows GD, Norman TR, and Davies B (eds.), Elsevier Science Publishers, Amsterdam, 1985, pp 47–54.
14. Hommer DW, Skolnick P, Paul SM: The benzodiazepine/GABA receptor complex and anxiety. In: *Psychopharmacology: The Third Generation of Progress,* Meltzer HY (ed), Raven Press, New York, 1977, pp 977–983.
15. Klein DF: Delineation of two drug-responsive anxiety syndromes. *Psychopharmacology* 5:397–408, 1964.

▬ G ▬

Use of Laboratory Tests in Clinical Psychopharmacology

The need for clinical chemistry support for diagnosis and treatment is generally less well established for psychiatry than for other medical specialties. Most diagnoses are based on subjective data, primarily the psychiatric history and mental status examination (Chapter 1E). Nevertheless, as a screening tool for organic disease, routine biochemistry screens are invaluable for evaluating psychiatric patients.

Hospital admissions will be routinely accompanied by a urinalysis, serum chemistry, and hematology. Outpatient and private practice settings also generally have access to laboratory support. Table 1G.1 lists laboratory tests that are recommended when starting psychoactive drug therapy. This list assumes that the patient is otherwise healthy, except for a mental illness requiring drug therapy. The presence of organic disease will likely increase the need for laboratory test monitoring. Baseline test values are useful when assessing suspected adverse drug reactions and predicting impairment in drug clearance.

The interpretation of biochemical test results in psychiatric patients is similar to that in other types of patients. This chapter reviews laboratory procedures, with specific applications in clinical psychopharmacology and some of the common clinical chemistry profiles. Only a brief overview can be given, and the reader is encouraged to consult standard references as needed for detailed information (1). Case examples are presented to illustrate laboratory test abnormalities encountered in psychoactive drug therapy monitoring.

VARIATIONS IN CLINICAL LABORATORY TESTING
Normal Ranges

The normal range for a test result refers to the mean value and two SDs on either side of the mean determined for that institution's specific laboratory in a healthy population who are free of disease. This range incorporates 95% of the values expected in healthy individuals. Thus, 2.5% of the population will be outside this range, above and below it. This distribution should be remembered as a potential explanation when investigating an aberrant test value in an otherwise healthy individual.

Often, there is an overlap between the values of a diseased population and those of healthy patients. Depending on the degree of this overlap, values can be false-negative (abnormal patients with normal data) and false positive (healthy patients with abnormal data). Most laboratories will update their normal ranges periodically as additional data from a healthy population are incorporated into the reference range. Ideally, normal ranges reflect high sensitivity and specificity. The sensitivity of a test refers to its ability to detect the presence of a disease when it is present. Specificity measures the ability of a test to indicate the absence of a disease when it is absent.

Laboratory Error

Interpretation of test results requires confidence in the validity of the data. When requesting laboratory tests, it is necessary to follow proper procedures for collection and storage of specimens for analysis. Most laboratories have written guidelines. Specimens collected at an inappropriate time or in an incorrect manner may be useless for interpretation. Table 1G.2 lists possible sources of laboratory error.

The issue of quality control is important in laboratory operations (2). The easiest way to verify an abnormal test result is to repeat the test. Similar results should enhance confidence in the data. The greater the abnormality, the more effort should be expended in determining the cause.

All laboratory methods should be accurate and precise. Accuracy is dependent upon calibration of the instrument with reliable standards. Precision refers to the reproducibility of results, that is, within the same day, on different days, and at different laboratories. A common measure of test performance in analyti-

Table 1G.1.
Recommended Laboratory Tests for Initiating Psychoactive Drug Therapy in Medically Healthy Patients

Drug Therapy	Thyroid Function	Renal Function	Hepatic Function	Hematological Profile	Cardiovascular Status	Others
Lithium	TSH strongly recommended	Minimum of serum creatinine and specific gravity	Not usually performed	CBC recommended	ECG if over 40 yr old or there is history of cardiac disease	Serum lithium if history is in doubt; history and recent physical
Cyclic antidepressants	Not usually necessary	Not usually necessary	Optional	Optional	ECG if over 40 yr old or there is history of cardiac disease	Serum drug concentration if history is in doubt; history and recent physical
Antipsychotics	Not usually necessary	Not usually necessary	Desirable	Desirable; required for clozapine	ECG if over 40 yr old or there is history of cardiac disease	History and recent physical
Carbamazepine	Not usually necessary	Not usually necessary	Desirable	Desirable	Not usually necessary	History and physical; serum electrolytes
Clonidine	Not usually necessary	Not usually necessary	Not usually necessary	Not usually necessary	ECG strongly recommended	History and recent physical
Methylphenidate	Not usually necessary	Not usually necessary	Desirable	Recommended	Recommended if there is history of cardiac disease	Height and weight; history and recent physical
Benzodiazepines	Not usually necessary	Not usually necessary	Desirable	Not usually necessary	Not usually necessary	History and physical

Table 1G.2.
Possible Sources of Laboratory Error Involving Blood Sampling

Sample collection	Incorrect container
	Use of gel separators
	Sample collected at an inappropriate time
	Incorrect label applied to container
	Wrong patient
	Exposure to temperature extremes
	Collection from site of drug injection
	Incorrect storage conditions
	Hemolysis due to shaking of tube or too small a needle used to draw sample
	Inadequate centrifugation/separation
	Inaccurate decanting or pipetting of serum
Patient variables	Unusual stress or exercise
	Incomplete collection (urinary voiding)
	Position (supine vs. standing)
	Hydration status
Analytical variables	Interferences from drugs or endogenous substances
	Altered procedure or new operator
	Technical problems
	Calibration inaccurate
	Use of outdated reagents

cal laboratory operations is the coefficient of variation, or CV. This statistic is determined by dividing the standard deviation from replicate measures of the same test sample by the mean value. The result is multiplied by 100. This gives a value, in a percentage, of the variability of the measurement. The CV is frequently calculated for both within-day variability of replicate samples and between-day variability. The CV should usually be less than 5% but is highly dependent upon the measurement being performed. Most laboratories will supply this type of quality control data upon request.

BIOCHEMICAL MULTITEST PROFILES

A multitude of biochemical tests are available to the clinician. Most institutions require a minimal number of tests upon admission. Both elevated and decreased values may have clinical significance, especially when correlated with the patient's history and physical examination. The value of routine biochemical tests has been questioned in the medical literature, with providing excessive information and contributing to the high cost of medical care cited as problems. Nevertheless, tests are invaluable when combined with the patient's history and physical examination in diagnosing disease. In psychiatry, biochemical tests are used to screen for medical illness and to rule out conditions that may present with psychiatric symptoms.

Blood Chemistry

Blood chemistry screens usually include serum electrolytes and some miscellaneous enzymes. Panels of 6, 12, or 18 tests are usually available. In some institutions, convenient groupings of tests representing specific organ functions can be ordered. Table 1G.3 lists the general normal concentration ranges for serum electrolytes and other routinely available blood chemistry values, along with some potential causes for abnormal results. A blood chemistry is desirable before starting most psychoactive drugs. The presence of occult disease is frequently first recognized in this manner.

Renal Function Tests

Urinalysis   A standard urinalysis consists of a visual examination, determination of urine pH and specific gravity, and a microscopic search for formed elements in the urine, such as red and white blood cells and the presence of bacteria. The presence of ketones and glucose is usually recorded.

Specific Gravity   The specific gravity represents the solute content of urine. The normal range is 1.020 to 1.025. This value is a rough indicator of the body's fluid and electrolyte balance, a major function of the kidney. The ability of the kidney to concentrate and dilute urine is influenced by antidiuretic hormone (ADH). Abnormalities in ADH regulation may be reflected by urine volume and content.

Protein   Normally, less than 150 mg of protein per day is excreted into the urine, mostly in the form of albumin that leaks through the glomerulus. This amount produces a trace or 1 + estimate of proteinuria. Persistent proteinuria of 2 + or greater may indicate the presence of renal disease.

Serum Creatinine   Creatinine is a metabolic byproduct of energy released from phosphocreatine, a skeletal muscle component. It is freely filtered at the glomerulus and not reabsorbed. The normal serum value is 0.5 to 1.3 mg/dl. Elevations above this amount suggest abnormal renal function. Clearance of creatinine is a good reflection of glomerular filtration rate. The normal is 125 ml/min for men and 110 ml/min for women. Several methods have been proposed to calculate creatinine clearance on the basis of serum creatinine concentration, age, sex, and weight (3). There are no substitutes for direct measurement, but such estimates are useful. Because many drugs are eliminated by renal clearance, the creatinine clearance often correlates with the degree of impairment in drug clearance in renal dysfunction.

Blood Urea Nitrogen   Urea is the major nitrogenous end product of protein metabolism and amino acid degradation. It is formed in the liver, distributed in total body water, and transported in the blood to the kidneys for elimination. The normal range in serum or plasma is 10 to 20 mg/dl. Along with creatinine, blood urea nitrogen (BUN) is used as an index of renal function. The BUN is affected by hydration status, protein intake, liver disease, and other factors (4).

Liver Function Tests/Other Enzymes

Bilirubin   Bilirubin is formed as a breakdown product of heme in the reticuloendothelial system. Most bilirubin is formed from catabolism of red blood cells. Bilirubin is carried in the plasma by albumin to the liver, where it is made soluble for excretion by hepatic conjugation with glucuronic acid. Conjugated bilirubin is also known as direct bilirubin. The measurement of total bilirubin represents both conjugated and the unconjugated forms.

The rate-limiting step in the body's elimination of bilirubin is its excretion into bile. When biliary excretion is blocked, the serum concentration of bilirubin rises. This occurs in liver diseases, such as hepatitis or cirrhosis, in which there

Table 1G.3.
Some Common Biochemical Tests and Potential Causes for Abnormal Results

Test (Normal Range)	Causes for Abnormal Results	
	Elevations	Decreases
Sodium (135–145 mEq/liter)	Dehydration Diabetes insipidus Cushing's syndrome Excess steroids Excess sodium intake	Cirrhosis Renal failure SIADH[a] Lung cancer Diarrhea
Potassium (3.5–5.0 mEq/liter)	Renal failure Hemolysis Excess supplements Acidosis Most diuretics Adrenal insufficiency	Diarrhea Diuretics Cushing's syndrome Insulin Laxative abuse Crash diets
Calcium (9–11 mg/dl; 4.5–5.5 mEq/liter)	Thiazide diuretics Multiple myeloma Hyperthyroidism Excess vitamin D Malignancies Paget's disease	Renal failure Malabsorption Pancreatitis Low albumin Loop diuretics Steroids
Chloride (100–106 mEq/liter)	Dehydration Renal failure Respiratory alkalosis Metabolic acidosis	Renal disease SIADH Respiratory acidosis Metabolic alkalosis Diuretics Crash diets Vomiting, diarrhea
Bicarbonate (23–28 mEq/liter)	Diuretics Cushing's syndrome Respiratory acidosis Metabolic alkalosis	Diabetic ketosis Renal failure Respiratory alkalosis Metabolic acidosis Diarrhea Salicylate toxicity
Phosphorus (3.2–4.3 mg/dl)	Renal impairment Hemolysis Diabetes mellitus Hyperthyroidism	Hyperparathyroidism Hypokalemia Liver cirrhosis Aluminum antacids
Uric acid (3.0–7.0 mg/dl)	Renal failure Diuretics Gout Malignancies High aspirin doses	Allopurinol Steroids Phenylbutazone Azathioprine
Glucose (70–110 mg/dl)	Diabetes mellitus Hepatic disease Cushing's syndrome Acute stress Steroids, ethanol Oral contraceptives	Excess insulin Addison's disease Malabsorption Starvation β-Blockers Severe liver disease

[a]SIADH, syndrome of inappropriate secretion of antidiuretic hormone.

are impairment of uptake and hepatic excretion of bilirubin (5). Clinical signs and symptoms of hyperbilirubinemia include jaundice, dark urine, clay-colored stools, nausea, vomiting, and right upper quadrant abdominal pain. Normal values are 1.0 mg/dl for total bilirubin and 0.4 mg/dl for direct bilirubin.

Albumin   Albumin is formed in the liver and is the major component of serum protein. The normal range is 3.5 to 4.5 gm/dl. Albumin functions to maintain intravascular osmotic pressure and as an important carrier protein in the blood, transporting fatty acids, amino acids, and hormones. It is the major drug binding protein for acidic drugs. Albumin serum concentration serves as an index of nutritional status and the chronicity of liver disease (6).

Alkaline Phosphatases   Alkaline phosphatases are enzymes involved in the hydrolysis of organic phosphate esters. The normal range is 2.0 to 4.5 Bodansky units/ml or 30 to 115 IU/liter. These enzymes are found in many tissues, with high concentrations in liver, bone, placenta, and the intestines. Elevations are associated with diseases of the liver or bone, or both. In hepatitis, alkaline phosphatase activities are frequently elevated two to five times greater than normal. Levels of 10 to 20 times normal may occur in Paget's disease, in hyperparathyroidism, or in malignancies (27).

Serum Glutamic Oxaloacetic Transaminase   Aspartate aminotransferase (AST) is the preferred name for glutamic oxaloacetic transaminase (SGOT), an intracellular enzyme involved in both amino acid catabolism and gluconeogenesis. The normal range is 5 to 40 IU/ml. AST is present in high concentrations in heart, liver, muscle, and renal tissue. Damage to any of these tissues results in elevation of serum AST. A related hepatic enzyme is alanine aminotransferase (ALT), formally serum glutamic pyruvic transaminase (SGPT), whose normal range is 5 to 40 IU/ml.

Lactic Dehydrogenase   Lactic dehydrogenase (LDH) is an enzyme involved in the oxidation of lactate to pyruvate, the final step in anaerobic glycolysis, an energy producing pathway. The normal range is 70 to 210 IU/liter. LDH is distributed in all tissues, so that an elevation does not indicate a specific damaged organ. Fractionation into isoenzymes, however, can be performed by some laboratories to determine the specific organ involved. Elevations must be interpreted with other clinical information (8).

Creatine Phosphokinase   Creatine phosphokinase (CPK) is an enzyme found primarily in muscle tissue (cardiac and skeletal) and in the brain. It is the first enzyme to rise after an acute myocardial infarction. CPK also rises in response to muscle injury. Intramuscular administration of diazepam, chlorpromazine, and other drugs will precipitate increases. Rhabdomyolysis, a rare complication of rapid intramuscular neuroleptization, is expected to be accompanied by increased CPK and myoglobin in the urine. Some data indicate that CPK is high in acute schizophrenia (9).

Thyroid Function Tests

Thyroid-stimulating Hormone   Thyroid-stimulating hormone (TSH) is the single most valuable test to assess thyroid functioning. The normal value is less than 10.0 μIU/ml. Other thyroid measures include serum triiodothyronine (T-3) uptake, total serum thyroxine assay (T-4), free T-4, and serum antithyroidglobulin titers. In hypothyroidism, which can present with symptoms suggesting the presence of depression, the T-4 and T-3 levels are usually decreased while the serum TSH is increased. Lithium can cause hypothyroidism in a significant percentage of patients. Hypothyroidism is prevalent in the elderly, and aged patients should be screened for evidence of hypothroidism before lithium therapy is begun. An elevated TSH value will usually accompany symptoms such as psychomotor retardation, weight gain, hair loss, or increased sensitivity to cold.

Hematology

Complete Blood Count A complete blood count (CBC) will typically consist of the red blood cell count, hemoglobin, hematocrit, and a white blood cell count differentiated into subtypes. Very often, erythrocyte indices are useful for assessing iron, folate, or other deficiencies. These indices include mean corpuscular volume and mean corpuscular hemoglobin concentration.

Red Blood Cells The normal value is 4.5 to 6.0 million cells/mm^3 for men and 4.0 to 5.5 million cells/mm^3 for women. Red blood cells are produced in the bone marrow and circulate with a life-span of approximtely 120 days before being destroyed by the reticuloendothelial system.

Hematocrit The hematocrit is a measure of the volume of packed red blood cells expressed as a percentage of whole blood volume. This parameter reflects whether red cell mass is appropriate for a person's needs. Any hematocrit outside the normal range should be investigated. The normal is 40 to 54% for men and 38 to 47% for women.

Hemoglobin Hemoglobin is the oxygen-carrying component of red blood cells (RBCs). The total concentration is determined by the total number of RBCs and the hemoglobin concentration in each cell. The normal value is 12 to 17 gm/dl for men and 11 to 15 gm/dl for women.

White Blood Cells The white blood cell (WBC) count represents the number of WBCs contained in 1 mm^3 of whole blood. The normal range is 4,000 to 11,000/mm^3. An increased WBC count is frequently a sign of infection; however, several psychoactive drugs may produce leukocytosis, the most prominent among which is lithium. Clozapine may decrease the WBC count, and a weekly CBC is recommended for the duration of therapy (Chapter 3C). A WBC differential is a listing of the various types of WBCs present in the peripheral blood. It is reported either as a percentage or as the number of each type per 100 total white cells.

Neutrophils These represent 50 to 75% of the WBCs and are the first cells to gather in response to an acute infection. Their number can be reduced by antipsychotic drugs and anticonvulsants. Immature neutrophils are referred to as bands that comprise up to 5% of the WBC count. They are increased in response to an acute bacterial infection. This effect is frequently referred to as a "shift to the left."

Lymphocytes These are the second most common circulating WBC type, comprising 17 to 43% of the total cell count. Two types of lymphocytes, T-cells and B-cells, are responsible for cell-mediated and humoral immunity functions.

Monocytes These cells are made in the bone marrow and are transported by the blood to tissues, where they become macrophages. The normal value is 1 to 10% of the WBC count.

Eosinophils The primary role of these cells is to inactivate mediators of inflammation released from mast cells. The number is typically increased in allergic reactions to drugs and in allergic disorders such as bronchial asthma.

Basophils The function of these cells is poorly understood. Normally, they compose up to 2% of the WBC count. Stress-associated increases in red and white cells occur.

PSYCHOACTIVE DRUG CONCENTRATION MEASUREMENTS

Analytical Methods

Drug and metabolite concentration measurements are becoming more widespread in the monitoring of psychoactive drug therapy. Correlations continue to be sought between drug concentrations in various body fluids and clinical response or toxicity. Purported therapeutic plasma concentration ranges have been proposed for most psychoactive drugs. The instrumentation and procedures used for quantitating antidepressants, antipsychotics, and other psychoactive drugs vary widely, depending upon the laboratory performing the tests.

Lithium   Lithium is an excellent example of the need for accurate and reliable analytical measurements (10). As an atom, lithium exists as a nucleus with three protons and three orbiting electrons. As an ion, the outermost electron is associated with some other atom, resulting in a net positive charge. When a solution containing lithium is sprayed into a flame, an electron absorbs energy and is displaced to a position of higher energy, further away from the nucleus. The initial phenomenon of the atom absorbing specific amounts of energy is the basis for the technique of atomic absorption spectrometry. The emission of energy in the form of light as the excited atom returns to the original energy level is the basis for flame photometry or flame emission spectrophotometry. Flame photometry is inherently the more sensitive of the two tests, but both methods are routinely used to quantitate lithium and both have a sensitivity level well below plasma concentrations encountered clinically. Both methods are reliable techniques that can be used interchangeably by knowledgeable technicians (11, 12).

Cyclic Antidepressants, Antipsychotics, and Benzodiazepines   Methods for quantitating cyclic antidepressants, antipsychotics, and benzodiazepines can be based on any of several widely utilized techniques (13–15). Chromatographic techniques have become popular in recent years. When a sample containing the drug of interest is dissolved into a moving fluid or flowing gas stream and passed under high pressure through a narrow-bore tube packed with a solid, the drug molecules will tend to separate from other components in a mixture. Quantitation then becomes a function of comparing the response of the drug in the unknown sample to prepared standards of known concentration, using a suitable method of detection (e.g., ultraviolet absorbance, fluorescence, electrochemical, or nitrogen detection). Methods based on liquid chromatography (LC) are supplanting gas chromatography (GC), but neither can be judged as being superior to the other. Thin layer chromatography is used for some applications, but its operation is tedious and less reliable than either LC or GC.

Other popular analytical methods are based on immunological principles and include radioimmunoassay and homogeneous enzyme-multiplied immunotechnique. Generally, the immunologically based methods are very sensitive, but frequently they have less specificity than chromatographic techniques. They are typically used for screening applications to detect the presence of drugs in urine or plasma, followed by quantitation with specific methods. When patients are taking multiple drugs, the potential exists for assay interferences. The analytical laboratory should be alerted to this possibility.

The radioreceptor assay is a recently developed analytical technique that determines the amount of receptor-active substances in a biological sample. It quantitates not only the amount of parent drug in a sample but also that of metabolites that have activity for the same receptor. This principle can be applied to several psychoactive drugs but has found the most application with the antipsychotics (16).

When applied to antipsychotic drug concentration measurements, the radioreceptor assay utilizes *in vitro* competition between active substances in the test sample and a radioactive isotope-labeled antipsychotic for receptor binding sites in a suspension of dopamine receptors extracted from calf brain tissues (17). Proponents of this assay offer several advantages. First, the assay measures only the effects of the free, non-protein bound drug so that problems with interindividual variations in plasma protein binding are avoided. Second, the effects of all active metabolites are measured together. However, this is an advantage only if the measured effect is therapeutically relevant. In addition, all active metabolites in plasma may not be present in the brain to exert an effect. Although the radioreceptor assay has been a valuable research tool, it has not yet brought about any substantial improvement in the monitoring of antipsychotic therapy (18).

DEXAMETHASONE SUPPRESSION TEST

Several biochemical tests have been proposed for use in evaluating patients for the presence of depression based on observations of neuroendocrine abnormalities present in the disorder (19). The dexamethasone suppression test (DST) has become the most widely investigated and applied of these tests. The initial enthusiasm that was generated for the DST in the early 1980s has waned somewhat, but the test is likely to become more valuable as its specificity continues to be defined through clinical research.

The DST is based on the premise that many severely depressed patients have a hypothalamic-pituitary-adrenal axis abnormality (20). This is manifested by an elevated basal plasma cortisol concentration, dysregulation of the normal plasma cortisol circadian rhythm, and failure to suppress plasma cortisol concentrations after the administration of dexamethasone, an exogenous cortisol-like substance.

Procedure

Dexamethasone (1 mg) is given orally as a tablet at 11 PM. The following day, up to three venous blood samples are collected, typically at 8 AM, 4 PM, and/or 11 PM. A serum cortisol level greater than 5 µg/dl for any of the blood samples is abnormal and represents a positive test. Abnormal test results may occasionally have values between 20 and 30 µg/dl.

Interpretation

The DST is thought to be useful in helping the clinician diagnose patients presenting with confusing or mixed clinical pictures (21, 22). Unfortunately, the test has low sensitivity for detecting depression (45 to 50%). This means that many people who are depressed will not have a positive test. Thus, the DST will fail to identify some patients with depression. Specificity, however, is high (85 to 90%). Thus, for most people who do not have depression, the test will be negative. A specificity of less than 100% means that some normal subjects will have a positive test.

The DST may be a useful tool for the practitioner involved in the diagnosis and treatment of mental illness. Several studies have shown that an abnormal DST reverts to normal when a depressed patient responds to therapy. However, the possibility of false-negative and false-positive results due to drug therapy and other conditions should be kept in mind in the interpretation of results. Table 1G.4 lists drugs and medical conditions that may interfere with the validity of the DST.

TSH RESPONSE TO TRH STIMULATION

The thyrotropin-releasing hormone (TRH) test has been widely investigated as a laboratory aid in the diagnosis of major depressive episodes (23, 24). TRH is a tripeptide found in the hypothalamus (see Chapter 1B). When released, it causes secretion of thyroid-stimulating hormone (TSH) from the anterior pituitary gland. Endocrinologists have long used the TRH test as a test of thyroid axis functioning.

Procedure

Synthetic TRH, in a 500-μg dose, is administered intravenously in the morning to the patient at bed rest after an overnight fast. Samples of plasma for measurement of TSH are collected at baseline and at 15, 30, 60, and 90 minutes after TRH administration. The maximal TSH response is calculated by substracting the baseline value from the maximal concentration recorded.

Interpretation

A blunted TSH response, defined as less than a 7-μIU/ml maximal change, to TRH has been noted in depression. Approximately 25% of patients with major depression demonstrate this blunted reponse. However, the TRH test has a rather low specificity. Some patients with other disorders, such as alcoholism, panic disorder, dysthymic disorder, mania, anorexia nervosa, and bulimia, have also shown this response.

PATIENT PROFILE NO. 1

Bone Marrow Suppression Secondary to Clozapine

History   Mr. B.A. is a 57-year-old former race car driver who has been institutionalized for the past 8 years with chronic schizophrenia. He has mild hypertension controlled with hydrochlorothiazide. His past psychiatric history includes numerous attempts at symptom control with antipsychotic drugs. He has recently been receiving haloperidol (60 mg/day); benztropine (1 mg b.i.d.); temazepam (30 mg h.s.); and antacid (30 ml) as needed. Two weeks ago, the antipsychotic and benztropine were discontinued. Two days later, he was started on clozapine (75 mg/day), which was increased over 1 week to 300 mg/day. On examination, his affect was subdued, and he appeared to be actively hallucinating. Blood pressure was 96/70 mm Hg, pulse was 84/min; and oral temperature was 99.6°F. His skin felt warm and dry.

Laboratory Profile   Total WBC count was 3800/mm^3 with a normal differential. Liver and renal tests were normal. Slight elevations were noted in serum calcium, cholesterol, total protein, albumin, and uric acid. Slight decreases were present in serum potassium and phosphate.

Discussion   Bone marrow suppression secondary to clozapine is discussed in Chapter 3C. The period of greatest risk for this adverse drug reaction is 6 weeks to 6 months after initiating therapy. This is the period when laboratory

Table 1G.4.
Interferences with the Dexamethasone Suppression Test

False-positive DST results are associated with:
  Phenytoin
  Barbiturates
  Pregnancy
  Glutethimide
  Serious infections and cancer
  Serious physical illness of any kind
  Unstable diabetes
  Carbamazepine
  Major trauma or surgery
  Extreme weight loss
  Alcohol abuse
  Rifampin
  Estrogens
  Anorexia nervosa
  Withdrawal of psychotropic drugs
False-negative results are associated with:
  Addison's disease
  High dose benzodiazepine treatment
  Corticosteroids

---

monitoring should be most intense. It is not uncommon for patients to have a transient decrease in WBCs with a normal differential. The WBC count should be monitored twice weekly if a fall is noted, as compared to baseline values. No change in therapy is necessary when the total WBC is above 3500/mm^3. When the total CBC falls below 3000/mm^3 or the granulocytes fall below 1500/mm^3 the drug should be discontinued. Prophylactic antibiotics should be avoided, but evidence of infection should be sought, and appropriate therapy should be instituted when needed. A potential hazard of sudden clozapine withdrawal is a supersensitivity psychosis. Treatment with other antipsychotics may be necessary.

Hypotension, hyperthermia, and tachycardia are common side effects of clozapine. The drug's cardiovascular effects are minimized if the initial dose is 75 mg/day or less, and the daily dose is then gradually increased. These effects often abate with continued therapy.

Thiazide diuretics may affect a number of laboratory tests. They inhibit the excretion of uric acid and may elevate serum calcium by diuresis of sodium and water. Dehydration can result in elevation of total protein, albumin, and other serum constituents. Hypokalemia is a common effect of diuretic therapy.

PATIENT PROFILE NO. 2
Cholestatic Sensitivity due to Phenothiazines

History   Mr. J.D. is a 33-year-old graduate student who presented with complaints of a severe sore throat, headache, and a history of right upper abdomen pain for several days. Three weeks previously he had been prescribed chlorpromazine (25 mg b.i.d.) for increasing anxiety and paranoia related to events surrounding his divorce proceedings.

On examination, oral temperature was 101.5°F; pulse was 105/min; and blood pressure was 125/90 mm Hg. He was noted to have scleral icterus with a white exudate of the tonsils. The liver was palpable below the right costal margin.

Laboratory Profile   Bilirubin, alkaline phosphatase, and AST (SGOT) were elevated. Decreases below normal were noted in total protein, albumin, and calcium.

Discussion   A cholestatic lesion of the liver can be induced by phenothiazine therapy (25). This adverse drug reaction is reflected by elevation of bilirubin, alkaline phosphatase, and AST. Other causes of elevated liver enzymes include alcoholic and infectious hepatitis. Cholestasis produces decreased excretion of AST and cholesterol. A mild decrease in albumin and total protein is caused by the hepatic disease. This can result in decreased calcium, as albumin is its principle plasma-binding protein. Hepatic enlargement is a typical clinical feature. Scleral icterus (yellow discoloration of the eyes) and jaundice, due to increased bilirubin, may be the first signs of this drug reaction.

PATIENT PROFILE NO. 3

Antithyroid Effects of Lithium Therapy

History   Mrs. A.W. has been hospitalized for 10 days because of recurrence of manic-depressive illness. She had received lithium carbonate (900 mg/day) until 3 days ago when the dosage was increased to 1200 mg/day after a 12-hour serum lithium concentration of 0.7 mEq/liter was measured. Routine admission laboratory values were obtained.

Laboratory Profile   TSH was increased. Thyroxine (T-4), triiodothyronine (T-3) resin uptake, and free thyroxine index were normal.

Discussion   Lithium prevents the release of thyroid hormones (26). This effect results in lower circulating thyroxine and T-3 levels that stimulate the release of thyrotropin-releasing hormone (TRH). This, in turn, promotes TSH release from the thyroid gland. Occasionally, a patient will show thyroid enlargement during chronic lithium therapy. Less frequently, symptoms of hypothyroidism will be present. Early symptoms consist of lethargy, constipation, and cold intolerance. Further symptoms may include intellectual decline, loss of appetite with modest weight gain, dry skin, aching muscles, and voice changes. Further evaluation of thyroid function may be performed with a TRH stimulation test. This would be expected to show an exaggerated TSH response. A decrease in T-4 is common to all causes of hypothyroidism. For patients without clinical symptoms, exogenous thyroid replacement therapy is usually unnecessary; however, some case reports suggest that untreated patients may be at increased risk for rapid cycling of affective disorders.

PATIENT PROFILE NO. 4

Haloperidol-associated Neuroleptic Malignant Syndrome

History   Mr. S.B. is a 38-year-old banker who has been hospitalized for 2 weeks after an acute psychotic episode. He has been treated with haloperidol (30 mg/day). At 5 AM, staff members found him lying on the floor unconscious. On physical examination, pulse was 95/min; blood pressure was 115/70 mm Hg; rectal temperature was 40°C; and respirations were rapid and shallow. His skin was damp, and a marked muscular rigidity was present in his lower limbs.

Laboratory Profile   Laboratory examinations revealed a total WBC of 21,000/ mm^3, with 7% bands. Elevations were found in serum creatine phosphokinase, AST, LDH, and alkaline phosphatase.

Discussion   The pathogenesis of the neuroleptic malignant syndrome, a potentially fatal adverse drug reaction, is poorly understood. The cardinal symptoms are hyperpyrexia, altered consciousness, muscular rigidity, and autonomic dysfunction (27, 28). The elevation in liver enzyme concentrations is a typical finding, as are serum creatine phosphokinase levels and a leukocytosis with a shift to the left. Treatment consists of discontinuing the offending drug and providing supportive therapy. Specific therapy may include anticholinergic agents, dantrolene, or bromocriptine.

REFERENCES

1. Henry JB (ed): *Todd-Sanford-Davidsohn Clinical Diagnosis and Management by Laboratory Methods*, ed 16, WB Saunders, Philadelphia, 1979.
2. Gerson B, Orsulak PJ: Clinical laboratory quality control: application to analysis of tricyclic antidepressants. In: *Clinical Pharmacology in Psychiatry*, Usdin E (ed), Elsevier, New York, 1981, pp 43–57.
3. Hull JH, Hak L, Koch GG, et al: Influence of range of renal function and liver disease on predictability of creatinine clearance. *Clin Pharmacol Ther* 29:516–521, 1981.
4. Kassier J: Clinical evaluation of kidney function-glomerular function. *N Engl J Med* 285:385–389, 1971.
5. Schmid R: Bilirubin metabolism in man. *N Engl J Med* 287:703–709, 1972.
6. Rothschild MA, Oratz M, Schreibner SS: Albumin synthesis. *N Engl J Med* 286:748–757, 816–821, 1972.
7. Kaplan MM: Alkaline phosphatase. *Gastroenterology* 62:452–468, 1972.
8. Wilkinson JH: Serum isoenzymes. *Crit Rev Clin Lab Sci* 1:599–637, 1970.
9. Meltzer HY, Ross-Stanton J, Schlessinger S: Mean serum creatine kinase activity in patients with functional psychoses. *Arch Gen Psychiatry* 37:650–655, 1980.
10. Cooper TB, Carroll BJ: Monitoring lithium dose levels: estimation of lithium in blood and other body fluids. *J Clin Psychopharmacol* 1:53–58, 1981.
11. Levy AL, Katz EM: Comparison of serum lithium determination by flame photometry and atomic absorption spectrophotometry. *Clin Chem* 16:840–842, 1970.
12. Lippman S, Regan WL, Manshadi M: Plasma lithium stability and a comparison of flame photometry and atomic absorption spectrophotometry analysis. *Am J Psychiatry* 138:1375–1377, 1981.
13. de Silva JAF: Benzodiazepine analysis: electron capture-GLC and ancillary techniques. In: *Clinical Pharmacology in Psychiatry*, Usdin E (ed), Elsevier, New York, 1981, pp 3–34.
14. Bertilsson L: Quantitative mass fragmentography: a valuable tool in clinical psychopharmacology. In: *Clinical Pharmacology in Psychiatry*, Usdin E (ed), Elsevier, New York, 1981, pp 59–71.
15. Ebert MH, Vunakis HV, Hawks R: Radioimmunoassays for psychotropic drugs. In: *Clinical Pharmacology in Psychiatry*, Usdin E (ed), Elsevier, New York, 1981, pp 73–93.
16. Innis RB, Snyder SH: Radioreceptor assay: techniques and applications to psychopharmacology. In: *Clinical Pharmacology in Psychiatry*, Usdin E (ed), Elsevier, New York, 1981, pp 103–120.
17. Creese I, Snyder SH: A simple and sensitive radioreceptor assay for antischizophrenic drugs in blood. *Nature* 270:180–182, 1977.
18. Ko GN, Korpi ER, Linnoila M: On the clinical relevance and methods of quantification of plasma concentrations of neuroleptics. *J Clin Psychopharmacol* 5:253–262, 1985.
19. Leonard BE: Neurotransmitter receptors, endocrine responses and the biological substrates of depression: a review. *Hum Psychopharmacol* 1:3–21, 1986.
20. Gold PW, Loriaux DL, Roy A, et al: Responses to corticotropin-releasing hormone in the hypercortisolism of depression and Cushing's disease: pathophysiologic and diagnostic implications. *N Engl J Med* 314:1329–1335, 1986.

21. Carroll BJ, Feinberg M, Greden JF, et al: A specific laboratory test for the diagnosis of melancholia: standardization, validation, and clinical utility. *Arch Gen Psychiatry* 38:15–22, 1981.
22. APA Task Force on Laboratory Tests in Psychiatry: The dexamethasone suppression test: an overview of its current status in psychiatry. *Am J Psychiatry* 144:1253–1262, 1987.
23. Gold MS, Pottash ALC, Extein I, et al: The TRH test in the diagnosis of major and minor depression. *Psychoneuroendocrinology* 6:159–169, 1981.
24. Loosen PT: The TRH-induced TSH response in psychiatric patients: a possible neuroendocrine marker. *Psychoneuroendocrinology* 10:237, 1985.
25. Hollister LE, Hall RA: Phenothiazine derivatives and morphologic changes in the liver. *Am J Psychiatry* 123:221–212, 1966.
26. Wilson WH, Jefferson JW: Thyroid disease, behavior, and psychopharmacology. *Psychosomatics* 26:481–492, 1985.
27. Caroff SN: The neuroleptic malignant syndrome. *J Clin Psychiatry* 41:79–83, 1980.
28. Birkhimer LJ, DeVane CL: The neuroleptic malignant syndrome: presentation and treatment. *Drug Intell Clin Pharm* 18:462–465, 1984.

2

Drug Therapy for Mood Disorders

The major mood disorders for which drug therapy will be monitored, described in Chapter 1, are mania and depression. Depression is the most common psychiatric condition that clinicians are likely to encounter in adult patients. According to the National Institute of Mental Health, 10 to 20 million people, or approximately 15% of the United States adult population, suffer from a serious depressive disorder in any given year. Of these, over 20,000 commit suicide annually. Unfortunately, many patients do not seek professional help. For those who do, the available therapies do not cure either mania or depression. However, they frequently improve the quality of life through decreasing hospital stay, reducing the number and severity of episodes, and increasing the length of time between episodes. With maintenance therapy, some patients are maintained in a long-term state of remission.

The response to treatment for mood disorders is frequently rewarding. Although the pathogenesis of these disorders is not known and thus the mechanism of action of the effective therapies is uncertain, the response of target symptoms is frequently good. However, for symptom control to be optimal, dosage regimen design is an important factor in each person's therapy. The principles of drug action outlined in Chapter 1 can aid in the selection and design of dosage regimens using the drugs to be described in detail in the present chapter.

When acute mania or suicidal depression is present, treatment of the mood disorders may require hospitalization. Manic patients are likely to be first treated with a major antipsychotic drug, such as haloperidol or chlorpromazine (Chapter 3), followed by lithium. For patients with unipolar depression, lithium may be useful acutely, but it is better for maintenance therapy or prophylaxis against the recurrence of a mood disorder. The tricyclic antidepressants, one of the newer cyclic antidepressants, a monoamine oxidase inhibitor, or carbamazepine will probably be chosen, and in that order, for treatment of acutely depressed patients. Overall, pharmacotherapy is an integral part of treating mood disorders. Nevertheless, all depressed patients need supportive psychotherapy, and some will be candidates for electroconvulsive therapy (ECT).

In the sections that follow, databases are presented for the prototype drugs used in treating mood disorders. Everyone who monitors psychoactive drug therapy needs to be familiar with lithium. In addition to its specific antimanic properties, lithium has numerous other uses and is frequently used in combination with other psychoactive drugs. Imipramine is the reference tricyclic antidepressant, and much of the information in its database will apply to other cyclic antidepressants. Trazodone represents the "second generation" of antidepressants, and mental health professionals should be acquainted with how its clinical pharmacology differs from that of the tricyclics. As will become apparent, much overlap occurs between the various cyclic antidepressants in relative indications, neurochemical actions, and side effects. There has been a resurgence of interest in the monoamine oxidase inhibitors (MAOIs) over the past few years. A knowledge of phenelzine, the prototype MAOI, is useful for understanding and monitoring antidepressant therapy. Finally, the benefits and limitations of alternatives to the prototype antidepressant line of therapy should be recognized.

A

Lithium Database

FORMULATIONS

Lithium carbonate tablets: 300 mg (8.12 mEq of lithium)
Lithium carbonate capsules: 300 mg (8.12 mEq of lithium)
Lithium carbonate tablets, sustained release: 300 mg (8.12 mEq of lithium); 450 mg (12.18 mEq of lithium)
Lithium citrate syrup: 8 mEq of lithium per 5 ml
Brand names: Lithium carbonate (Roxane); Eskalith (SKF); Lithonate (Rowell); Lithane (Miles Pharmaceuticals); Lithotabs (Rowell); Lithobid (Ciba)

BASIC PHARMACOLOGY

Lithium, with an atomic weight of 6.94, is the lightest of all solid elements. Lithium is commercially available as either the carbonate or the more water-soluble citrate salt. Both have a slight saline taste. Tissues of various plants and animals have been found to contain lithium, but no necessary physiological function of this alkali metal is known. A striking fact about lithium is its chemical similarity to sodium and potassium. This similarity suggests that lithium may interact with these electrolytes or with magnesium and calcium in various physiological functions. Interference by lithium in ionic membrane transport functions is a proposed mechanism of action of lithium. Other postulated mechanisms responsible for lithium's efficacy in treating mood disorders include inhibition of the intracellular enzyme adenylate cyclase and cyclic adenosine monophosphate-mediated processes in the body, blockade of the development of supersensitive neuronal receptors, and effects on prostaglandin synthesis (1).

When administered to young, healthy subjects, lithium lacked an appreciable effect on peripheral measures of noradrenergic, serotonergic, and dopaminergic neurotransmission (2). This finding contrasts with other reports that lithium alters monoamine activity in patients. Thus, lithium may have a corrective action on neurotransmitter abnormalities that are present in patients with mood disorders but not in healthy subjects. Current thought favors an effect of lithium on membrane transport systems and/or modulation of hyperactive neurons as the most likely mechanisms of its therapeutic action. Lithium's expected effects on various standard laboratory tests are outlined in Table 2A.1.

Table 2A.1.
Expected Physiological Effects from Lithium Therapy[a] for Monitoring

Parameter	Drug Effect
Thyroid function	
T-4, T-3	Decreases noted within 4 mo with reversal to pretreatment levels within 12 mo of continuous therapy
TSH	Persistent increases noted within 4 mo of beginning therapy
Cardiovascular status	
ECG	Depression of T-waves at upper end of therapeutic concentrations; rarely, inversion
Heart rate, blood pressure	No changes expected in healthy patients
Renal function	
Serum creatinine and clearance, BUN	Normal values should not change in most adults over several years; children have been followed for 3 to 5 yr without changes; values will deteriorate markedly in toxic states.
Urine output	Frequent increases above 2 liters/24 hr correlating with duration of therapy; may begin soon after beginning therapy and frequently, but not always, parallels polydipsia.
Hepatic function	
AST (SGOT), ALT (SGPT)	No effect expected on hepatic enzymes
Hematology status	
CBC	Significant but innocuous leukocytosis within 1 to 3 wk, reversible within 1 wk off of lithium
Neuroendocrine status	
Dexamethasone suppression test	No effects expected
Fasting blood glucose	Short-term (1 yr) decrease, but no chronic effects expected; increases should prompt further patient assessment.

[a]Abbreviations: T-4, serum thyroxine; T-3, serum triiodothyronine; TSH, thyroid-stimulating hormone; ECG, electrocardiogram; BUN, blood urea nitrogen; AST, asparate aminotransferase; SGOT, serum glutamic oxaloacetic transaminase; ALT, alanine aminotransferase; SGPT, serum glutamic pyruvic transaminase; CBC, complete blood count.

PHARMACOKINETIC PROPERTIES

Lithium is commonly administered orally, although parenteral and rectal formulations have been investigated in European countries. The absorption of lithium from the gastrointestinal tract is rapid and is virtually complete within 6 to 8 hours, regardless of the salt form administered. Peak plasma concentrations occur within 30 minutes to 2 hours after a dose. The sustained release formulations will produce lower peak serum lithium concentrations, occurring within 4 to 12 hours after administration (see Chapter 1D, Fig. 1D.10), and bioavailability studies have suggested more variability in their completeness of absorption, as compared to rapid release products (3). Complete absorption is reflected by less than 1% of an oral lithium dose normally recoverable in the stool.

Lithium is distributed into most body tissues and fluids. An initial distribution volume corresponds to the extracellular fluid space, with a steady-state final volume of distribution of approximately 80 to 120% of body weight (0.8 to 1.2 liters/kg). The lithium concentration in brain, thyroid gland, and saliva at steady state may exceed that in plasma. Concentrations in heart, lung, kidney, and muscle tissue are similar to those in plasma. The erythrocyte concentration is usually less than in plasma or whole blood, and a ratio of the two has been suggested to be clinically useful for monitoring compliance and predicting efficacy. Unfortunately, a large variability in erythrocyte to plasma ratios has been found according to sex, age, and diagnostic category, suggesting that such measures have no practical value (4).

Some data suggest that patients with a previous history of mania demonstrate increased lithium retention, as compared to various control groups. This observation stresses the need for close monitoring in acutely ill patients.

Lithium is not bound to plasma proteins or metabolized but is nearly completely removed from the body by renal clearance mechanisms. Approximately 95% of a single lithium dose is eliminated in the urine. Lithium is freely filtered by the renal glomeruli, with about 80% of the filtered lithium reabsorbed by the proximal renal tubules. Lithium renal clearance is about 20% of creatinine clearance, with typical values falling between 10 and 40 ml/min. The terminal elimination half-life of lithium usually ranges between 18 to 24 hours in young adults and approaches 30 to 36 hours in elderly patients. One report has suggested that a prolongation of lithium half-life occurs with extended therapy (5). This report emphasizes the need to monitor lithium therapy continually when it is used chronically. A summary of lithium's pharmacokinetic parameters is presented in Table 2A.2

INDICATIONS

Lithium is approved by the Food and Drug Administration (FDA) for treatment of acute mania and for prophylaxis of bipolar affective disorder. Numerous, well-controlled studies have shown that lithium induces improvement or remission in greater than 70% of patients with acute mania. Placebo-controlled trials have also shown that it is effective in manic-depressive patients in preventing both manic and depressive episodes (6, 7). Lithium has also been tried in a variety of other psychiatric disorders, with varying degrees of success.

Unipolar and Bipolar Depression

Although lithium has been shown to have antidepressant properties in individual cases (8, 9), evidence does not warrant routine use of lithium over conventional antidepressant pharmacotherapy or ECT. Lithium may be of benefit in patients who are refractory to or intolerant of the standard antidepressant medications. Several studies indicate that lithium may augment standard antidepressant therapy, and it can be added to an antidepressant regimen with appropriate monitoring at most any point in therapy (10).

Schizophrenia and Schizoaffective Disorders

Although several uncontrolled studies indicate that patients with schizophrenia respond positively to lithium (11), the clinical evidence is not conclusive,

Table 2A.2.
Pharmacokinetic Parameters of Lithium

Parameter	Range
Peak concentration from a single 600-mg dose of lithium carbonate	0.45 to 0.85 mEq/liter
Time of peak concentration	0.5 to 2 hr for rapid release tablets; 4 to 12 for delayed release
Total body clearance	Equal to renal clearance
Renal clearance	10 to 40 ml/min
Hepatic clearance	None
Elimination half-life	18 to 24 hr in young adults; 30 to 36 hr in elderly
Plasma protein binding	None
Volume of distribution	0.8 to 1.2 liter/kg
Therapeutic range:	
Antimanic	0.8 to 1.4 mEq/liter
Prophylaxis	0.4 to 1.0 mEq/liter

and lithium is not approved for treatment of these disorders. Lithium, when combined with a neuroleptic, may be useful in patients who do not respond adequately to an antipsychotic drug alone. Schizophrenic or schizoaffective patients who respond to lithium may in reality be atypical manic-depressives, and such response indicates the need for careful diagnosis.

Aggression/Emotional Instability in Children/Adults

Several studies indicate that lithium may have a stabilizing effect in children and adolescents who have periodic mood and behavior disturbances (12, 13). In adults, lithium has diminished impulsive, aggressive behavior not associated with psychosis (14, 15).

Drug Abuse

Although a number of animal studies suggest that lithium antagonizes certain effects of amphetamines, morphine, and cocaine, the efficacy of lithium in treating these disorders in humans has not been established. However, lithium may be beneficial in cases of drug abuse that are secondary to a primary mood disorder.

Hyperthyroidism

A common side effect of lithium therapy is inhibition of thyroid hormone release; thus, it has been tried as a treatment for hyperthyroidism and metastasizing thyroid cancer (16).

Granulocytopenia

Lithium administration is frequently accompanied by leukocytosis. The rise in leukocyte count generally appears during the 1 week after treatment, continues throughout the treatment period, and disappears when lithium is discontinued. Not surprisingly, lithium has thus shown some efficacy in treating cancer chemotherapy-induced granulocytopenia (17).

Migraine and Cluster Headache

Lithium has been used in a number of uncontrolled trials in treating headache. The drug seems to be most promising in treating chronic cluster headache (18).

DOSAGE REGIMEN DESIGN

Before starting therapy it is desirable to have obtained some standard laboratory test results (see Tables 1G.1 and 2A.1). Complete baseline studies would include a complete blood count, urinalysis, the common biochemical tests, baseline tests of thyroid function, and an electrocardiogram (ECG). Minimal testing should include renal and thyroid function studies. The urinalysis may provide evidence of acute or chronic renal disease, and the thyroid tests provide a baseline against which any subsequent impairment of thyroid function can be measured. For all patients, especially those over 60 years of age, a serum creatinine or creatinine clearance test is highly desirable.

Lithium is similar to the tricyclic antidepressants in that the onset of full therapeutic effect is slow. Commonly, a latency in the appearance of full therapeutic effects may be 2 weeks or longer. Therefore, in treating moderate or severe manic episodes, antipsychotic drugs are often started along with lithium to control hyperactivity and agitation. Haloperidol is highly regarded for this use and is discussed in Chapter 3B.

Depending on the patient's clinical needs, age, weight, and renal function, doses may range between 600 and 2400 mg/day. However, measurements of plasma concentrations are heavily relied upon for assessing both the dose required for satisfactory treatment of an acute manic episode and the adequacy of maintenance treatment. Serum concentrations of lithium correlate much better with clinical effects of lithium than does dose.

THERAPEUTIC DRUG MONITORING

For control of manic episodes, the target serum concentration is usually 0.8 to 1.4 mEq/liter. Initial doses are generally 600 to 900 mg/day, depending on the size and age of the patient. Roughly, steady-state conditions for the selected dose level will be reached in 5 to 7 days, at which time a determination of serum lithium should be done. Concentration measurements should be taken 12 hours after a dose, regardless of the dosage schedule, i.e., whether the daily dose is divided into two, three, or four doses, as the concentration versus effect data in the literature reflect this interval (3). The plasma concentration of lithium should be checked often (e.g., at weekly intervals) during the first 4 weeks of therapy. Less intensive monitoring for stable patients is usually sufficient thereafter.

It is generally agreed that lithium therapy should only be undertaken when it is possible to measure serum (or plasma) lithium concentrations. The variability in clearance among individuals is much greater than the ratio of toxic to therapeutic plasma concentration, so empirical dosing should always be accompanied by therapeutic drug monitoring to prevent toxicity. This reflects lithium's low therapeutic index (see Chapter 1D and Fig. 1D.3). The goal for maintenance therapy is to maintain serum lithium at the lowest possible concentration compatible with maintaining the patient in a symptom-free remission.

The therapeutic concentration range for lithium refers to the limits between which typical lithium responders are distributed. Based on clinical experience, the therapeutic range of lithium falls between 0.4 and 1.4 mEq/liter when a blood (plasma or serum) sample is collected 12 hours after a dose at steady state. For the same clinical effect, some patients, especially the elderly, will require concentrations only in the lower part of the range, near 0.4 to 0.8 mEq/liter; for others, a serum concentration corresponding to the same degree of symptom improvement may need to be near the upper limit of the therapeutic range.

Clinical experience shows that patients in an acute manic state, require and tolerate a higher serum lithium level than do patients in a euthymic state. This is not definitively proven. Serum lithium concentrations as high as 2.00 mEq/liter have been used during acute mania, but this level should not be necessary, and attempts should be made to keep the treatment concentrations below 1.4 mEq/liter. Although a serum lithium concentration of 1.4 mEq/liter is not intrinsically dangerous, it may herald the onset of intoxication. If serum concentrations are above 1.4 mEq/liter, lithium determinations should be repeated to evaluate whether toxicity is impending. The dose should be lowered whenever possible to result in a reduced body burden of lithium, as reflected by a lower serum concentration.

The efficacy of lithium in preventing recurrences of manic-depressive disorder is unquestioned. The decision to use lithium chronically depends on such factors as the frequency and severity of previous episodes and the willingness to comply with lithium therapy and monitoring. Anyone with a frequency of one or more episodes of illness per year would be considered a candidate for maintenance treatment. There is a strong clinical impression that serum lithium concentrations in the range of 0.4 to 0.8 mEq/liter will be sufficient for successful maintenance therapy of most patients.

In using serum lithium concentrations in monitoring therapy, two assumptions are inherent. First, that the serum concentration is reproducible within a patient who is taking chronic therapy and, second, that results are comparable between patients. These assumptions are violated if the timing of blood samples for lithium determination is not maintained constant both for the same patient and for different patients. By convention, blood samples for lithium determination are drawn 12 hours after the dose, regardless of the number of doses per day. If sampling is performed much sooner than 12 hours after a dose, there is a likelihood that sampling will occur during the absorption and distribution phases, when concentrations are changing rapidly (see Fig. 1D.2 for desipramine). This error can lead to problems of reproducibility within the same patient. If samples are drawn more than 12 hours after a dose, the results are less comparable between patients. As the accepted therapeutic concentration range for lithium assumes that sampling will be performed 12 hours after a dose (3), only by following a similar sampling protocol can patient data be considered meaningful, when compared to the accepted therapeutic range. Some additional factors to consider when interpreting serum lithium concentrations are discussed below.

Accuracy of Assay Method Employed

Generally, both the flame photometer and flame emission spectrophotometer have sufficient accuracy for lithium determinations (19) (see Chapter 1G). What is more important than the analytical method used is that the testing laboratory maintain a rigorous quality control program. Typically, between day reproducibility, as reflected by a calculated coefficient of variation, should be less than 5%.

Bioavailability of the Lithium Preparation

It can generally be assumed that lithium preparations are at least 85 to 95% absorbed. If a patient switches from one preparation to another, differences in total absorption may show up as increased or decreased steady-state serum lithium concentrations. Although such variations are not expected to be great, lithium serum concentration should be rechecked whenever a change is made in dosage formulation.

Once Daily versus Multiple Daily Doses

Serum concentrations resulting from the use of sustained release preparations may vary from what was measured when a patient was previously using conventional release tablets (see Chapter 1D, Fig. 1D.10). Theoretical simulations suggest that the greater the frequency of administration, the lower the measurable 12-hour lithium concentration (3). This difference is an artifact of dosage regimen design, as the total systemic exposure should not change when the same total daily dose is administered, regardless of how frequently it is divided during the day (3).

Concurrent Therapy/Drug Interactions

Any factor that affects renal function, including dietary sodium intake and excretion, will probably affect lithium renal clearance also. This includes vigorous exercise, pregnancy, dietary changes, and drug interactions. Drug interactions with lithium are discussed below and outlined in Table 2A.3.

CONTRAINDICATIONS—WARNINGS—PRECAUTIONS

The use of lithium should not be undertaken lightly. As stated previously, lithium toxicity is closely related to serum levels and can occur at therapeutic doses. Facilities for serum lithium determinations are required to monitor therapy. The risk/benefit considerations in preventing the recurrence of bipolar disorder heavily favor the use of lithium for many patients. However, lithium should generally not be given to patients with significant myocardial or cardiovascular disease or in the presence of severe renal disease, organic brain disease, or pregnancy (see below).

Renal damage from long-term lithium therapy is a controversial issue. Morphological changes with glomerular and interstitial fibrosis and nephron atrophy have been reported in patients who underwent chronic lithium therapy for many years (20). However, similar lesions have been found in patients before beginning lithium therapy, so lithium cannot be regarded as specifically nephrotoxic. Nevertheless, the dose of lithium should be kept low to minimize the uncertain risk that long-term lithium use may result in renal damage.

DRUG INTERACTIONS

Any therapy or condition that affects renal function will probably alter renal lithium clearance. Acetazolamide, theophylline, and mannitol, all of which increase glomerular filtration rate, can substantially increase the renal clearance of lithium (21, 22). Lithium clearance will decrease in the presence of concurrently administered thiazide diuretics, and the serum lithium concentration will increase. This result is predictable from pharmacokinetic considerations (Equa-

Table 2A.3.
Drug Interactions with Lithium

Interacting Drug	Mechanism/Effect/Management
Carbamazepine or haloperidol	Rare neurotoxicity from an unknown mechanism; closely monitor patients receiving these combinations.
Ibuprofen or indomethacin	Decreased lithium clearance possibly from inhibition of renal prostaglandin synthesis; result is increased serum lithium; adjust lithium dose or consider using aspirin.
Naproxen	Decreased lithium clearance by unknown mechanism; monitor lithium serum concentration closely.
Iodide salts	Additive effects in causing hypothyroidism; discontinue iodide salts or give thyroid replacement if needed.
Furosemide, ethacrynic acid or bumetanide	Possible elevated serum lithium from decreased renal excretion; adjust lithium dose if needed.
Theophylline	Increased renal excretion of lithium; monitor serum levels and adjust dose if needed.
Thiazide diuretics	Decreased renal excretion of lithium results in elevated lithium levels, which can lead to serious toxicity; use of a loop diuretic may be preferable.

tion 19 in Chapter 1D). When therapy with one of the above drugs must be combined with lithium, a dosage modification of lithium will probably be required to offset a change in lithium clearance if serum concentrations are to remain undisturbed.

Indomethacin has been reported to increase plasma lithium concentrations from 30 to 50% (23). Other nonsteroidal anti-inflammatory agents may have a similar effect (24). Aspirin is the preferred anti-inflammatory drug for use in many patients because of its absence of an effect on lithium excretion (25).

Isolated case reports suggest an increase in the toxicity of lithium from combined therapy with carbamazepine (26), methyldopa (27), phenytoin (28), and haloperidol (29), although this latter combination is frequently used safely together. Whenever the addition of another drug is made to a drug therapy regimen of lithium, the serum lithium concentration should be checked more frequently in the initial stages of therapy. Table 2A.3 outlines the major drug interactions of lithium to monitor.

ADVERSE REACTIONS—OCCURRENCE AND MANAGEMENT

The use of lithium can be associated with numerous side effects. Minor lithium intolerance is reflected by side effects that are usually mild, transient, and completely reversible. They occur most commonly at the onset of treatment and after dosage increments. These effects usually abate with continued treatment. When gastrointestinal intolerance occurs with lithium carbonate products, the use of lithium citrate or a sustained release preparation may alleviate some of the distress. Table 2A.4 summarizes the side effects of lithium according to severity. The most frequent are thirst, polyuria, nocturia, tremor, and diarrhea (30).

Table 2A.4.
Side Effects of Lithium

Mild and Usually Transient
  Nausea, abdominal discomfort, mild diarrhea
  Polydipsia, polyuria
  Fine hand tremor
  Muscular weakness, fatigue, lethargy
  Generalized discomfort
Suggesting Early or Moderate Lithium Toxicity
  Severe GI distress—nausea, vomiting, severe diarrhea
  Anticholinergic-like symptoms—blurred vision, dry mouth
  Muscular weakness
  Coordination impairment, ataxia
  Confusion, drowsiness, irritability
Acute or Severe Lithium Toxicity
  Impairment of consciousness, stupor, coma
  Neuromuscular asymmetries—nystagmus
  Coarse tremor
  Epileptiform seizures
  Hyperreflexia
  Slurred speech, vertigo, somnolence
  Arrhythmias, hypotension, peripheral circulatory failure
  Respiratory depression

The treatment of moderate toxicity is to withhold lithium and restart at previous nontoxic doses when symptoms clear and serum concentrations have substantially decreased. If untreated, severe toxicity can lead to convulsions, coma, and death (31).

Lithium can contribute to a variety of dermatological problems. Most common are maculopapular rashes and acneiform and follicular eruptions. Many of these problems may spontaneously remit or require temporary cessation of lithium administration. The exacerbation of psoriasis may require that lithium use be stopped altogether (32).

Lithium can cause several rare side effects. Inappropriate secretion of antidiuretic hormone (SIADH) (33) has been reported to occur with lithium, as well as with tricyclic antidepressants, tranylcypromine, bupropion, and carbamazepine. Hyponatremia and other electrolyte abnormalities are often correctable by fluid restriction.

MANAGEMENT OF OVERDOSE

If lithium is taken in excessive amounts (sometimes as an intentional overdose) or if renal mechanisms fail to eliminate it properly, the serum concentration may rise above 2.0 mEq/liter, and symptoms of lithium toxicity will invariably be present. Early symptoms are sluggishness, lethargy, tremor or muscle twitchings, ataxia, slurred speech, vomiting, and diarrhea. With increasing toxicity, the patient lapses into a coma, with hyperactive deep reflexes, muscle tremors, fasciculations, and seizures. Severe electrolyte changes can occur, with consequent cardiac impairment; death may be due to cardiac arrhythmias. Treatment consists of discontinuing the drug and applying the supportive measures usually used with patients in coma. Maintaining normal fluid and electrolyte balance is essential. Increasing excretion of lithium by forced alkaline diuresis or with osmotic diuretics such as mannitol has been effective. As lithium is a simple ion, it is dialyzed readily. Both peritoneal and hemodialysis have been effective, but the former should be used only if hemodialysis facilities are not available. The relatively small volume of distribution of lithium, as compared to that of other psychoactive drugs, means that more of the body burden of drug is available in the systemic circulation for removal by dialysis methods.

USE IN RENAL AND/OR HEPATIC DISEASE

As lithium is eliminated completely unmetabolized, few special considerations apply to lithium use in hepatic disease. As predicted by Equation 18 in Chapter 1D, its total body clearance and, therefore, average steady-state plasma concentration should be unaffected by a reduction in hepatic function. However, severe hepatic disease will eventually affect renal function. Whenever an intercurrent illness or therapeutic intervention may affect renal function or electrolyte balance, more vigilant plasma concentration monitoring is recommended.

Lithium was used in thousands of patients before it was discovered that structural renal damage might be a consequence of its use (20). This knowledge stimulated rethinking of the practice of dosing lithium just below the onset of toxicity and altered therapeutic goals to adjust dosing to the lowest possible plasma concentration compatible with remission of symptoms. The risk of precipitating renal insufficiency at therapeutic concentrations is low and, with proper monitoring, lithium can be administered to patients with preexisting renal disease, even patients with end-stage renal disease undergoing intermittent hemodialysis.

USE IN CHILDREN AND ADOLESCENTS

Safety and efficacy for use of lithium in children under 12 have not been established. As discussed above, lithium is finding increasing usefulness in children (12). Aggressive conduct disorder and bipolar disorder are potential uses. As with adults, renal function should be closely monitored (34).

USE IN THE ELDERLY

As the elderly have an age-associated decrease in renal function, frequently not reflected by increased serum creatinine (35), lithium should be used cautiously in this population, with frequent serum concentration monitoring. The suggested baseline laboratory tests for beginning lithium therapy (see above; Table 1G.1) are especially important to perform in elderly patients. Lithium therapy should be started gradually in doses of 150 mg of lithium carbonate two or three times a day. The serum concentration required to treat a manic episode is between 0.7 to 1.0 mEq/liter, and it is seldom necessary to achieve the concentrations of 1.2 mEq/liter or higher that may be needed in younger adults. The incidence of some side effects, such as tremor, may be greater in patients above the age of 60.

USE IN PREGNANCY

Of all psychoactive agents potentially indicated during pregnancy, lithium seems to require the most caution. Women are more prone than men to develop manic-depressive illness, with the illness typically beginning during the childbearing years. Lithium crosses the placenta and distributes into the fetus.

Although some controversy exists (36), the prevailing opinion is that lithium is teratogenic. Information from the International Registry of Lithium Babies (37) suggests that the maximal frequency of congenital malformations does not substantially exceed the expected incidence in the non-lithium treated population; however, the apparent overrepresentation of severe and often fatal cardiovascular problems, particularly Ebstein's anomaly, indicates the need for extreme caution in the use of this drug in pregnant or potentially pregnant women. If the patient plans to become pregnant, lithium ideally should be discontinued until after the first or second trimester of pregnancy. For some women, the risk of an affective episode if lithium is withdrawn may outweigh the risks of continuing the drug. Alternative treatments, such as antipsychotic and antidepressant drugs, carbamazepine, or a benzodiazepine, may be preferable in some women.

Fetal exposure to lithium during the first trimester probably increases the possibility of malformation. Echocardiographic screening can be used to visualize the heart as early as 16 weeks of gestation. Such screening is recommended in mothers exposed to lithium.

During pregnancy there are increases in the clearance of orally administered drugs that are primarily cleared by renal mechanisms. This is probably due to increases in renal plasma flow and glomerular filtration rate. Lithium clearance and serum concentrations return to prepregnancy values after delivery and may require dosage adjustments. Lithium is readily transferred to the nursing infant through breast milk, in which it has a concentration of about one-third that in serum (38). These infants may show no effects or may have toxic reactions. Breast feeding by mothers taking lithium is contraindicated.

PATIENT INFORMATION

It is essential that patients receiving lithium be told of the importance of adherence to the prescribed treatment regimen. Noncompliance is a major factor leading to recurrence of symptoms, hospital readmissions, and disruption of family life (39). Patients can be told to take their doses after meals or with food or milk to minimize gastrointestinal irritation. The signs of mild toxicity (Table 2A.4) should be explained to patients and their caregivers, and they should be instructed to discontinue therapy and notify their physician if these signs of toxicity occur: severe diarrhea, vomiting, mild ataxia, or lack of coordination and muscular weakness. Patients should be told to avoid nonprescription (over-the-counter) analgesic drugs, such as ibuprofen, and other nonsteroidal anti-inflammatory drugs, and not to make major changes in their diet or salt intake.

REFERENCES

1. Baldessarini RJ: Drugs and the treatment of psychiatric disorders. In: *The Pharmacological Basis of Therapeutics*, Gilman AG, Goodman LS, Rall TW, Murad F (eds), MacMillan, New York, 1985, pp 387–445.
2. Rudorfer MV, Karoum F, Ross RJ, Potter WZ, Linnoila M: Differences in lithium effects in depressed and healthy subjects. *Clin Pharmacol Ther* 37:66–71, 1985.
3. Amdisen A, Carson SW: Lithium. In: *Applied Pharmacokinetics: Principles of Therapeutic Drug Monitoring*, Evans WE, Schentag JJ, Jusko WJ (eds), Applied Therapeutics, San Francisco, 1986.
4. Cooper TB, Simpson GM: Kinetics of lithium and clinical response. In: *Psychopharmacology: A Generation of Progress*, Lipton MA, DiMascio A, Klein KF (eds), Raven Press, New York, 1978, pp 923–931.

5. Goodnick PJ, Fieve RR, Meltzer HL, Dunner DL: Lithium elimination half-life and duration of therapy. *Clin Pharmacol Ther* 29:47–50, 1981.
6. Prien RF, Klett CJ, Caffey EM Jr, et al: Lithium carbonate and imipramine in prevention of affective episodes. *Arch Gen Psychiatry* 29:420–425, 1973.
7. Kane JM, Quitkin FM, Rifkin A, Ramos-Lorenzi JR, Nayak DD, Howard A: Lithium carbonate and imipramine in the prophylaxis of unipolar and bipolar II illness. *Arch Gen Psychiatry* 39:1065–1069, 1982.
8. Mendels J: Lithium in the treatment of depression. *Am J Psychiatry* 133:373–378, 1976.
9. Worrall EP, Moody JP, Peet M, Dick P, Smith A, Chambers C, Adams M, Naylor GJ: Controlled studies of the acute antidepressant effects of lithium. *Br J Psychiatry* 135:255–262, 1979.
10. Price LH, Conwell Y, Nelson JC: Lithium augmentation of combined neuroleptic-tricyclic treatment in delusional depression. *Am J Psychiatry* 140:318–322, 1983.
11. Miller FT, Libman H: Lithium carbonate in the treatment of schizophrenia and schizoaffective disorder: review and hypothesis. *Biol Psychiatry* 14:705–711, 1979.
12. Jefferson JW: The use of lithium in childhood and adolescence: an overview. *J Clin Psychiatry* 43:174–177, 1982.
13. Campbell M, Fish B, Korein J, Shapiro T, Collins P, Koh C: Lithium and chlorpromazine: a controlled crossover study of hyperactive severely disturbed young children. *J Autism Childhood Schizophrenia* 2:234–263, 1972.
14. Sheard MH, Marini JL, Bridges CI, Wagner E: The effect of lithium on impulsive aggressive behavior in man. *Am J Psychiatry* 133:1409–1413, 1976.
15. Shader RI, Jackson AH, Dodes LM: The antiaggressive effects of lithium in man. *Psychopharmacology* 40:17–24, 1974.
16. Temple R, Berman M, Robbins J, Wolff J: The use of lithium in the treatment of thyrotoxicosis. *J Clin Invest* 51:2746–2756, 1972.
17. Lyman GH, Williams CC, Preston D: The use of lithium carbonate to reduce infection and leukopenia during systemic chemotherapy. *N Engl J Med* 302:257–260, 1980.
18. Ekbom K: Lithium for cluster headache: review of the literature and preliminary results of long-term treatment. *Headache* 21:132–139, 1981.
19. Cooper TB, Carroll BJ: Monitoring lithium dose levels: estimation of lithium in blood and other body fluids. *J Clin Psychopharmacol* 1:53–58, 1981.
20. Hestbech J, Hansen HE, Amdisen A, et al: Chronic renal lesions following long-term treatment with lithium. *Kidney Int* 12:205–213, 1977.
21. Perry PJ, Calloway RA, Cook BL, Smith RE: Theophylline precipitated alterations of lithium clearance. *Acta Psychiatr Scand* 69:528–537, 1984.
22. Jefferson JW, Greist JH, Baudhuin M: Lithium: interactions with other drugs. *J Clin Psychopharmacol* 1:124–134, 1981.
23. Frolich JC, Leftwich R, Ragheb M, Oates JA, Reimann I, Buchanan D: Indomethacin increases plasma lithium. *Br Med J* 1:1115–1116, 1979.
24. Reimann IW, Frolich JC: Effects of diclofenac on lithium kinetics. *Clin Pharmacol Ther* 30:348–352, 1981.
25. Reimann IW, Diener U, Frolich JC: Indomethacin but not aspirin increases plasma lithium ion levels. *Arch Gen Psychiatry* 40:283–286, 1983.
26. Chaudhry RP, Waters BGH: Lithium and carbamazepine interaction: possible neurotoxicity. *J Clin Psychiatry* 44:30–31, 1983.
27. Osanloo E, Deglin JH: Interaction of lithium and methyldopa. *Ann Intern Med* 92:433–434, 1980.
28. Maccallum WAG: Interaction of lithium and phenytoin. *Br Med J* 280:610–611, 1980.
29. Cohen WJ, Cohen NH: Lithium carbonate, haloperidol, and irreversible brain damage. *JAMA* 230:1283–1287, 1974.
30. Johnston BB, Dick EG, Naylor GJ, Dick DAT: Lithium side effects in a routine lithium clinic. *Br J Psychiatry* 134:482–487, 1979.
31. Hansen HE, Amdisen A: Lithium intoxication. *Q J Med* 186:123–144, 1978.
32. Deandrea D, Walker N, Mehlmauer M, White K: Dermatological reactions to lithium: a critical review of the literature. *J Clin Psychopharmacol* 2:199–204, 1982.
33. Bartter FC, and Schwartz WB: The syndrome of inappropriate secretion of ADH. *Am J Med* 42:790–806, 1967.

34. Khandelwal SK, Varma VK, Murthy RS: Renal function in children receiving long-term lithium prophylaxis. *Am J Psychiatry* 141:278–279, 1984.
35. Rowe JW, Andres R, Tobin JD, Norris AH, Shock NW: The effect of age on creatinine clearance in men: a cross-sectional and longitudinal study. *J Gerontol* 31:155–163, 1976.
36. Silverman JA, Winters RW, Strande C: Lithium carbonate therapy during pregnancy: apparent lack of effect upon the fetus. *Am J Obstet Gynecol* 109:934–936, 1971.
37. Schou M, Goldfield MD, Weinstein MR, Villeneuve A: Lithium and pregnancy. I. Report from the register of lithium babies. *Br Med J* 2:135–136, 1973.
38. Schou M, Amdisen A: Lithium and pregnancy. III. Lithium ingestion by children breast fed by women on lithium treatment. *Br Med J* 2:138, 1973.
39. Connelly CE, Davenport YB, Nurnberger JI Jr: Adherence to treatment regimen in a lithium carbonate clinic. *Arch Gen Psychiatry* 39:585–588, 1982.

B

Imipramine Database

FORMULATIONS

Imipramine hydrochloride tablets: 10 mg, 25 mg, 50 mg
Imipramine hydrochloride capsules: 125 mg, 150 mg, 200 mg
Imipramine hydrochloride injection: 25 mg/ml
Brand names: Tofranil (Geigy); Janimine (Abbott); SK-Pramine (SKF); various generic brands

BASIC PHARMACOLOGY

Imipramine (IMI) (Fig. 2B.1) and the related tricyclic antidepressants have actions on various central nervous system receptors. Of primary interest in studying imipramine's mechanism of antidepressant effect has been its ability to block the reuptake of serotonin and norepinephrine (NE) into presynaptic nerve terminals. This pharmacological effect occurs immediately with acute administration, but there may be a delay of up to several weeks in alleviating depressive symptoms. Related to the above effects on monoamine neurotransmitters is imipramine's ability to cause a subsensitivity of β-adrenergic receptor sites and a decrease in whole body NE turnover after chronic administration. The effect on NE turnover occurs over the course of days or weeks, more in harmony with the improvement in depressive symptoms. This delayed effect is thought to be related to IMI's mechanism as an antidepressant (1). Other actions include anticholinergic and antihistaminic effects. These properties of IMI are shared by most cyclic antidepressants, although to differing degrees, and are further discussed in Chapter 2E.

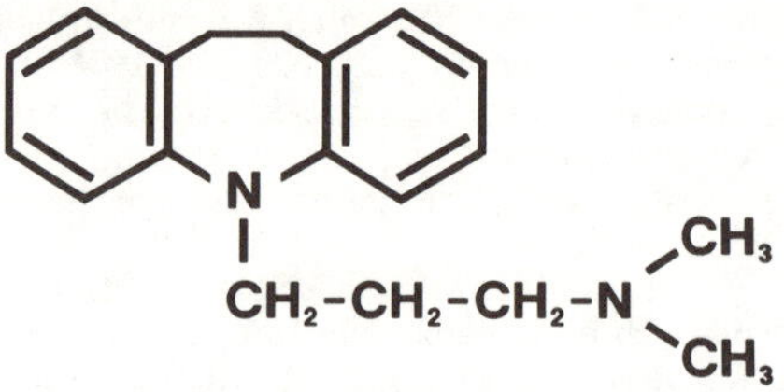

Figure 2B.1.   Chemical structure of imipramine.

When administered to healthy volunteers, IMI frequently produces sedation, a slight fall in blood pressure accompanied by an increased pulse rate, and, occasionally, a feeling of lightheadedness. Orthostatic hypotension may be present upon standing, and the subject may complain of blurred vision and dry mouth. These effects are also produced in depressed patients but tend to dissipate, especially the drowsiness and anticholinergic effects, upon continued daily administration. Rapid eye movement (REM) sleep (see Chapter 4E) is suppressed during therapy but returns to baseline after drug administration is stopped. IMI's expected effects on various standard laboratory tests are outlined in Table 2B.1.

PHARMACOKINETIC PROPERTIES

The important pharmacokinetic properties of IMI are summarized in Table 2B.2. After oral administration, imipramine is absorbed in the alkaline environment of the intestines. The rate of appearance of drug in the blood is rapid. Pharmacokinetic studies frequently report measurable plasma concentrations within 15 minutes after an oral dose (2). Peak concentrations are observed 2 to 8 hours after a single dose. Although not thoroughly studied, administration of food has been found to have little effect on imipramine absorption. In one report, a standardized meal had no effect on imipramine absolute bioavailability, peak concentration attained after an oral dose, or the time between administration and the occurrence of peak plasma concentration (3). These findings suggest that IMI can be conveniently administered with meals without affecting its total absorption.

The systemic bioavailability of imipramine is low (Table 2B.2) (4). Comparison of the area under the concentration versus time curve (AUC) for oral and intravenous doses of imipramine in the same subjects indicated an availability of drug between 30 and 70%. Nevertheless, studies that have determined the urinary excretion of IMI metabolites indicate that oral absorption is nearly complete (2). This discrepancy can be explained by a high degree of presystemic elimination. When absorbed from the gastrointestinal (GI) tract, a high proportion of IMI passing through the liver is metabolized on its way to the general circulation. This effect contributes to the highly variable systemic bioavailability after oral doses and pronounced differences in steady-state concentrations among patients taking the same milligram or milligram per kilogram daily dose (5). Interpatient variability in steady-state concentration is large, with a reported 30-fold difference in concentration from the same administered daily dose, an effect unpredictable from patient appearance, demographics, or intuitive expectations.

Imipramine is a lipophilic drug and therefore distributes widely throughout the body organs. Steady-state volumes of distribution approach 30 times body

Table 2B.1.
Expected Physiological Effects from Imipramine Therapy for Monitoring[a]

Parameter	Drug Effect
Cardiovascular status	
Heart rate	Frequent increase of up to 10 beats/min persisting throughout therapy
ECG	Prolonged QRS greater than 100 msec when plasma concentrations exceed 1000 ng/ml; reduced T-wave amplitude, rarely at usual plasma concentrations
Blood pressure	Orthostatic hypotension is common in up to 20% of treated patients.
Renal function	
Serum creatinine and clearance, BUN	Normal values should not change in most adults.
Hepatic function	
AST (SGOT), ALT (SGPT), alkaline phosphatase	Transient benign increases may occur during 1st mo. Substantial increases accompanied by increases in bilirubin should prompt further assessment of liver function. Imipramine- and desipramine-associated hepatitis has been reported.
Hematology status	
CBC	Rare, transient increases in eosinophils; decreases in leukocytes; trivial decreases in platelet count
Neuroendocrine status	
DST, plasma cortisol	Therapy not expected to interfere with DST; frequent normalization of DST with successful antidepressant therapy
Other tests	
EEG	Decreased REM sleep

[a]For abbreviations, see Table 2A.1. DST, dexamethasone suppression test; EEG, electroencephalogram.

weight (Table 2B.2) and show considerable intersubject variation. The extensive distribution of imipramine in tissues partly explains why hemodialysis and hemoperfusion have been largely unsuccessful in removing significant amounts of IMI from the body after overdosage (6). At any time, only a small fraction of the steady-state amount of imipramine in the body is actually circulating in the plasma, despite the high degree of plasma protein binding (Table 2B.2).

Imipramine and the other tricyclic antidepressants are extensively metabolized drugs. Renal clearance accounts for elimination of less than 5% of administered doses in the urine as unchanged drug (2). The major metabolic pathways include oxidation and conjugation; N-oxidation and dealkylation are minor pathways. After oral administration of imipramine, the demethylated metabolite, desmethylimipramine (desipramine), is produced in the liver. Two additional biotransformation products result from hydroxylation at the 2-carbon positions, 2-hydroxyimipramine (2-OH-IMI) and 2-hydroxydesipramine (2-OH-DMI). Several minor metabolites are produced, and glucuronide conjugation occurs extensively before urinary excretion.

Desipramine (DMI) was introduced for clinical use as a separate antidepressant shortly after imipramine. Like imipramine, DMI is well absorbed from the

Table 2B.2.
Pharmacokinetic Parameters of Imipramine

Parameter	Range
Bioavailability	Nearly complete absorption; total bioavailability reduced from extensive presystemic elimination to 30 to 70%
Time of peak concentration after single dose	Between 2 and 8 hr
Plasma protein binding	85 to 96%
Volume of distribution	10 to 30 liters/kg
Total plasma clearance	30 to 100 liters/hour
Renal clearance	Negligible
Elimination half-life	6–28 hours, increasing with age after adulthood
Active metabolites	Desipramine, 2-hydroxyimipramine, 2-hydroxy-desipramine
Steady-state metabolite-to-parent concentration ratio	DMI:IMI average of 1.5 2-OH-IMI:IMI average of 0.2 2-OH-DMI:DMI average of 0.5
Therapeutic range for antidepressant effect	180 to 350 ng/ml of combined imipramine plus desipramine in adults; 120 to 250 ng/ml in children

gastrointestinal tract and distributes widely throughout the body. DMI has a longer half-life than imipramine and frequently accumulates in plasma during imipramine therapy to concentrations greater than those of imipramine (Table 2B.2). Therefore, plasma drug concentration monitoring of IMI must also consider the role of DMI. During DMI therapy, a small but clinically insignificant amount of methylation to IMI can occur in vivo.

The 2-hydroxy metabolites of IMI and DMI have been investigated (5). Although they are generally present in measurable quantities in the plasma during IMI therapy (Table 2B.2) and have pharmacological effects similar to those of IMI and DMI, the bulk of research data thus far suggests that measuring their plasma concentrations does not improve the correlation between concentration and therapeutic efficacy.

INDICATIONS

Imipramine is FDA approved for the relief of symptoms of depression and depression accompanied by anxiety. In addition, IMI is the only tricyclic antidepressant with a specific FDA approval for the treatment of enuresis. Imipramine and other tricyclic antidepressants have been tried with some success for various mental and medical disorders listed in Table 2B.3.

Imipramine's use for depression, especially endogenous depression, is its primary indication. These patients will frequently have sleep disturbances, diurnal mood variation, loss of weight and libido, and psychomotor retardation, the neurovegetative signs not consistently present in less ill patients. Of endogenously depressed patients, 60 to 70% should respond well to IMI.

For depressed patients presenting with delusions, there is controversy over whether electroconvulsive therapy should be considered as the treatment of choice (7, 8). The more severe an illness, the more easily recognizable is clinical improvement, and this is true for depression. Therefore, it may be more diffi-

Table 2B.3.
Conditions for Which Imipramine or Tricyclic Antidepressants May Have Beneficial Effects

Condition	Efficacy Monitoring Parameters
Anorexia nervosa	Weight gain; improvement in appetite, self-concept
Attention deficit disorder	Decrease in distractibility; increased attention span; improved behavior
Bulimia nervosa	Decreased binging episodes
Enuresis	Decreased bed or daytime wetting frequency
Encopresis	Reduction in soiling
Posttraumatic stress disorder	Decreased startle response, anxiety, rumination, nightmares
Panic disorder	Decreased anxiety; fewer panic episodes; less avoidance behavior
Migraine headache	Decreased frequency or intensity or duration
Obesity	Weight loss, decreased craving, self-control
Peptic ulcer disease	Decreased epigastric pain, GI distress
Premature ejaculation	Reports of improved sexual performance

cult to perceive improvement in patients with milder forms of depression without a good assessment of premorbid functioning. However, nonendogenous, or neurotic, depression also responds well to imipramine therapy (9). Schizophrenic patients frequently have a high incidence of depressive symptoms during a postpsychotic state. This syndrome can be confused with akinesia, but IMI has produced good improvement in these patients' affective states (10).

Imipramine has been shown to be effective for treatment of panic disorder. The onset of significant effectiveness may be slow, but 60 to 90% of patients can be expected to show some improvement.

DOSAGE REGIMEN DESIGN

Pharmacotherapy with imipramine is best begun by giving small initial doses. This practice may be beneficial to test drug acceptability and to accustom the patient to the occurrence of side effects, which often dissipate in a few days. A pharmacokinetic test dose may be given, and samples may be collected to predict the maintenance dose for a targeted steady-state concentration. This procedure is generally limited to research settings.

The initial recommended imipramine dose is 50 to 75 mg/day administered as a single daily dose at bedtime. For some patients, especially the elderly and patients with anxiety, 25 to 50 mg/day is appropriate. Patients should be told that some side effects may appear, including dry mouth, constipation, and sleepiness. They should also be told that these symptoms mean that the drug is working but that symptoms of depression may not begin to improve markedly for 7 to 14 days. A change in sleep pattern is usually the first symptom of improvement and may be noticeable in 1 or 2 days. This effect probably relates more to a direct effect on sleep parameters, rather than an effect from alleviating depression. An improvement in energy and motor activity may begin in the 1st week; however, the characteristic dysphoric mood of depression may take weeks to disappear completely. As improvement begins, patients should be monitored for suicide risks. This is a time in which unanticipated suicide attempts frequently occur.

If improvement has been substantial 4 to 7 days after initiating therapy and the patient seems well, imipramine should be continued for a month. If the patient is still depressed after the 1st week, the night dose can be increased, and a small morning dose can be added. The total dosage can be increased by 25 to 50 mg every 1 to 3 days until 150 mg/day is reached. The entire dose can still be given at night.

For a patient who does not show significant clinical improvement in one or more depressive symptoms after 1 week at 150 mg/day, it is appropriate to titrate further dosage increases if there are no medical contraindications or manifestations of toxicity. A plasma concentration measurement, as discussed below, may be helpful at this time. The maximal dose of imipramine is usually 250 to 300 mg/day. An exception is when a patient does not display intolerable side effects, and a plasma concentration measurement yields a value below the purported therapeutic range. At the end of 4 weeks of therapy at 150 mg/day or greater, most patients will have improved. For those who have not, dosage should be continued at 150 to 300 mg/day for another 3 weeks. Alternatively, another pharmacological therapy may be considered useful (Chapter 2F).

Imipramine should be continued for some months after moderately depressed patients improve. As a general rule it should be continued for as long as the symptoms had been present before treatment began, before attempting to reduce the dosage. This should be done gradually, one tablet a week to watch for a recurrence. If depression recurs, the original dosage should be reinstituted. Generally, imipramine should be continued for about 3 months after remission of a major depressive episode. In some patients with longstanding symptoms, 6 months of therapy is needed.

When IMI is used to treat panic disorder, dosage should be started low, 10 to 25 mg/day, and increased no more rapidly than 25 to 50 mg/week. These patients frequently experience psychomotor activation when dosed according to recommendations for treating depression. Side effects can be prominent, and drop-out rates from treatment are high. Panic attacks generally show more response at lower doses than does agoraphobia. Increasing daily doses above 200 mg can be expected to yield only minimal additional benefits for panic patients.

When discontinuing imipramine after continuous therapy for 2 weeks or longer, it is prudent to taper the dosage downward. A gradual reduction in dosage will minimize withdrawal symptoms. This phenomenon consists of flu-like symptoms such as nausea, vomiting, diarrhea, chills, sweating, headache, and malaise. A cholinergic rebound from withdrawal of muscarinic blockade has been hypothesized to be responsible. These symptoms usually disappear within a week.

THERAPEUTIC DRUG MONITORING

Approximate steady-state concentrations of imipramine will occur within four to five half-lives (Table 2B.2) or after 4 to 7 days of receiving a constant daily dosage. It is likely that some elderly patients will require a longer time before reaching steady-state conditions because a longer average half-life in this population, as compared to that of young adults (5), means a longer period of drug accumulation in the body. There is little reason to check the steady-state imipramine concentration for most patients who show adequate clinical response after 2 to 4 weeks of therapy. However, for patients who do not respond adequately, especially on a dose of 150 mg/day or more, a steady-state plasma concentration measurement may be helpful.

Steady-state concentrations of imipramine are determined as a minimal concentration at the end of a dosage interval. The recommended time for sampling is the early morning, before the first dose of the day, approximately 12 hours after the previous dose. Blood for plasma or serum concentration should be taken from an antecubital vein in tubes that have been shown not to introduce artifactual changes in measured concentrations because of the presence of a plasticizer or gel separator (5, 14).

Several large studies have indicated that a therapeutic concentration range exists for imipramine (11–13). Concentrations of 180 ng/ml or greater for combined imipramine plus desipramine concentrations have been associated with a positive outcome of antidepressant therapy. Nevertheless, some patients will respond below this concentration range, and some will not respond at any concentration. Thus, the therapeutic range of 180 to 350 ng/ml represents a target to achieve before labeling a patient a nonresponder and seeking alternative therapy. Doses can be adjusted with the assumptions that linear pharmacokinetics exists (see Chapter 1D) and that plasma concentrations will increase proportionally. Studies of the hydroxylated metabolites of imipramine and desipramine have shown that measuring plasma concentrations of these drugs does not improve confidence in applying IMI's therapeutic range.

When patient progress is satisfactory, including absence of unacceptable side effects, no adjustment in dose is necessary unless plasma concentrations are excessive. Steady-state concentrations greater than 350 ng/ml support the need for close monitoring to recognize signs of toxicity, such as anticholinergic delirium (16). When dosage changes produce therapeutic concentrations, at least 4 weeks should elapse with continuous dosing before changing therapy. The reported therapeutic concentration range for imipramine was the most robust 2 to 4 weeks after patients had been taking a constant dosage for 1 to 3 weeks.

CONTRAINDICATIONS—WARNINGS—PRECAUTIONS

It should be remembered that many depressed patients will be suicidal. Unfortunately, the tricyclic antidepressants can be fatal in overdose and, therefore, a large prescription quantity should be avoided in outpatients. The dose of IMI producing fatalities is highly variable. A child has died from an ingestion as low as 350 mg, and adults have survived overdosages between 5 and 10 gm (17).

Patients with open-angle glaucoma can be safely treated with IMI, but those with angle closure should have a referral to an ophthalmologist. IMI has the potential to aggravate glaucoma, especially narrow angle, as its anticholinergic effects can precipitate acute symptoms. In patients over the age of 40, a history of "halos" around lights associated with eye pain should prompt an ophthalmic examination.

During maintenance therapy of patients with bipolar (manic-depressive) disorder, imipramine may accelerate the switch from depression to mania. Monitoring for symptoms of hypomania would be appropriate in these patients. Lithium may be a useful addition to the therapy of these patients but may not always prevent the switch process from occurring (15).

Table 2B.4.
Drug Interactions with Imipramine

Interacting Drug	Effect
Barbiturates	Hepatic enzyme induction results in decreased imipramine plasma concentrations.
Methylphenidate, chloramphenicol, phenothiazines, cimetidine, oral contraceptives	Increased plasma concentration through hepatic enzyme inhibition
Thyroid hormone	Possibly increased antidepressant efficacy through an unknown mechanism
Dicumarol	Increased hypoprothrombinemic effect by an unknown mechanism
Clonidine, guanethidine	Decreased antihypertensive effect
Sympathomimetics (epinephrine, phenylephrine)	Enhanced α-adrenergic effects
Monoamine oxidase inhibitors	Increased adverse drug effects are possible. Close monitoring is mandatory. Allow 7 days between starting either one after discontinuing the other, or both may be started together (see Chapter 2D).

DRUG INTERACTIONS

Table 2B.4 provides a list of some drugs that interact with imipramine. Many of these interactions are mediated by enzyme induction or inhibition and may not require any action on the therapist's part other than an increased vigilance for side effects.

As a highly metabolized drug, IMI could be expected to interact with cimetidine because of its inhibition of hepatic microsomal enzymes and its ability to decrease hepatic blood flow. When coadministered with cimetidine in a pharmacokinetic study, imipramine's hepatic clearance was reduced and its elimination half-life was increased. This suggests that, with continuing treatment, IMI would take a longer time to achieve steady-state concentration, and steady-state would be higher than therapy without cimetidine. Although this situation may have no clinical consequences, it points out the need to monitor the total therapy of patients, as other drugs may alter the dose response relationships for antidepressant therapy by increasing or decreasing their plasma concentration.

The combined administration of imipramine and phenothiazines is a situation in psychiatry of combining two useful drugs that interact pharmacokinetically. A mutual metabolic inhibition can occur with this drug combination. Nelson et all (18) found that, among 30 patients taking similar milligram-per-kilogram doses of desipramine (DMI), 15 who also took an antipsychotic drug had mean steady-state DMI concentrations that were twice as high. The interaction between antipsychotics and tricyclic antidepressants suggests that IMI doses should be appreciably reduced if IMI is added to a regimen that already includes an antipsychotic and that the addition of an antipsychotic to an IMI regimen could potentially result in increased side effects.

Table 2B.5.
Expected Side Effects of Imipramine Therapy

Effect	Rare	Less Common	More Common
Dry mouth			X
Blurred vision		X	
Gastrointestinal disorders		X	
Nausea		X	
Vomiting		X	
Drowsiness			X
Ataxia		X	
Disorientation	X		
Decreased energy			X
Headache		X	
Musculoskeletal complaints		X	
Blood pressure decrease		X	
Tachycardia		X	

ADVERSE REACTIONS—OCCURRENCE AND MANAGEMENT

Imipramine's side effects can be grouped into three categories: autonomic, cardiac, and miscellaneous. Through its actions on the parasympathetic nervous system, IMI may cause ciliary muscle paralysis, alteration in bladder sphincter tone, decreased salivation, and altered gastrointestinal motility. Blurred vision is rarely serious and frequently dissipates in about 1 week. Dose reduction may be helpful if the problem continues. Urinary retention and micturition difficulties, if troublesome, can be treated with bethanechol (Urecholine, 10 to 25 mg three times a day), by decreasing dosage, or by changing to another cyclic antidepressant with less anticholinergic (muscarinic receptor) activity (Chapter 2E, Table 2E.2). Dry mouth will appear in a high proportion of imipramine treated patients and can be helped by increasing fluid intake and use of sugarless candy. Constipation may be reduced by the use of a psyllium containing bulk laxative. In monitoring this side effect, it is worth remembering that some cases of constipation in the elderly have led to paralytic ileus.

Postural hypotension occurs frequently with IMI and cannot be predicted on the basis of the patient's age, drug dose, or plasma concentration (19). The best predictor of orthostatic hypotension during treatment is previous orthostatic problems before therapy. A sinus tachycardia (increase of about 10 beats/min) will commonly occur, and some patients will note palpitations. Imipramine has a direct quinidine-like effect on cardiac muscle and may prolong the PR interval and widen the QRS complex (Table 2B.1). Miscellaneous effects include weight gain, the appearance of rashes, and, rarely, jaundice. The expected side effects of imipramine are summarized in Table 2B.5.

MANAGEMENT OF OVERDOSE

The manifestations of imipramine overdose are extensions of their anticholinergic, cardiac, and central effects. Flushed, hot, dry skin may be present along with dilated pupils, decreased gastrointestinal motility, and urinary retention. Consciousness may fluctuate from excitation and agitation to sedation and coma. Seizures are common in comatose patients. Hypotension may be present because of α-blockade, decreased cardiac output, and myocardial depression. Arrhythmias may occur. Unfortunately, there is no specific antidote to imipramine or other tricyclic poisoning. The use of physostigmine to reverse the anticholinergic cardiovascular abnormalities is controversial and is not recommended. The principles of supportive care are appropriate: decrease absorption and provide treatment for complications as they occur.

For the person with sinus tachycardia as the only symptom, no treatment may be necessary. If the patient presents shortly after ingestion and is asymptomatic, ipecac can be administered to induce emesis. Activated charcoal or gastric lavage may be helpful. This can be repeated in 4 to 6 hours. The anticholinergic effects of imipramine may cause part of the unabsorbed dose to remain in the GI tract for up to 18 hours. Thus, relavage should be considered. In severe overdosage, hemodialysis and forced diuresis are not effective because of the high tissue concentrations and low renal clearance. Agitation or convulsions are appropriately treated with 5 to 10 mg of diazepam intravenously or with equivalent doses of lorazepam, while monitoring for respiratory depression. Alkalinization with sodium bicarbonate may help reduce the incidence of cardiac arrhythmias. Other therapies used for arrhythmias include phenytoin in a dose of 100 mg infused intravenously over 3 minutes and propranolol in a dose of 0.1 mg/kg intravenously every 2 to 5 minutes. If untreated, cardiac toxicity can progress from sinus tachycardia to A-V conduction disturbances to supraventricular tachycardia, followed by ventricular arrhythmias, profound bradycardia, and asystole. Intravenous physostigmine salicylate has been reported to reverse some of the symptoms of imipramine poisoning, but it has not proven to be as lifesaving as first reports had suggested (30).

Monitoring of an imipramine overdose should include observation for at least 4 to 6 hours for the asymptomatic patient. Usually, evidence of toxicity will appear within this time. A serious overdose can be indicated by a plasma concentration of greater than 1000 ng/ml and/or a QRS interval of greater than 100 msec (20). However, some normal people will have a QRS duration greater than 100 msec. Coma usually disappears gradually and is not in itself life-threatening. However, cardiac arrests have occurred up to 5 days after an overdose. ECG monitoring should be continued whenever there is doubt about the seriousness of an overdosage.

USE IN RENAL AND/OR HEPATIC DISEASE

The renal clearance of imipramine is low, with less than 5% of a dose excreted as unmetabolized drug in the urine. However, most drug metabolites, by nature of the reactions that formed them, are more water-soluble than their precursors. Therefore, imipramine's metabolites could be expected to undergo more renal excretion. This implies that, in patients with renal dysfunction, metabolites may accumulate in plasma because of a lower renal clearance, even though plasma concentrations of IMI seem safe. Sutfin et al (2) found that, after a single imipramine dose, approximately 8% was excreted as free 2-hydroxydesipramine and 33% as imipramine or desipramine glucuronide conjugates. The appreciable renal clearance of unconjugated 2-hydroxydesipramine implies that accumulation might occur in chronic renal failure and alter the apparent dose-concentration relationship.

Conventional wisdom suggests that liver disease should impair drug metabolism. However, the three major determinants of hepatic clearance, i.e., plasma protein binding, blood flow, and microsomal enzyme activity (see Chapter 1D), may be altered such that no change, or even an increase in clearance, can occur. IMI clearance is increased in some alcoholics. This fact suggests that difficulty in treating depressed patients who are alcoholic may be compounded by altered metabolism, probably because of augmented hepatic enzyme activity. Nevertheless, dosing should be performed cautiously in these patients. Because of cirrhotic changes, excessive alcohol use will eventually compromise hepatic metabolic ability for a variety of drugs. When IMI dosing is required in patients who have either hepatic or renal disease, plasma concentration monitoring is recommended.

USE IN CHILDREN AND ADOLESCENTS

Imipramine is useful for the treatment of enuresis in children. The necessary dosage usually does not exceed 75 mg/day. In contrast to the treatment of depression, response often occurs early in therapy, sometimes on the first night after a dose (22). Children should be monitored for the same side effects as occur in adults.

Abruptly discontinuing IMI in children can be associated with withdrawal symptoms and should be avoided. Skipping even a single day's dosage can result in withdrawal symptoms in some children. When daily doses for any indication exceed 3.5 mg/kg, ECG monitoring and, if possible, plasma concentration measurements should be used. Preskorn et al (21) indicated that depressed children responded to IMI in a range of 125 to 225 ng/ml, a concentration range overlapping, but lower than, what many adults require for depression.

USE IN ELDERLY

The elderly are especially prone to the anticholinergic side effects of imipramine. Plasma concentrations of tricyclics above 450 ng/ml are generally unnecessary and may predispose a patient to anticholinergic delirum (16). Dosage increases should be slower in these patients. In addition, recent evidence suggests that nonlinearity of imipramine metabolism may occur in some elderly patients. Bjerre et al (23) demonstrated disproportional increases in desipramine plasma concentrations after increases in IMI dosage. It seems that the enzymatic pathways for further metabolism of DMI become saturated before those responsible for converting IMI to DMI. Dugas and Bishop reported a case of nonlinearity with a patient receiving desipramine (24).

USE IN PREGNANCY

Animal studies indicate that imipramine is capable of causing fetal deformities and delayed teratogenic effects. DeVane and Simpkins (25) reported no change in the number of rat pups born per litter after maternal imipramine exposure; however, a 20% reduction in birth weight and an increase in infant mortality were found. The effect of the decreased birth weight led to persistent growth retardation in both male and female offspring. This type of data is difficult to extrapolate to humans.

Data from several international surveillance groups do not support an increased incidence of human birth defects with tricyclic drugs (26). Withdrawal symptoms manifested by breathlessness, cyanosis, and tachypnea occurred in an infant whose mother had been taking desipramine (27). There are also case reports of infants who had seizures after being born to mothers taking imipramine (28).

Sovner and Orsulak reported finding imipramine and desipramine in breast milk in concentrations similar to that in plasma (29). The clinical significance of imipramine and other cyclic antidepressants in breast milk has not been determined.

The use of imipramine and the other tricyclic antidepressants should be avoided in pregnancy. Although recommendations have indicated that these drugs are relatively safe, the recent animal data showing that imipramine disrupts hypothalamic organization during fetal development suggest the need for avoiding this drug in pregnancy if possible.

PATIENT INFORMATION

Patients should be told not to expect rapid symptom relief and that several weeks may be necessary, accompanied by dosage adjustments, before the full benefits of this therapy are known. Patients should be told that minor side effects related to anticholinergic actions may occur, particularly at the beginning of therapy, but that they often dissipate later.

REFERENCES

1. Linnoila M, Karoum F, Calil H, et al: Alteration of norepinephrine metabolism with desipramine and zimelidine in depressed patients. *Arch Gen Psychiatry* 39:1025–1028, 1982.
2. Sutfin TA, DeVane CL, Jusko WJ: The analysis and disposition of imipramine and its active metabolites in man. *Psychopharmacology* 82:310–317, 1984.
3. Abernethy DR, Divell M, Greenblatt DJ, et al: Absolute bioavailability of imipramine: influence of food. *Psychopharmacology* 83:104–106, 1984.
4. Gram LF, Christiansen J: First-pass metabolism of imipramine in man. *Clin Pharmacol Ther* 17:555–563, 1975.
5. DeVane CL: Cyclic antidepressants. In: *Applied Pharmacokinetics: Principles of Therapeutic Drug Monitoring*, ed 2, Evans WE, Schentag JJ, Jusko WS (eds), Applied Therapeutics, San Francisco, 1986, pp 852–909.
6. Pentel PR, Bullock ML, DeVane CL: Hemoperfusion for imipramine overdose: elimination of active metabolites. *J Toxicol Clin Toxicol* 19:239–248, 1982.
7. Glassman A, Kantor S, Shostak M: Depression, delusions, and drug response. *Am J Psychiatry* 132:716–719, 1975.
8. Quitkin F, Rifkin A, Klein DF: Imipramine response in deluded depressive patients. *Am J Psychiatry* 135:806–811, 1978.
9. Simpson GM, Lee JH, Cuculic Z, Kellner R: Two dosages of imipramine in hospitalized endogenous and neurotic depressive. *Arch Gen Psychiatry* 33:1093–1102, 1976.
10. Siris SG, Morgan V, Fagerstrom R, Rifkin A, Cooper MA: Adjunctive imipramine in the treatment of postpsychotic depression. *Arch Gen Psychiatry* 44:533–539, 1987.
11. Reisby N, Gram LF, Beck P, et al: Imipramine: clinical effects and pharmacokinetic variability. *Psychopharmacology* 54:263–272, 1977.
12. Glassman AH, Perel JM, Shostak, M, et al: Clinical implications of imipramine plasma levels for depressive illness. *Arch Gen Psychiatry* 34:197–204, 1977.
13. Glassman AH, Schildkraut JJ, Orsulak PJ, et al: Tricyclic antidepressant blood level measurements and clinical outcome: an APA task force report. *Am J Psychiatry* 142:155–163, 1985.
14. Orsulak PJ, Sink M, Weed J: Blood collection tubes for tricyclic antidepressant drugs: a reevaluation. *Ther Drug Monit* 6:444–448, 1984.
15. Wehr TA, Goodwin FK: Rapid cycling in manic-depressives induced by tricyclic antidepressants. *Arch Gen Psychiatry* 36:555–559, 1979.
16. Preskorn SH, Simpson S: Tricyclic-antidepressant-induced delirium and plasma drug concentration. *Am J Psychiatry* 139:822–823, 1982.

17. Bickel MH: Poisoning by tricyclic antidepressant drugs. *Int J Clin Pharmacol* 11:145–176, 1975.
18. Nelson JC, Jatlow PI, Bock J, et al: Major adverse reactions during desipramine treatment, relationship to plasma drug concentrations, concomitant antipsychotic treatment, and patient characteristics. *Arch Gen Psychiatry* 39:1055–1061, 1982.
19. Glassman AH, Bigger JT, Giardina EV, et al: Clinical characteristics of imipramine-induced orthostatic hypotension. *Lancet* 1:468–472, 1979.
20. Spiker DG, Weiss AN, Chang SS, et al: Tricyclic antidepressant overdose: clinical presentation and plasma levels. *Clin Pharmacol Ther* 18:539–546, 1975.
21. Preskorn SH, Weller EB, Weller RA: Depression in children: relationship between plasma imipramine levels and response. *Clin Psychiatry* 43:450–453, 1982.
22. DeVane CL, Walker RD, Sawyer WP, Wilson JA, et al: Concentrations of imipramine and its metabolites during enuresis therapy. *Pediatr Pharmacol* 4:245–251, 1984.
23. Bjerre M, Gram LF, Kragh-Sørensen P, et al: Dose-dependent kinetics of imipramine in elderly patients. *Psychopharmacology* 75:354–357, 1981.
24. Dugas JE, Bishop DS: Nonlinear desipramine pharmacokinetics: a case report. *J Clin Psychopharmacol* 5:43–45, 1985.
25. DeVane CL, Simpkins JM: Possible teratogenic effects of imipramine in the rat. In: *Clinical Pharmacology in Psychiatry*, Dahl SG, Gram LF, Paul SM, Potter WZ (eds), Springer-Verlag, Berlin, 1986, pp 174–178.
26. Banister P, Dafoe C, Smith ESO, Miller J: Possible teratogenicity of tricyclic antidepressants. *Lancet* 1:838–839, 1972.
27. Webster PAC: Withdrawal symptoms in neonates associated with maternal antidepressant therapy. *Lancet* 2:318–319, 1973.
28. Eggermont E, Raveschat J, DeVene V, et al: The adverse influence of imipramine on the adaptation of the newborn infant to extrauterine life. *Acta Pediatr Belg* 26:197–204, 1972.
29. Sovner R, Orsulak PJ: Excretion of imipramine and desipramine in human breast milk. *Am J Psychiatry* 136:451–452, 1979.
30. Burks JS, Walker JE, Rumack BH, Ott JE: Tricyclic antidepressant poisoning: reversal of coma, choreoathetosis, and myoclonus by physostigmine. *JAMA* 230:1405–1407, 1974.

▬ C ▬

Trazodone Database

FORMULATIONS

Trazodone hydrochloride tablets: 50 mg, 100 mg, 150 mg
Brand names: Desyrel (Mead Johnson); Dotazone (Major), various generic brands

BASIC PHARMACOLOGY

Trazodone is a triazolopyridine derivative (Fig. 2C.1) that represents a new structural class of cyclic antidepressants. Of the marketed antidepressants, trazodone possesses the highest degree of sedative effects and the least anticholinergic activity. Although proven to be an effective antidepressant (1), trazodone is inactive in many of the standard animal tests that screen for antidepressant potential (2). For example, it is inactive in the prevention of

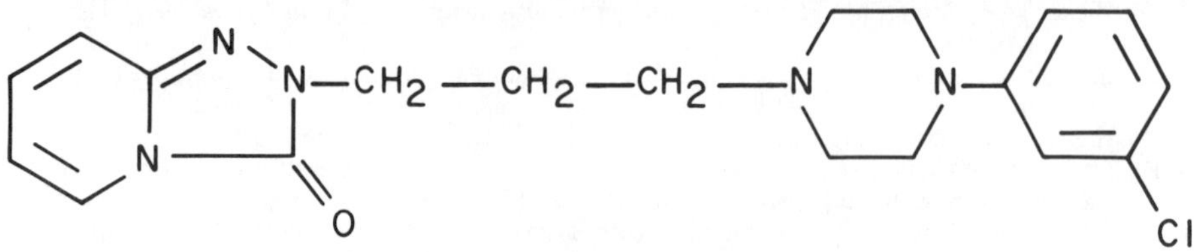

Figure 2C.1.   Chemical structure of trazodone.

reserpine-induced ptosis, L-DOPA or yohimbine potentiation, and rodent models of behavioral despair. Trazodone is not a monoamine oxidase inhibitor. Despite these novel actions, trazodone shares some neurochemical effects typical of other antidepressants (3). Pretreatment of rats with trazodone inhibited the serotonin depleting effects induced by fenfluramine. Trazodone also stimulated release of norepinephrine and has potent presynaptic α-adrenergic blocking activity.

At low doses, trazodone acts in laboratory animals as a serotonin (5-HT) antagonist; at high doses, it behaves as a serotonin agonist. The agonist activity observed after tradodone dosing to rats is delayed for 20 to 30 minutes. This leads to speculation that a trazodone metabolite may be responsible for the serotonin agonist effects rather than there being a dual neurochemical effect by trazodone (4).

Trazodone is extensively metabolized, and three major metabolites have been identified: trazodone-N-oxide, oxatriazolepyridin propionic acid (OPTA), and m-chlorophenylpiperazine (m-CPP). Both the N-oxide and OPTA metabolites are inactive as 5-HT reuptake inhibitors or 5-HT agonists. However, the m-CPP metabolite is a more potent 5-HT agonist than is trazodone. In trazodone-treated rodents, the plasma concentration of m-CPP was less than that of trazodone while at the same time the m-CPP concentration in brain tissue exceeded that of trazodone (5) (see Chapter 1D, Fig. 1D.13). This phenomenon suggests that the antidepressant actions of trazodone may be mediated by a combination of effects of the drug with its metabolite. In this regard, trazodone is similar to many of the tricyclics, which are biotransformed to metabolites with potent central nervous system actions.

Trazodone is commercially available as the hydrochloride salt and is marketed in various strengths. It has a bitter taste, but most formulations are film coated. When administered to healthy volunteers or depressed patients, trazodone induces a pronounced sedative effect but a lack of anticholinergic related complaints. The sedation caused by trazodone produces a longer period of drowsiness in the elderly, as compared to younger adults. This effect may be partly related to slower elimination of trazodone in the older population (6, 7). The expected effects of trazodone on common biochemical tests are listed in Table 2C.1.

PHARMACOKINETIC PROPERTIES

Trazodone is well absorbed after oral administration. The relative bioavailability, using an intravenous dose for comparison, was found to vary between 72 and 91% (7). Some of the reduction from complete absorption may be related to the presystemic elimination of trazodone. The rate of trazodone absorption seems to be influenced by food. The peak concentration was lower and delayed

Table 2C.1.
Expected Physiological Effects from Trazodone Therapy for Monitoring[a]

Parameter	Drug Effect
Cardiovascular status	
Heart rate	Occasional tachycardia accompaning orthostasis
ECG	Rare intracardiac conduction disturbances
Blood pressure	Hypotension upon chronic therapy in susceptible individuals, more frequent in elderly but less frequent or severe than with tricyclic drugs
Renal function	
Serum creatinine and clearance, BUN	Normal values should not change in most adults
Hepatic function	
AST (SGOT), ALT (SGPT), alkaline phosphatase	No changes expected other than minor increases within normal limits
Hematology status	
CBC	Occasional minor decreases in leukocytes and neutrophils, clinically insignificant unless below normal limits
Neuroendocrine status	
Plasma prolactin	Both increases and decreases reported, but little change is to be expected.
DST, plasma cortisol	Therapy not expected to interfere with DST; frequent normalization of DST with successful antidepressant therapy

[a]For abbreviations, see Table 2B.1.

when trazodone was taken in the nonfasting state. Even though food may decrease the rate of absorption, the total amount of trazodone absorbed may remain the same. Peak plasma trazodone concentration usually occurs between 30 minutes and 3 hours after an oral dose. Patients complaining of excessive drowsiness during this time suggests that side effects may be related to absorption rate. To minimize this complaint, the drug may be administered at more frequent intervals during the day or with food in an attempt to decrease the peak concentration.

Trazodone's volume of distribution (V_D) is lower than that of the tricyclic antidepressants, in the range of 1.0 to 2.0 liters/kg. However, in obese subjects, the V_D is increased, resulting in an increased half-life for elimination (note Equation 17, Chapter 1D). As obese subjects have no alteration in body clearance of trazodone, as compared to that of leaner subjects (7), dosage selection in obese patients should consider ideal body weight rather than total body weight. A heavy individual may have no better ability to clear trazodone from the body than a lighter patient.

Peak levels are in the 0.3 to 1.0 μg/ml range after oral doses. These values are higher than those of plasma concentrations produced from the same dose in milligrams of the tricyclics and are reflective of differences in distribution and elimination properties between the drugs.

Table 2C.2.
Pharmacokinetic Parameters of Trazodone

Parameter	Range
Bioavailability	70 to 90%
Time of peak concentration after single dose	0.5 to 3 hours
Plasma protein binding	89 to 95%
Volume of distribution	1.0 to 2.0 liters/kg; increased in obesity
Total plasma clearance	120 to 200 ml/min
Renal clearance	Negligible
Elimination half-life	3 to 14 hours
Active metabolites	m-Chlorophenylpiperazine
Steady-state plasma metabolite-to-parent concentration ratio	Less than 1.0
Therapeutic range for antidepressant effect	Inadequately defined

The concentration time curve after a trazodone dose demonstrates a biphasic elimination, with a terminal half-life of 3 to 14 hours (7). In the elderly, especially elderly men, the half-life is prolonged. In most patients, steady-state accumulation should occur in less than 1 week with chronic dosing. A summary of trazodone's pharmacokinetic properties is given in Table 2C.2.

INDICATIONS

Trazodone is FDA-approved for treatment of depression. This indication can be further defined as "major depressive disorder," as described in DSM-III-R (see Chapter 1F). Controlled clinical trials, including double-blinded studies, have been conducted in both depressed inpatients and outpatients (1). Improvement in depression is similar to that observed with the prototype tricyclic antidepressants, imipramine and amitriptyline, with a reported complete remission rate of 46 to 70%. As occurs with all available antidepressants, some patients will be relative nonresponders and might benefit from an alternative therapy (see Chapter 2E).

Trazodone has been tried for indications other than depression. It was of limited value for treatment of schizophrenia (8, 9). Trazodone apparently posesses antianxiety properties but cannot be recommended as a first line of therapy (9). In one study (10), 17 chronic alcoholics were given 100 mg of trazodone per day upon abrupt discontinuance of alcohol. Anxiety, depression, and tremors were all decreased significantly in 3 to 5 days. These effects suggest that trazodone was partly effective in ameliorating the alcohol withdrawal syndrome, but other confirmatory data are not available. At present, trazodone should be reserved for patients with significant depression or depression accompanied by anxiety.

DOSAGE REGIMEN DESIGN

The recommended daily dose of trazodone is 150 to 600 mg divided into two or more doses. The initial daily dose for most patients is 50 to 150 mg. Twenty-five to 50 mg can be added every 3 to 4 days until 450 mg is reached. This is the recommended maximal daily dose for outpatients; however, for inpatients, up to 600 mg/day can be given.

Drowsiness or sedation will probably begin on the 1st day of therapy and continue. This effect may be an advantage for patients with significant psychomotor agitation or a disadvantage for patients whose usual daytime activities require full alertness. Later in treatment, daytime sedation may be minimized by administering the majority of the daily dose at bedtime. One study that compared single nighttime and divided daily dosage administration found equivalent therapeutic efficacy for the two dosage regimens (10). Some caution is warranted with patients who may be known to experience pavor nocturnus, or night-terrors, as single nightly doses of antidepressants have worsened this condition. This side effect has not been reported with trazodone.

Some degree of response to trazodone therapy should occur within 2 weeks for most patients; however, as with the tricyclic antidepressants, some patients may require 4 weeks or more of drug therapy for optimal response. The first symptoms to improve frequently are anxiety and sleep disturbance.

Similar considerations apply for maintenance therapy with trazodone, as with the tricyclic antidepressants. The decision as to whether to continue a patient on trazodone after the remission of depressive symptoms will depend upon such factors as the patient's history of recurrences, their severity, and the willingness of the patient to cooperate with continued therapy. As with most all psychoactive drugs, trazodone should not be discontinued abruptly; rather, a gradual tapering over a week or more is recommended. For patients who have received continuous therapy over a period of months, clinical logic would suggest discontinuing the drug over a period of several weeks.

THERAPEUTIC DRUG MONITORING

The therapeutic range for trazodone is uncertain. Few clinical trials have reported trazodone serum concentrations and correlation to either clinical response or toxicity. Daily doses of trazodone in the range of 150 to 450 mg/day seem to produce plasma concentrations in the range of 500 to 1500 ng/ml. Based on preliminary data, clinical response to trazodone has been observed when plasma concentrations were generally greater than 750 ng/ml and less than 1500 ng/ml. Plasma for therapeutic drug monitoring should be collected 8 to 12 hours after a dose in steady-state conditions. The half-life of trazodone is prolonged in elderly men and in obese persons, so these patients may require one or two additional days to achieve steady state.

CONTRAINDICATIONS—WARNINGS—PRECAUTIONS

Although trazodone may cause some cardiac side effects, principally tachycardia, orthostasis, and, rarely, conduction disturbances, its use is associated with fewer and less severe cardiac effects than use of the traditional tricyclic antidepressants (11). Trazodone should not be administered to any patient with a recent myocardial infarction. In patients with cardiac disease, caution should be exercised. Arrhythmias have occurred in some patients with preexisting cardiac disease who took trazodone.

The effects of trazodone treatment for a week on the blood pressure response to tyramine, in comparison to the effects of placebo, were similar (12). This is in contrast to the effects of imipramine on systolic blood pressure after tyramine administration, an effect mediated by norepinephrine. The main cardiovascular effects of trazodone to monitor are blood pressure and pulse rate. Complaints of dizziness should be sought in any patient with a history of orthostasis. Several reports suggest that trazodone may elevate serum digoxin levels. Digoxin concentrations should be monitored when this combination of drugs is used.

Some unipolar depressed patients have been reported to develop manic symptoms when treated with trazodone (13). Thus, trazodone does not preclude this phenomenom, but it may be similar to the tricyclic antidepressants in having a propensity to initiate the switch process in occasional bipolar depressed patients.

Trazodone has been tested in patients with open angle glaucoma and found to decrease intraocular pressure (2). However, studies have not been reported in glaucoma patients with depression receiving chronic trazodone therapy, so caution should be exercised with these patients. As with the tricyclics, those patients with angle-closure disease may be at risk for increased intraocular pressure. However, given trazodone's lack of anticholinergic effects, it may be an appropriate alternative to tricyclic antidepressants in glaucoma patients who have had difficulty in the past with antidepressant therapy.

DRUG INTERACTIONS

Trazodone does not block catecholamine reuptake like the tricyclic antidepressants, so it should have less propensity to exaggerate the effects of monoamine oxidase inhibitors. Such interactions have not been reported, but it is prudent to allow a lapse between starting or stopping a monoamine oxidase inhibitor and any other antidepressant.

The sedation that occurs with trazodone suggests that other central nervous system depressants, including alcohol, should be used cautiously with trazodone (14). Enhanced sedative effects could be expected in patients receiving antihistamines, and outpatients should be appropriately cautioned about activities that require a high degree of concentration.

Trazodone may affect the blood pressure response to clonidine or α-methyldopa (15). All patients taking antihypertensive medications should be closely monitored for changes in blood pressure during concomitant trazodone therapy. Trazodone did not interfere with the cerebral actions of L-DOPA in rodents (16), but its clinical effects in patients with Parkinson's disease have not been reported.

ADVERSE REACTIONS—OCCURRENCE AND MANAGEMENT

Drowsiness or dizziness is the most frequently reported side effect of trazodone. Table 2C.3 lists the common side effects and their anticipated frequency of occurrence.

Even placebo treated patients experience side effects during clinical trials, and some complaints can be expected from most patients. However, the severity of side effects from trazodone can be expected to be less than with the prototype tricyclic antidepressants. Side effects are rarely severe enough to require discontinuance of therapy.

The appearance of priapism as a severe side effect of trazodone was unexpected (17). Antipsychotics, but not tricyclic antidepressants, had been reported previously to cause this adverse reaction. This side effect in male patients occurs as a prolonged painful erection, probably as a result of unusual α-receptor sensitivity in susceptible patients. The condition may require surgical intervention, which has attendant morbidity. A complaint of unusual erectile activi-

Table 2C.3.
Expected Side Effects of Trazodone Therapy

Effect	Rare	Less Common	More Common
Dry mouth			X
Blurred vision		X	
Gastrointestinal disorders		X	
Nausea		X	
Vomiting		X	
Drowsiness			X
Ataxia		X	
Disorientation	X		
Decreased energy			X
Headache		X	
Musculoskeletal complaints		X	
Blood pressure decrease	X		
Tachycardia	X		
Priapism	X		

ty should be viewed with suspicion as a prodromal symptom of priapism, and the drug should be stopped immediately. Other sexual problems of both antidepressants and antipsychotics include erectile dysfunction, ejaculatory problems, and changes in libido. No single drug stands out as being the worst offender in causing these problems.

MANAGEMENT OF OVERDOSE

There is no specific antidote for overdosage of trazodone. Treatment is supportive and symptomatic. Given its smaller volume of distribution than the tricyclic antidepressants, dialysis procedures may be more effective in removing trazodone from the body, but this has not been confirmed. Limited overdose experience with trazodone suggests a greater degree of safety, as compared with the tricyclics (18).

USE IN RENAL AND/OR HEPATIC DISEASE

No specific dosage adjustment is recommended for trazodone in the presence of renal impairment. Given its negligible clearance by renal mechanisms, decreased renal function should not result in greater accumulation of drug. However, this principle may not hold for metabolites (see Chapter 1D). As the renal clearance of the active metabolite m-CPP is not known, caution should be exercised with trazodone dosing in patients with severe renal impairment.

In patients with alcoholic or other liver diseases that commonly compromise hepatocellular function, the clearance of trazodone can be expected to be impaired and its half-life to be prolonged. Smaller doses would be appropriate for these patients, and their care should be accompanied by close clinical monitoring.

USE IN CHILDREN AND ADOLESCENTS

Trazodone therapy has not been reported in children less than 18 years old. Given the experience and safety record of tricyclic antidepressants in adolescents, there seems to be little clinical advantage of using trazodone in this population except for greater safety in overdose situations.

USE IN ELDERLY

Trazodone kinetics have been observed to be altered in the elderly. After a single oral dose (7), the terminal half-life was significantly prolonged and the total body clearance was decreased in elderly men. Initial doses should be reduced by at least one-third in this population. The time until steady state will be prolonged; thus, dosage changes should be made less frequently to allow complete accumulation at each dose level and to assess tolerance and clinical effects. The high degree of sedation produced by trazodone will be a consideration in many elderly patients.

USE IN PREGNANCY

Trazodone is classed as pregnancy category C. This means that there are no controlled studies in women to document the drug's safety. Trazodone has been claimed to be free of gross teratogenic effects on the basis of limited animal studies (19), but there is increasing evidence that subclinical teratogenic effects occur in animals treated with several psychoactive drugs, including antidepressants (20). The use of trazodone in pregnant or nursing women should be restricted to those patients whose anticipated benefits far outweigh the risk of discontinuing therapy.

PATIENT INFORMATION

Patients should be told not to take trazodone with alcohol, barbiturates, or other central nervous system depressants (antihistamines, over-the-counter sedatives, etc.). They should also be warned about the effects of drowsiness on the ability to operate machinery, drive an automobile, or perform any hazardous task that requires sustained attention. The degree of drug-induced impairment in mental and/or physical ability may be underestimated by patients, especially during the initial stages of drug therapy. The possibility of priapism occurring during therapy should be discussed, and patients should be told to report any unusual symptoms.

REFERENCES

1. Bryant SG, Ereshefsky L: Antidepressant properties of trazodone. *Clin Pharm* 1:406–416, 1982.
2. Brogden RN, Heel RC, Splight TM, et al: Trazodone: a review of its pharmacological properties and therapeutic use in depression and anxiety. *Drugs* 21:401–419, 1981.
3. Clements-Jewery S, Robson PA, Chidley LJ: Biochemical investigations into the mode of action of trazodone. *Neuropharmacol* 19:1165–1173, 1980.
4. Caccia S, Ballabio M, Samanin R, Zanini MG, Garattini S: (−)-*m*-Chlorophenyl-piperazine, a central 5-hydroxytryptamine agonist, is a metabolite of trazodone. *J Pharm Pharmacol* 33:477–478, 1981.
5. Miller RL, DeVane CL: Analysis of trazodone and *m*-chlorophenylpiperazine in plasma and brain tissue by high-performance liquid chromatography. *J Chromatogr* 374:388–393, 1986.
6. Bayer AJ, Pathy MSJ, Ankier SI: Pharmacokinetic and pharmacodynamic characteristics of trazodone in the elderly. *Br J Clin Pharmacol* 16:371–376, 1983.
7. Greenblatt DJ, Friedman H, Burstein ES, et al: Trazodone kinetics: effect of age, gender, and obesity. *Clin Pharmacol Ther* 42:193–200, 1987.
8. Cassano GB: Trazodone in schizophrenia. In: *Trazodone: A New Broad-Spectrum Antidepressant*, Gershon S, Rickels K, Silvestrini B (eds), Excerpta Medica, Amsterdam, 1980, pp 75–82.
9. Rawls WN: Trazodone. *Drug Intell Clin Pharm* 16:7–13, 1982.

10. Brooks D, Prothero W, Bouras N, Bridges PK, Jarman CMB, Ankier SI: Trazodone—a comparison of single night-time and divided daily dosage regimens. *Psychopharmacology* 84:1–4, 1984.
11. Himmelhoch JM: Cardiovascular effects of trazodone in humans. *J Clin Psychopharmacol* 1:76S–81S, 1981.
12. Larochelle P, Hamet P, Enjalbert M: Responses to tyramine and norepinephrine after imipramine and trazodone. *Clin Pharmacol Ther* 26:24–30, 1979.
13. Warren M, Bick PA: Two case reports of trazodone-induced mania. *Am J Psychiatry* 141:1103–1104, 1984.
14. Warrington SJ, Ankier SI, Turner P: An evaluation of possible interactions between ethanol and trazodone or amitriptyline. *Br J Clin Pharmacol* 18:549–557, 1984.
15. van Zwieten PA: Inhibition of the central hypotensive effect of clonidine by trazodone: a novel antidepressant. *Pharmacology* 15:331–335, 1977.
16. Lisciani R, Baldini A, Ciottoli G: Behavioral study on the interactions between trazodone and L-dopa. *Pharmacol Res Commun* 11:265–272, 1979.
17. Scher M, Krieger JN, Juergens S: Trazodone and priapism. *Am J Psychiatry* 140:1362–1363, 1983.
18. Root I, Ohlson GB: Trazodone overdose: report of two cases. *J Anal Toxicol* 8:91–94, 1984.
19. Suzuki Y: Teratogenicity and placental transfer of trazodone. In: *Modern Problems of Pharmacopsychiatry*, Ban T, Silverstrini B (eds), S. Karger, Basel, 1974, 87–94.
20. DeVane CL, Simpkins JW: Possible teratogenic effects of imipramine in the rat. In: *Clinical Pharmacology in Psychiatry*, Dahl SG, Gram LF, Paul SM, Potter WZ (eds), Springer, Berlin, 1986, pp 174–178.

D

Phenelzine Database

FORMULATIONS

Phenelzine tablets: 15 mg
Brand name: Nardil (Parke-Davis)

BASIC PHARMACOLOGY

Monoamine oxidase enzymes are present in many organs of the body. In the brain they degrade various neurotransmitters, including epinephrine and norepinephrine. Thus, the monoamine oxidase inhibitors (MAOIs) act by effectively enhancing the action and altering the balance of important neurotransmitters in the central nervous system (see Chapter 1B). In an as yet unknown manner, this relates to their mechanisms of action as antidepressants.

Phenelzine (Fig. 2D.1) is representative of the nonselective MAOI. This terminology is used to reflect the increasing selectivity of the newer drugs in this class. Traditionally, the MAOIs have been divided into the hydrazine (phenelzine, isocarboxazid) and nonhydrazine (tranylcypromine, pargyline, deprenyl, clorgyline) derivatives. A further distinction is whether they reversibly or irreversibly inhibit monoamine oxidase (MAO).

Recently, it has been discovered that MAO exists in two forms (1, 2). These are referred to as type A and type B. The major difference in these subtypes is

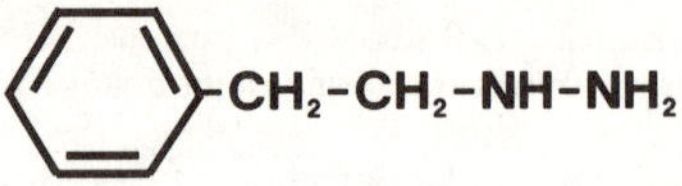

Figure 2D.1.   Chemical structure of phenelzine.

Table 2D.1.
Types of Monoamine Oxidase, Their Substrates, and Inhibitors

	Type of Enzyme	
	Type A	Type B
Substrates		
Serotonin	+	
Phenylethylamine		+
Norepinephrine	+	
Dopamine		+
Tyramine	+	+
Inhibitors		
Clorgyline	+	
Deprenyl		+
Harmaline	+	
Pargyline		+
Tranylcypromine	+	+
Phenelzine	+	+
Isocarboxazid	+	+

the substrates with which they preferentially interact. An added complexity is that their distribution in the body is nonhomogeneous. This knowledge has stimulated drug development to avoid one of the most difficult problems of using MAOIs (3). Nonselective inhibition of MAO can lead to hypertensive reactions when excessive tyramine or other catecholamines are consumed in the diet (4). Some drugs currently in clinical trials can prolong the action of important endogenous catecholamines, yet avoid potentially hazardous reactions by not inhibiting the specific MAO responsible for metabolism of interacting amines. Table 2D.1 lists the major MAOIs and the preferred substrates according to type of enzyme. Because tyramine can be destroyed by MAO type B, administering a MAOI specific for type A could increase the neurotransmission of serotonin or norepinephrine while still allowing excessive tyramine to be eliminated by type B, thus avoiding its systemic effects on blood pressure.

The MAOIs have low affinity for muscarinic receptors. Thus, they usually cause little in the way of anticholinergic side effects. They also are not antihistaminic. When administered to healthy, depressed patients, phenelzine usually causes a slight decrease in blood pressure. The expected effects on various standard laboratory tests are outlined in Table 2D.2.

PHARMACOKINETIC PROPERTIES

The pharmacokinetic properties of phenelzine are not well described in the biomedical literature. In urine, phenelzine sulfate is a major excretion product. The half-life of phenelzine, calculated from urinary excretion data in five patients, averaged slightly less than 1 hour (5). Phenelzine causes irreversible MAO inhibition, and, thus, the drug's pharmacokinetics are likely to correlate with its clinical effects in a complex manner.

Table 2D.2.
Expected Physiological Effects from MAOI Therapy for Monitoring[a]

Parameter	Drug Effect
Cardiovascular status	
Heart rate	Slight decrease of approximately 5 beats/minute
ECG	Occasional decreased QTC intervals with normal QRS intervals
Blood pressure	A reduction occurs frequently, especially decreased systolic blood pressure upon standing; an enhanced pressor sensitivity to tyramine and sympathomimetic drugs occurs early in therapy and may persist for weeks after therapy is stopped.
Renal function	
Serum creatinine and clearance, BUN	No changes expected
Hepatic function	
AST (SGOT), ALT (SGPT), alkaline phosphatase	Hepatocellular damage is rare but has been reported in a few patients. No changes are expected outside normal limits.
Hematology status	
CBC	Leukopenia has been reported but is rare.
Neuroendocrine status	
DST, plasma cortisol	May normalize with successful therapy
Fasting blood glucose	MAOIs may lower blood glucose and improve glucose tolerance.

[a]For abbreviations, see Table 2B.1.

Phenelzine is a basic amine with a structure similar to that of other drugs that are acetylated during metabolism. This pathway is suggested to be an important route of disposition for phenelzine, although an acetyl metabolite has not yet been identified in humans. The ability to acetylate drugs is genetically controlled, and this pharmacogenetic characteristic can be typed as fast or slow. Slow drug acetylators would have higher plasma concentrations of parent drug and lower concentrations of acetylated metabolites. This patient characteristic could result in therapeutic drug responses at lower drug doses (6, 7). Such a phenomenon has been observed with isoniazid, hydralazine, and procainamide, other drugs metabolized by acetylation. Therefore, several studies have attempted to determine whether differences in phenelzine clinical response occur according to acetylator phenotype. The results have been equivocal (8). Nevertheless, it has been suspected that slow acetylators would respond quicker or have a greater number of side effects than fast acetylators. However, the present data do not yet support phenotyping patients as an aid to selecting phenelzine dosage.

INDICATIONS

Phenelzine is FDA-approved for treatment of depressed patients clinically characterized as atypical, nonendogenous, or neurotic. These patients often

Table 2D.3.
Target Symptoms Suggested for Monitoring Antidepressant Response in Atypical or Endogenously Depressed Patients

Atypical	Endogenous
Difficulty initiating sleep	Early morning awakening
Hypersomnia	Diminished sleep
Weight gain	Weight loss
Food craving	Loss of appetite
Agoraphobia	Psychomotor retardation
Panic experiences	Loss of energy
Hypochondriasis	Suicidal ideation
Obsessive traits	Constriction of interests
Psychic anxiety	
Somatic anxiety	

have mixed anxiety and depression and phobic or hypochondriacal features. Thus, the target symptoms for monitoring clinical response will differ somewhat from the classical symptoms of endogenous depression. Table 2D.3 compares typical clinical features of these two types of depressed patients. There is current research activity in further defining this heterogenous group of patients (9, 10).

Phenelzine should rarely be the first antidepressant drug of choice, except in patients with atypical depression. Rather, it may be more suitable for use with patients who have failed to respond to either one or more cyclic antidepressants or lithium. Overall, the low degree of cardiac toxicity and apparent absence of central anticholinergic toxicity with phenelzine, as compared to those factors in the tricyclics, may be considered an advantage in some patients.

Reviews of controlled trials of MAOIs, including phenelzine, suggest an improvement rate of approximately 70%. This is similar to the improvement seen with tricyclic antidepressants. Perhaps more importantly, it should be understood that MAOI responders may have different clinical features than have tricyclic responders (11, 12). There is less conclusive evidence of phenelzine's usefulness with severely depressed patients with endogenous features (32, 33).

Phenelzine has several unapproved uses. The antiphobic effects of phenelzine have been well demonstrated, and the drug is most likely to be the agent of choice in the treatment of agoraphobia and social phobias (13, 14). Phenelzine is equal to or better than imipramine in the treatment of panic disorder. Limited research indicates that MAOIs, especially phenelzine, may be used successfully in patients with migraine headache refractory to other treatment (15). Phenelzine has also been effective in the treatment of bulimia (16).

In recent years, there has been wider recognition of posttraumatic stress disorder (PTSD), especially in Vietnam War veterans. These patients frequently have generalized anxiety and panic attacks (17). A favorable response has been noted in patients treated with phenelzine to relieve the anxiety and depressive symptoms associated with PTSD (18). As phenelzine depresses REM sleep in animals and humans, it can be expected to decrease dream activity. Target symptoms may include nightmares and flashbacks when one is monitoring phenelzine therapy in patients with PTSD.

DOSAGE REGIMEN DESIGN

Recommended doses for most patients are 45 to 75 mg daily, or 1 mg/kg, in three divided doses. In some patients, doses in the range of 45 to 60 mg/day will be effective. However, there is a wide variability in response to standard doses. Up to 90 mg/day, in the absence of limiting side effects, is recommended before treatment with phenelzine is abandoned as unsuccessful.

A suggested initial dose is 15 mg at bedtime. This can be increased by 15 mg at 2-day intervals to reach 45 mg by the end of the 1st week. Patients with panic disorder are very sensitive to the activating effects of antidepressants, including phenelzine, and dosage should be started low and increases must be made slowly.

Many depressed patients will not achieve optimal benefit at a dose below 45 mg/day. At this dose level, there is risk of exposing patients to side effects without accruing substantial antidepressant effects. By the end of 2 weeks, if side effects are absent, a dose of 60 mg/day can be reached and maintained. Once-daily dosing may be used. By the end of 5 weeks, if no significant improvement in symptoms has occurred, the dose can be increased further. A gradual increase is recommended, perhaps by alternating doses of 60 and 75 mg/day.

Some lag in response usually exists, but many responsive patients can be expected to show improvement by 2 weeks, just as occurs with tricyclic-responsive patients. By the end of 6 weeks of therapy, the response should be greater than at 2 weeks. Depressed mood, thought content, and especially anxiety are symptoms to monitor that show improvement over time (Table 2D.3). Too rapid reduction of phenelzine dosage during maintenance therapy, especially during the first 6 months after remission of an acute illness, can result in return of symptoms (19). Abruptly stopping phenelzine can result in REM sleep rebound with insomnia and nightmares.

THERAPEUTIC DRUG MONITORING

There are presently no guidelines for using plasma concentration as an aid to guide phenelzine therapy. Plasma concentrations from therapeutic doses are in the low nanogram-per-milliliter range and are therefore difficult to quantitate. The most useful aid to guiding dosage has been the degree of platelet MAO inhibition. The hypothesis stimulating these investigations has been that peripheral MAO inhibition would reflect brain MAO inhibition. Robinson et al (20) found a dose-related degree of MAO inhibition between phenelzine doses of 30 and 60 mg/day. Their work and that of others (21) suggests the need for achieving at least 85% platelet MAO inhibition to achieve a substantial clinical effect. Some research data suggest that patients whose baseline MAO activity is relatively high respond well to MAOIs. Unfortunately, few laboratories are equipped to measure MAO inhibition, and the degree of laboratory difficulty with this procedure, along with low demand, makes it unlikely to achieve widespread utilization. However, the data emphasize that dosage requirements may be up to 90 mg/day for some patients.

CONTRAINDICATIONS—WARNINGS—PRECAUTIONS

Phenelzine is contraindicated in patients with pheochromocytoma, congestive heart failure, or a known hypersensitivity to the drug. Phenelzine should be avoided in patients who must take concurrent sympathomimetic amines,

Table 2D.4.
Drug Interactions with Monoamine Oxidase Inhibitors

Interacting Drug	Effect
Amine-containing foods	Increased blood pressure; possible hypertensive crisis; can occur up to several weeks after discontinuing the MAOI
Anorexiants and other sympathomimetics: Amphetamine Ephedrine Fenfluramine Methylphenidate Pseudoephedrine Phenylpropranolamine	Elevated blood pressure with possible hypertensive crisis and intracranial hemorrhage can occur. This combination activates large quantities of endogenous catecholamines.
Guanethidine	The antihypertensive effect of this drug may be decreased by an unknown mechanism.
Insulin, sulfonylureas	An increased hypoglycemic effect may occur.
Levodopa	Enhanced effects of levodopa; possible hypertensive crisis
Meperidine, dextromethorphan	Cardiovascular instability, hyperpyrexia, agitation, and death have occurred.
Tricyclic antidepressants	The effects of both drugs can be increased, leading to enhanced clinical and/or toxic effects (see text).

guanethidine, or meperidine or who have diets high in tyramine content. These drug-drug and drug-food interactions are explained below.

Like other antidepressants, phenelzine may precipitate a manic reaction in patients with bipolar disorder (22). As lithium has been successfully used in combination with phenelzine (23), it may be useful to prevent rapid cycling in susceptible patients.

Patients have developed pyridoxine (vitamin B_6) deficiency while taking phenelzine. Patients who complain of numbness of the hands, shock-like feelings in the spine, or other symptoms suggesting a neurological origin, may have this problem. Treatment is easily accomplished with supplemental dietary pyridoxine. The recommended dose is 300 mg daily.

DRUG INTERACTIONS

Drug interactions may occur frequently with the MAOIs. The most serious interactions result in drastic changes in blood pressure. Hypertensive crises have been associated with concomitant therapy with several drugs (4, 24, 25). The mechanism is usually related to combined effects on catecholamine stimulation of adrenergic receptors. These and other interactions are summarized in Table 2D.4. Patients receiving phenelzine should be warned that many over-the-counter (OTC) cough and cold remedies contain drugs that interact with the MAOIs. Phenylpropanolamine, a principle ingredient of many OTC nasal decongestants and appetite suppressants, should be strictly avoided.

Inhibition of MAO prevents gastrointestinal and liver metabolism of pressor amines found in some foods and beverages. This interaction potentiates their ability to release norepinephrine from adrenergic neurons. Table 2D.5 lists diet-

Table 2D.5.
Dietary Restrictions Recommended for Patients Taking Phenelzine

Foods high in tyramine content that must be avoided
  Cheese, especially aged cheese (Limburger, Gouda, Edam, Cheddar)
  Foods containing cheese (pizza, fondue, many Italian dishes)
  Wine, particularly Chianti and red wines in general
  Fermented or aged foods, especially meats or aged fish (pepperoni, summer
    sausage, pickled herring)
  Broad bean pods
  Chicken or beef liver
  Yeast extracts
Foods with moderate tyramine content that are best avoided
  Other alcoholic beverages (gin, vodka, whiskey)
  Avocados
  Yogurt
  Bananas
  Raisins, figs
  Soy sauce
Foods relatively low in tyramine content that can be consumed in moderate
    amounts
  Bread
  Cottage and cream cheese
  Chocolate
  Coffee, tea, and caffeine-containing beverages
  Other fresh fruits

ary restrictions for patients receiving phenelzine. Foods high in tyramine content should be avoided at least 1 day before and for 2 weeks after taking phenelzine (34, 35).

Of particular interest is the interaction between MAOIs and tricyclic antidepressants. This combination of drugs has been implicated in causing hypertensive crises, but they can be used safely and advantageously together (36). When transferring a patient from a cyclic antidepressant to a MAOI, a medication-free interval of at least 1 week should be allowed. The MAOI should be initiated using half the normal dose for the first 4 to 6 days of therapy. A less common situation arises when a patient who has failed a trial with a MAOI needs to be treated with a cyclic antidepressant. A drug-free interval after discontinuing the MAOI may be less necessary but is still desirable. If the MAOI has been administered for less than 1 week, then the cyclic antidepressant can be started immediately at low dose after discontinuing the MAOI. If the MAOI has been administered for more than 3 weeks, then a 1-week interval should be allowed between the two drugs. Approximately 1-week or longer is required for MAO to be regenerated after chronic therapy with a MAOI.

In refractory depressed patients, an initial combination of a MAOI and cyclic antidepressant can be used. Phenelzine is preferred over tranylcypromine. Some drug-free interval should be allowed if the patient has been taking either a tricyclic antidepressant or a MAOI for more than 1 week. The drugs can be started simultaneously, using smaller than usual doses of each. A recommended dose is 10 mg of a tertiary tricyclic (amitriptyline or imipramine), with increments in weekly intervals of 10 mg/day. This combination may be quickly effective.

Patients taking phenelzine or other MAOIs should have their therapy discontinued 2 to 3 weeks before anesthesia (37). Sympathomimetic amines are frequently used in surgery to control blood pressure and may interact to precipitate a hypertensive crisis. In addition, MAOIs interact with meperidine in a similar manner. Morphine that has not been implicated in such an interaction and would be a preferred narcotic analgesic to control severe pain. Other interactions with skeletal muscle relaxants suggest the need to avoid MAOIs when surgery must be performed. Caution should also be exercised when patients who have received MAOIs are to be treated with electroconvulsive therapy.

ADVERSE REACTIONS—OCCURRENCE AND MANAGEMENT

The most serious reactions to phenelzine include changes in blood pressure, and hypertensive crisis is the most important of these. These reactions are characterized by some or all of the following symptoms: occipital headache that may radiate frontally, palpitation, neck stiffness or soreness, nausea, vomiting, sweating, dilated pupils, and photophobia. Either tachycardia or bradycardia may be present. Intracranial bleeding has occurred in association with the increase in blood pressure. Blood pressure should be observed frequently to detect evidence of any pressor response in patients receiving phenelzine (Table 2D.2) or other drugs (Table 2D.4). The hypertensive response can occur after a single dose. Management includes discontinuing phenelzine, administration of phentolamine (up to 5 mg intravenously), and management of fever. However, it should be appreciated that phenelzine, when taken alone, is more likely to produce a hypotensive, rather than a hypertensive, response. The common side effects of MAOIs are listed in Table 2D.6. In comparison to imipramine (Chapter 2B), phenelzine produces about the same frequency of side effects. However, a greater number of phenelzine patients may have to discontinue therapy because of the severity of side effects.

MANAGEMENT OF OVERDOSE

Hospitalization for severe overdosage is recommended. The initial symptoms may be misleadingly minimal, progressing in severity over 24 hours. A mixed clinical picture of stimulation and central nervous system depression can exist. Excitement, irritability, tachypnea, and tachycardia may be present. Tendon reflexes can be exaggerated, and hypotension or hypertension is possible. Severe hypertension may be treated with an α-adrenergic blocking agent. Intravenous phentolamine (5 mg) is frequently recommended. All pressor agents used for hypotension must be used with extreme caution, as they can be potentiated by MAOI therapy. Treatment is largely symptomatic and should follow standard guidelines for drug overdosage. This would include maintenance of fluid and electrolyte balance, as well as sodium bicarbonate in doses up to 3 mEq/kg/hr for acidosis. Treatment for overdosage may be required for several days. Dialysis procedures may be valuable, but little documentation is available for their recommendation. Deaths have occurred from phenelzine overdoses of 25 to 100 mg/kg.

Table 2D.6.
Expected Side Effects of Phenelzine Therapy

Effect	Rare	Less Common	More Common
Dry mouth			X
Nausea			X
Headache		X	
Constipation			X
Blurred vision		X	
Orthostatic hypotension			X
Hypertensive reaction		X	
Dizziness			X
Ataxia	X		
Muscle cramps		X	
Weakness, fatigue			X
Agitation		X	
Insomnia		X	
Excitement or hypomania		X	
Sexual dysfunction (anorgasmia, impotence)			X
Lupus-like skin reaction	X		

USE IN RENAL AND/OR HEPATIC DISEASE

No routine dosage adjustment is recommended in the presence of renal failure (28). In patients with a history of severe liver disease, phenelzine should be avoided, as liver toxicity with the nonhydrazines (tranylcypromine) seems to be very rare. Phenelzine has caused an idiosyncratic hepatic injury (38). Factors suggesting the need for careful monitoring include female sex, advanced age, and a history of alcohol abuse.

USE IN CHILDREN AND ADOLESCENTS

Major affective disorders are becoming increasingly recognized in children and adolescents. The use of MAOIs in these groups has not received systematic study, and phenelzine is not recommended for patients less than 16 years old.

USE IN THE ELDERLY

There has been a clinical impression that MAOIs are more toxic than tricyclic antidepressants in the elderly. However, several studies support the safety and efficacy of these drugs in aged patients (29, 30). There seems to be an increase in MAO activity in the brain correlating with age up to age 80 years. The plasma concentration of phenelzine, but not the rate of drug acetylation, has been reported to increase with age (31). Overall, evidence indicates that phenelzine may be safely and effectively used in the elderly with no more expectation of severe side effects than with the tricyclic drugs. Although the elderly may be particularly prone to orthostatic hypotension, this side effect also occurs frequently with the tricyclic antidepressants.

USE IN PREGNANCY

For years, many psychiatrists feared and avoided the use of MAOIs. The feeling was that these agents were less effective and more toxic than the tricyclic drugs. Consequently, by the late 1960s, the MAOIs had nearly disappeared from use. It is not surprising, then, that little is known about their effects on the fetus.

One study has indicated that phenelzine has the ability to cross the rat placenta. Lisinski et al (26) examined the influence of phenelzine on serotonin levels in the placenta and fetus and found increases in both tissues. Excessive serotonin is known to have a lethal effect on the rat fetus by provoking abortion in early pregnancy and causing necrosis of the fetus in the second half of pregnancy; therefore, any increase in the levels may intensify this action. Based on these minimal animal data and principles of good clinical practice, it seems prudent to avoid MAOIs in pregnant women.

One report noted an increased risk of malformations associated with MAOI use during the first trimester of pregnancy (27). Twenty-one mother-child pairs exposed to MAOIs were monitored, but details of the three cases exposed to phenelzine were not available.

No data are available regarding phenelzine's presence in breast milk. It can be presumed that drugs such as phenelzine, which pass readily into the central nervous system, must be lipid-soluble enough to pass into breast milk and should be avoided in mothers who breast feed.

PATIENT INFORMATION

Patients should be alerted to the possible seriousness of drug-drug and drug-food interactions. They should be instructed in dietary precautions (Table 2D.5) and told to avoid all other medications without first consulting a knowledgeable professional. Patients should also be told of the common side effects (Table 2D.6) that may occur and informed about the lag in response time.

REFERENCES

1. Pickar D, Murphy DL, Cohen RM, Campbell IC, Lipper S: Selective and nonselective monoamine oxidase inhibitors. Behavioral disturbances during their administration to depressed patients. *Arch Gen Psychiatry* 39:535–540, 1982.
2. Donnelly CH, Murphy DL: Substrate and inhibitor-related characteristics of human platelet monoamine oxidase. *Biochem Pharmacol* 26:853–858, 1977.
3. Potter WZ, Murphy DL, Wehr TA, Linnoila M, Goodwin FK: Clorgyline. A new treatment for patients with refractory rapid-cycling disorder. *Arch Gen Psychiatry* 39:505–510, 1982.
4. Cuthbert MJ, Greenberg MP, Morley SW: Cough and cold remedies: A potential danger to patients on monoamine oxidase inhibitors. *Br Med J* 1:404–407, 1969.
5. Johnstone EC: The urinary excretion of phenelzine. *Br J Clin Pharmacol* 6:185–188, 1978.
6. Tyrer P, Gardner M, Lambourn J, Whitford M: Clinical and pharmacokinetic factors affecting response to phenelzine. *Br J Psychiatry* 136:359–365, 1980.
7. Ravaris CL, Robinson DS, Ives JO, Nies A, Bartlett D: Phenelzine and amitriptyline in the treatment of depression. *Arch Gen Psychiatry* 37:1075–1080, 1980.
8. Rose S: The relationship of acetylation phenotype to treatment with MAOIs: a review. *J Clin Psychopharmacol* 2:161–164, 1982.
9. Davidson JRT, Miller RD, Turnbull CD, Sullivan JL: Atypical depression. *Arch Gen Psychiatry* 39:527–534, 1982.
10. Paykel ES, Parker RR, Penrose RJJ, Rassaby ER: Depressive classification and prediction of response to phenelzine. *Br J Psychiatry* 134:572–581, 1979.
11. Kay DWK, Garside RF, Fahy TJ: A double-blind trial of phenelzine and amitriptyline in depressed out-patients. A possible differential effect of the drugs on symptoms. *Br J Psychiatry* 123:63–67, 1973.
12. Ravaris CL, Nies A, Robinson DL, et al: A multiple-dose controlled study of phenelzine in depression-anxiety states. *Arch Gen Psychiatry* 33:347–350, 1976.

13. Sheehan DV, Claycomb JB, Kouretas N: Monoamine oxidase inhibitors: prescription and patient management. *Int J Psychiatry Med* 10:99–120, 1980.

14. Mountjoy M, Roth RF, Garside F, et al: A clinical trial of phenelzine in anxiety depressive and phobic neuroses. *Br J Psychiatry* 131:486–492, 1977.

15. Anthony M, Lance JW: Monoamine oxidase inhibition in the treatment of migraine. *Arch Neurol* 21:263–268, 1969.

16. Walsh BT, Stewart JW, Wright L, Harrison W, Roose SP, Glassman AH: Treatment of bulimia with monoamine oxidase inhibitors. *Am J Psychiatry* 139:1629–1630, 1982.

17. Birkhimer LJ, DeVane CL, Muniz CE: Post traumatic stress disorder: characteristics and pharmacologic response in the veteran population. *Compr Psychiatry* 26:304–310, 1985.

18. Hodgen GL, Cornfield RB: Treatment of traumatic war neurosis with phenelzine. *Arch Gen Psychiatry* 38:440–445, 1981.

19. Davidson J, Raft D: Use of phenelzine in continuation therapy. *Neuropsychobiology* 11:191–194, 1984.

20. Robinson DS, Nies A, Ravaris CL, et al: Clinical pharmacology of phenelzine. *Arch Gen Psychiatry* 35:629–635, 1978.

21. Georgotas A, Mann J, Friedman E: Platelet monoamine oxidase inhibition as a potential indicator of favorable response to MAOIs in geriatric depressions. *Biol Psychiatry* 16:997–1001, 1981.

22. Mattsson A, Seltzer RL: MAOI-induced rapid cycling bipolar affective disorder in an adolescent. *Am J Psychiatry* 138:677–680, 1981.

23. Nelson JC, Byck R: Rapid response to lithium in phenelzine nonresponders. *Br J Psychiatry* 141:85–86, 1982.

24. Elis J, Laurence DR, Mattie H, Prichard BNC: Modification by monoamine oxidase inhibitors of the effect of some sympathomimetics on blood pressure. *Br Med J* 2:75–78, 1967.

25. Lloyd JTA, Walker BRH: Death after combined dexamphetamine and phenelzine. *Br Med J* 2:168, 1965.

26. Lisinski J, Kurzepa S, Samojlik E: Influence of phenelzine on 5-hydroxytryptamine levels in rat placenta and fetuses. *Am J Obset Gynecol* 97:249–251, 1967.

27. Heinonen OP, Slone D, Shapiro S: *Birth Defects and Drugs in Pregnancy,* Publishing Sciences Group, Littleton, ms, 1977, pp 322–334.

28. Bennett WM, Aronoff GM, Morrison G, et al: Drug prescribing in renal failure: dosing guidelines for adults. *Am J Kidney Dis* 3:155–193, 1983.

29. Ashford JW, Ford CV: Use of MAO inhibitors in elderly patients. *Am J Psychiatry* 136:1466–1467, 1979.

30. Georgotas A, Kim M, Hapworth W, et al: Monoamine oxidase inhibitors and affective disorders in the elderly. *Psychopharmacol Bull* 19:662–665, 1983.

31. Robinson DS: Monoamine oxidase inhibitors and the elderly. In: *Age and the Pharmacology of Psychoactive Drugs,* Raskin A, Robinson DS, Levine J (eds), Elsevier-North Holland, Amsterdam, 1981, pp 151–162.

32. Paykel ED, Rowan PR, Parker RR, Bhat AV: Response to phenelzine and amitriptyline in subtypes of outpatient depression. *Arch Gen Psychiatry* 39:1041–1049, 1982.

33. Quitkin FM, McGrath P, Liebowitz MR, Stewart J, Howard A: Monoamine oxidase inhibitors in bipolar endogenous depressives. *J Clin Psychopharmacol* 1:70–74, 1981.

34. Neil JF, Licata SM, May SJ, Himmelhoch JM: Dietary noncompliance during treatment with tranylcypromine. *J Clin Psychiatry* 34:50–56, 1979.

35. McCabe B, Tsuang MT: Dietary consideration in MAO inhibitor regimens. *J Clin Psychiatry* 43:178–181, 1982.

36. Ananth J, Luchins D: A review of combined tricyclic and MAOI therapy. *Compr Psychiatry* 18:221–230, 1977.

37. Janowsky EC, Risch C, Janowsky DS: Effects of anesthesia on patients taking psychotropic drugs. *J Clin Psychopharmacol* 1:14–20, 1981.

38. Bonkovsky HL, Blanchette PL, Schned AR: Severe liver injury due to phenelzine with unique hepatic deposition of extracellular material. *Am J Med* 80:689–692, 1986.

E
Intraclass Comparisons of Antidepressants and Mood Stabilizers

Lithium is the best established antimanic drug available. It has calming effects on excited behavior that are not shared by the antipsychotics, although members of this drug class are frequently used in the initial treatment of acute mania. Rubidium is another element from the Ia group of the periodic table of elements. It has been tested for psychoactive properties, but the results have not held much promise (1). It is doubtful that a more useful antimanic drug than lithium will be found without first defining the pathophysiology of the mood disorders.

Lithium has been compared in clinical trials to the tricyclic drugs for its antidepressant properties. Data from VA cooperative studies (2) and other trials (3, 4) have shown lithium to be as good as a tricyclic in maintaining remission of depression, but imipramine or another cyclic antidepressant remains superior for treatment of an active depressive episode.

It is reasonable to expect that drugs acting on γ-aminobutyric acid (GABA), one of the major inhibitory neurotransmitters in the central nervous system (Chapter 1B), might be antimanic in addition to being anticonvulsant. Carbamazepine, sodium valproate, and clonazepam seem beneficial in the treatment of bipolar affective disorder. The full extent of their indications is still being defined (5–7).

The drugs available for use as antidepressants represent diverse chemical classes. The best known are listed in Table 2E.1. Until recently, the tricyclic antidepressants constituted the majority of available antidepressants. Imipramine, the prototype, was introduced into clinical practice in the late 1950s. Soon thereafter, amitriptyline appeared, followed by slight chemical variations in the form of desipramine, nortriptyline, doxepin, and protriptyline. Several other tricyclic antidepressants have since become available in the United States and elsewhere. These drugs all possess essentially the same pharmacological actions, including the ability to cause reuptake inhibition of monoamines and blockade of muscarinic, histaminic, and α-adrenergic receptors (8), although to differing degrees.

The tricyclic drugs are widely believed to vary little in clinical effectiveness, although patients may respond to a particular drug and not another. There have been several studies, largely equivocal in their results, attempting to define predictive characteristics of patient responses to specific tricyclics (9, 10). The major differences in the cyclic antidepressants are in their relative ability to affect certain neurotransmitters more than others, their molar potency, and their side effect profiles. These effects are compared in Table 2E.2 and form one basis for selection of initial drug therapy.

Table 2E.1.
Classification of Proven and Experimental Antidepressants and Their Usual Daily Doses

Medication	Daily Dose Range (mg)
Monoamine oxidase inhibitors	
Phenelzine	30–90
Tranylcypromine	30–50
Isocarboxazid	20–30
Clorgyline	5–10
Deprenyl	5–15
Cyclic antidepressants	
Monocyclics	
Bupropion	150–450
Fluvoxamine	50–300
Dicyclics	
Fluoxetine	20–80
Tricyclics	
Amitriptyline	50–300
Clomipramine	50–300
Desipramine	50–300
Doxepin	50–300
Imipramine	50–300
Nortriptyline	50–200
Protriptyline	15–60
Trimipramine	50–300
Tetracyclics	
Maprotiline	50–200
Oxaprotiline	50–150
Heterocyclics	
Adinazolam	30–90
Alprazolam	3–10
Amoxapine	150–450
Carbamazepine	400–1600
Trazodone	50–600

The major pharmacokinetic properties for individual drugs are listed in Table 2E.3. As a group, the cyclic antidepressants are characterized by high hepatic and low renal clearances, extensive plasma protein and tissue binding, and high volumes of distribution. The combination of a high volume of distribution and a high systemic clearance confers half-lives on most of the drugs in a convenient range of 6 to 24 hours. This characteristic has been used as a justification for once-daily dosing. The large volume of distribution of these drugs reflects a high degree of drug penetration to tissues, including sites of action in the central nervous system, and a poor dialyzalibity in treatment of intentional or accidental overdosage.

Not unexpectedly, the drugs that have received the most research attention have the best defined therapeutic plasma concentration ranges. These findings are discussed below, and the most important are summarized in Table 2E.4.

Table 2E.2.
Pharmacological Comparison and Relative Side Effect Profile for Some Prominent
Cyclic Antidepressants

Drug	Predominant Neurotransmitter Effect	Sedation Potential	Muscarinic Blockade	Orthostatic Hypotension
Amitriptyline	Serotonin	High	High	High
Amoxapine	Norepinephrine	Weak	Weak	Weak
Bupropion	Dopamine	Weak	Weak	Weak
Doxepin	Norepinephrine	High	Moderate	Moderate
Desipramine	Norepinephrine	Moderate	Moderate	Moderate
Fluoxetine	Serotonin	Weak	Weak	Weak
Imipramine	Serotonin	High	High	High
Maprotiline	Norepinephrine	Moderate	Weak	Moderate
Nortriptyline	Norepinephrine	Moderate	Moderate	Moderate
Protriptyline	Norepinephrine	Weak	Moderate	Moderate
Trimipramine	Serotonin	High	High	High
Trazodone	Serotonin	High	Weak	Weak

In the 1970s, several antidepressants were marketed that differed substantially in structure when compared to the traditional tricyclics. These so-called "second generation" antidepressants are better classified according to a simple nomenclature related to the number of ring systems contained within each structure (12) (Table 2E.1). They differ from the tricyclics mainly in their side effect profiles, as they are similar in clinical efficacy (13). The most important agents are discussed below.

The remaining group of antidepressants is the monoamine oxidase inhibitors. Isocarboxazid is infrequently used clinically and, although pargyline is available, it is labeled for use as an antihypertensive. Clorgyline and deprenyl, two selective inhibitors, are not yet available and are undergoing clinical trials (14, 15).

INDIVIDUAL AGENTS
Traditional Anticonvulsants

Carbamazepine   Carbamazepine (CBZ) demonstrates a remarkable structural resemblance to the tricyclic antidepressants (Fig. 2E.1; compare imipramine in Fig. 2B.1) It is an anticonvulsant agent with prominant antimanic properties (16, 17). It serves as an alternative for patients who are unable to tolerate lithium's side effects or who respond to lithium poorly. CBZ does not produce marked sedation or neuroleptic side effects. Patients with a rapid cycling disorder seem to respond well. CBZ may also be useful to ameliorate aggressive and violent behavior and may be useful for patients with schizoaffective disorders.

Slow increases in dosage are recommended, starting with 200 mg/day and increasing up to 1000 mg/day according to the clinical response. The effective dose range is between 400 and 1600 mg/day. A plasma concentration range of 6 to 12 µg/ml correlates to CBZ's anticonvulsant effects, but a strong correlation of CBZ response with plasma concentration in mania has not been reported. Nevertheless, it seems unnecessary to exceed a steady-state plasma concentration of 8 to 12 µg/ml to achieve good antimanic effects.

CBZ is an inducer of hepatic microsomal enzymes (see Table 1D.5). After 2 or more weeks of therapy, plasma concentrations of CBZ frequently decrease

Table 2E.3.
Pharmacokinetic Parameters of Cyclic Antidepressants

Drug	Oral Availability	Volume of Distribution (liters/kg)	Total Body Clearance (liters/hr)	Elimination Half-life (hr)	Fraction Unbound in Plasma	Active Metabolites
Alprazolam	0.95	1–2	6–140	7–18	0.30	α-Hydroxy
Amitriptyline	0.3–0.6	6–36	19–72	9–46	0.03–0.15	Nortriptyline
Bupropion	0.9	27–60	120–180	10–20	0.20	Hydroxybupropion
Carbamazepine	0.7–0.8	0.8–1.4		10–30; 12^a	0.15–0.35	10,11-Epoxide
Clomipramine	0.4–0.6	9–25	23–122	15–60	0.02–0.10	Desmethyl
Desipramine	0.3–0.6	20–60	78–168	12–28	0.08–0.27	2-Hydroxy
Doxepin	0.2–0.5	10–30	41–60	8–25	0.15–0.32	Desmethyl
Fluoxetine	0.95	12–42	6–42	120 +	0.06	Norfluoxetine
Imipramine	0.2–0.7	10–25	32–102	6–28	0.04–0.37	Desipramine
Maprotiline	0.8	16–32	17–34	27–50	0.12	Desmethyl
Nortriptyline	0.5–0.7	15–23	17–79	18–56	0.07–0.13	10-Hydroxy
Protriptyline	0.7–0.9	15–30	8–23	54–120	0.01–0.10	Desmethyl
Trazodone	0.7–0.9	0.8–1.5	7–12	4–13	0.05–0.11	m-Chlorophenylpiperazine

^{a}Carbamazepine induces its own metabolism, and patients on chronic therapy will have a decreased half-life.

Table 2E.4.
Recommendations for Using Cyclic Antidepressant Plasma Concentration Monitoring

Drug	Concentration Range (ng/ml)	Effect
Imipramine	180–350	This range of combined imipramine plus desipramine concentrations has correlated well in several studies with antidepressant effect in endogenous depression.
	Over 500	Behavior toxicity may occur; there is rarely any justification to exceed this combined concentration.
	Over 1000	Has frequently correlated with severe systemic toxicity requiring medical support; range also applies to other tricyclics.
Nortriptyline	50–150	Range best associated with antidepressant effects in endogenous depression
Amitriptyline	120–250	This combined amitriptyline plus nortriptyline concentration is the target for antidepressant effect.
	Over 500	Frequently associated with anticholinergic delirium
Desipramine	115–250	Target concentration for antidepressant effect

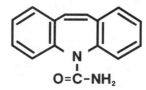

Figure 2E.1.   Chemical structure of carbamazepine.

because of autoinduction, at which time a dosage increase may be necessary to maintain effective plasma concentrations. This enzyme induction effect will enhance the clearance of other commonly used psychoactive drugs, including haloperidol and other antipsychotic agents (18).

CBZ must be monitored for side effects. Aplastic anemia and agranulocytosis, rarely resulting in death, have occurred. The appearance of a patient with an infection, fever, sore throat, or petechia should alert the clinician to possible hemotological toxicity.

Carbamazepine can produce a vasopressin-like antidiuretic effect resulting in hyponatremia. This risk may be increased by low baseline serum sodium when the patient begins therapy. Table 2E.5 lists the expected physiological effects of CBZ with hemotological guidelines for when to discontinue the drug.

Clonazepam   Clonazepam, an anticonvulsant benzodiazepine, has also been tried for mood stabilization (19). Doses in acutely manic patients, up to 40 mg/day, are substiantially higher than the 2 mg/day usually needed for control of seizures. The drug is more sedating than carbamazepine but, if proven effective, could be a safer alternative than lithium or carbamazepine. In doses of 1.5 to 6.0 mg/day it has shown good antipanic effects.

Table 2E.5.
Expected Physiological Effects from Carbamazepine Therapy for Monitoring[a]

Parameter	Drug Effect
Cardiovascular status	
Heart rate	No cardiac instability expected; less effect on
ECG	producing orthostatic hypotension than either
Blood pressure	MAOIs or tricylics. Rare reports of heart block;
	decreases in pulse rate should be evaluated.
Renal function	
Serum creatinine and	No changes expected
clearance, BUN	
Hepatic function	
AST (SGOT), ALT	Transient elevations may occur; some cases of
(SGPT), alkaline	hepatotoxicity have been reported. Baseline indices
phosphatase	should be obtained; expect increases in 2–3 weeks.
Hematology status	
CBC	Regular lowering of white count can be expected. Discontinue therapy under any of the following conditions:
	WBC $< 3000/mm^3$
	Neutrophils $< 1500/mm^3$
	Erythrocytes $< 4.0 \times 10^6\ mm^3$
	Hematocrit $< 32\%$
	Platelets $< 100,000/mm^3$
Neuroendocrine status	
DST, plasma cortisol	False positives can occur. Carbamazepine causes escape from dexamethasone suppression. Carbamazepine enhances vasopressin function and hyponatremia may occur.

[a]For abbreviations, see Table 2B.1.

Valproic Acid   Valproic acid is an anticonvulsant indicated for simple and complex absence seizures. Reports have also suggested that valproate has effects in manic patients similar to those seen with acute lithium therapy (20). It has been reported to be moderately useful in schizoaffective disorder (21). There is much less experience with this drug than with carbamazepine.

Dosage is 1000 to 1500 mg/day, starting with 250 to 500 mg/day. Periodic liver function tests are recommended, as hepatotoxicity has been reported. Other side effects are gastrointestinal in origin, principally nausea, vomiting, and anorexia. Anticholinergic and sedative effects are minor.

Benzodiazepines

Adinazolam   Experience with alprazolam documented that benzodiazepines may have specific antidepressant properties, in addition to their effects on the anxiety associated with depression. The triazolobenzodiazepines seem to possess properties not shared by the larger, previously marketed group of benzodiazepines (22). For example, alprazolam, but not diazepam, prevented the upregulation of β-adrenergic receptors induced by reserpine. Adinazolam, the aminoalkyl derivative of alprazolam, is currently in clinical trials and will be the first benzodiazepine with the specific indication for treatment of depression

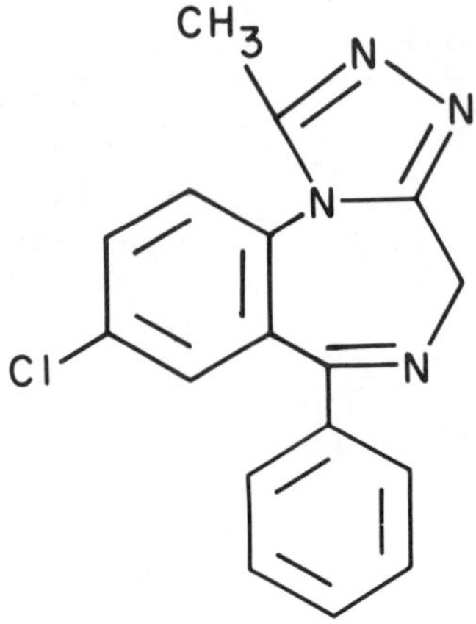

Figure 2E.2.   Chemical structure of alprazolam.

(23). Sedation is likely to be modest, and other side effects are likely to be minor. Tolerance, dependence, and withdrawal reactions have not been reported. A short elimination half-life may require multiple daily dosing or formulation in a sustained-release preparation to avoid symptom reemergence between doses.

Alprazolam   Among the benzodiazepines, alprazolam has been most extensively tested for its antidepressant potential (24, 25) (Fig. 2E.2). Its FDA-approved indications are anxiety and anxiety associated with depression. In clinical trials of depressed patients, dosage has been generally higher than required for antianxiety effects (4 to 10 mg/day). Alprazolam has distinct antidepressant effects equivalent to those of standard tricyclic drugs in controlling acute symptoms for up to 6 weeks, but the efficacy of long-term therapy for maintaining remission of depression is unsubstantiated.

Alprazolam has been conclusively proven to have antipanic effects and is potentially useful for other anxiety disorders, including posttraumatic stress disorder and obsessive-compulsive disorder. Dosage should be started low, approximately 1.5 mg/day or less, regardless of indication. Reports of difficulty in discontinuing the drug suggest the need for gradual tapering of the dose over an extended period (see discussion in Chapter 4C).

Cyclic Antidepressants

Amitriptyline   Sedation and a high degree of anticholinergic side effects are problematic when using amitriptyline (Table 2E.2). For a patient with a history of a previous response to the drug, it will be the preferred choice for retreatment. However, for many patients, imipramine remains a more suitable first choice among the tricyclic drugs (Chapter 2B). A positive relationship between plasma amitriptyline concentration and response has been noted in several trials (11). A therapeutic plasma concentration range is 120 to 250 ng/ml for amitriptyline, combined with the concentration of its metabolite nortriptyline. However, several large studies that have found no usable relationship between amitriptyline plasma concentration and clinical efficacy for treatment of depression. The determination of plasma amitriptyline concentrations is indicated in selected patients who are nonresponders and when noncompliance or anticho-

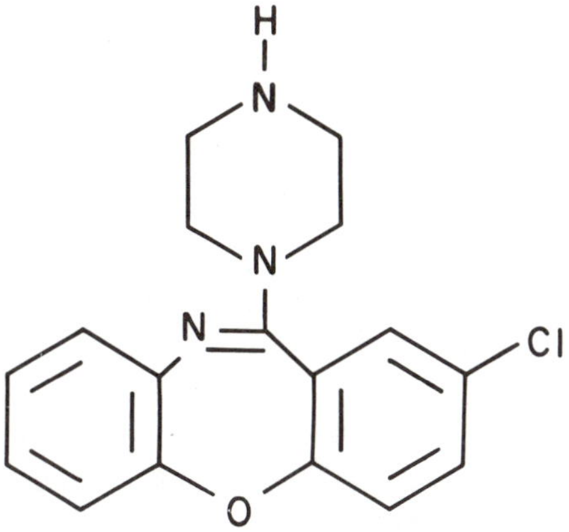

Figure 2E.3.   Chemical structure of amoxapine.

linergic toxicity is suspected. Concentrations greater than 450 ng/ml have been highly correlated with anticholinergic delirium (26).

Amoxapine   Amoxapine is a heterocyclic antidepressant (Fig. 2E.3), which, coincidentally, is the demethylated metabolite of loxapine, an antipsychotic agent (Chapter 3). An active metabolite, 7-hydroxyamoxapine, possesses dopamine receptor blocking action. This property suggests a mechanism by which amoxapine produces akathisia and other extrapyramidal side effects more typical of the antipsychotic class of drugs (27). Patients receiving amoxapine should be monitored for unusual movements. The Abnormal Involuntary Movement Scale (AIMS) or the Simpson-Angus scales for Extrapyramidal Symptoms (EPS), have proved to be valuable tools for this purpose (28). Amoxapine has efficacy similar to that of imipramine. Initial reports of a rapid onset of action have been viewed with skepticism. The drug's clinical pharmacokinetics are not well enough defined to allow recommendation of a target therapeutic plasma concentration range.

Cases of amoxapine overdosage have been complicated by acute renal failure and rhabdomyolysis. Hydration status should be monitored closely in the event of overdosage.

Bupropion   This long-awaited monocyclic antidepressant (Fig. 2E.4) has several clinical advantages, as compared to the tricyclic antidepressants, which suggest that it may be a first choice for some patients (29, 30). It lacks any appreciable anticholinergic or sedative effects, and it is probably the safest among all of the cyclic antidepressants, with the exception of alprazolam, for patients with cardiac disease. Orthostatic hypotension occurs to a much lesser degree than with the tricyclic antidepressants. Bupropion produces little or no weight gain or impairment in sexual functioning. However, it has the major drawback of occasionally provoking unexpected generalized seizures. The risk is increased when dosage is escalated sharply, and dosage should be kept under 450 mg for most patients and below 600 mg/day for all patients. Monitoring parameters for this side effect include prodromal signs of seizure activity, including complaints of nervousness, an exaggerated startle response, and psychomotor irritability. Treatment consists of intravenous diazepam or phenytoin and discontinuation of bupropion. As bupropion's active metabolites have half-

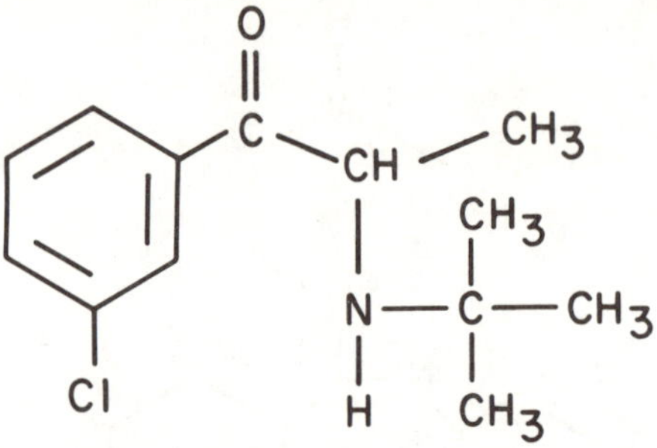

Figure 2E.4.   Chemical structure of bupropion.

lives of greater than 24 hours (31), monitoring should be continued for several days after the drug is stopped.

Bupropion has not received extensive investigation for the presence of a therapeutic plasma concentration range. Golden et al (32) found a curvilinear relationship between antidepressant effect and plasma concentration of hydroxybupropion (HB), bupropion's principal active metabolite. HB concentrations greater than 1250 ng/ml were associated with poor clinical outcome. High metabolite concentrations causing toxic effects involving dopaminergic systems may be related to psychotic reactions seen in occasional patients (33).

Unlike two other antidepressants, imipramine and phenelzine, bupropion lacks efficacy for treatment of panic disorder with phobias. This may be related to its prodopaminergic effects.

Clomipramine   Clomipramine is similar in structure, effect, and side effects to imipramine. The drug's potent effects on serotonin may relate to its clinical efficacy in depression. Also, there is evidence that it produces a better response in patients with obsessive-compulsive disorder (OCD) than do other cyclic antidepressants or standard anxiolytics (34). It may therefore be expected to alleviate anxiety in depressed patients. Clomipramine may well become the drug of choice in OCD and should become available in the United States in 1990. In well controlled studies, it has demonstrated marked antipanic effects. Daily doses are similar to those of the other major tertiary amine tricyclic drugs (Table 2E.1).

The response to clomipramine in OCD may be slow, requiring 4 to 6 weeks. Sometime a relapse in symptoms has been noted at 4 weeks, followed by further improvement. The overall improvement rate can be expected to be better than 50%. Patients should not be expected to become free of symptoms; however, their symptoms become less bothersome. Ironically, more symptoms may be reported as improvement occurs. Unfortunately, pharmacotherapy must be continuous for improvement to be sustained.

Desipramine   As the major imipramine metabolite, desipramine has several clinical advantages over its precursor. It is less anticholinergic and sedating. In particular, it is favored as a pharmacological probe in animal and human studies because it possesses the most selective actions on norepinephrine of the available cyclic antidepressants. A plasma concentration range associated with therapeutic effects is between 115 and 250 ng/ml (11); however, this therapeutic range is not as well established as that of imipramine. Studies in people between 60 and 80 years of age have shown that, for optimal antidepressant effect, these patients seem to require plasma concentrations in the same range

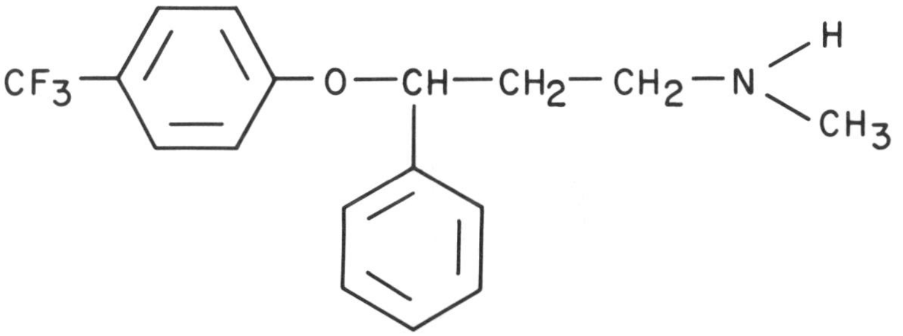

$$CF_3-\bigcirc-O-CH-CH_2-CH_2-N\overset{H}{\underset{CH_3}{\diagdown}}$$

Figure 2E.5. Chemical structure of fluoxetine.

as are used with younger adults. However, an increased risk of side effects exists for the elderly.

Doxepin Doxepin has been purported to have a lower degree of cardiac toxicity than other tricyclic antidepressants. However, much of the primary data responsible for this impression was obtained in animal studies, using doses that may not have afforded an ideal comparison with other drugs. This drug is cardiotoxic in overdosage and produces all of the side effects typical of the tricyclic class. Monitoring parameters are similar to those of imipramine.

Fluoxetine Fluoxetine (Fig. 2E.5) is a selective inhibitor of serotonin uptake with antidepressant effects comparable to those of the tricyclics (35). This neurochemical action suggests that fluoxetine may also be beneficial in the treatment of obsessive-compulsive disorder, but data from double-blind clinical trials to support this use have not yet appeared. Other unapproved uses of fluoxetine for which some data suggestive of efficacy exist include the treatment of obesity, decreasing food craving, and the treatment of alcohol abuse. Its use in the treatment of panic attacks seems to be accompanied by a high incidence of side effects, notably anxiety resembling overstimulation.

Fluoxetine and its active metabolite, norfluoxetine, have half-lives in the range of 7 and 14 days, respectively, a departure from the disposition kinetics of the previously marketed cyclic antidepressants. Thus, steady-state concentrations will not occur for several weeks of continuous dosing. The drug has shown only weak anticholinergic side effects. Common side effects include nausea, nervousness, and insomnia. Rare cases of excessive stimulation, when combined with monoamine oxidase inhibitors (MAOIs), have recently been reported. Such combinations are best avoided at present. Previous reports described a similar "serotonin syndrome" when L tryptophan was administered to patients along with a MAOI.

Recent reports have documented fluoxetine to provoke unexpected seizures in occasional patients. Whether this adverse reaction is dose-related is unknown. The long half-life of fluoxetine and its active metabolite suggest that dosage increases should be made no more frequently than every 1 to 2 weeks to allow full accumulation to steady state. Overall, the drug's advantages of low sedative potential and a lack of anticholinergic and cardiovasculer effects suggest that it could be the first choice of antidepressants for many patients.

Maprotiline This drug is the first available tetracyclic (Fig. 2E.6). Its initial impression of producing a faster onset of therapeutic benefit, as compared to that of the tricyclics, has not been born out with experience (36). In addition, there is a general impression that seizure activity, as a drug side effect, is more

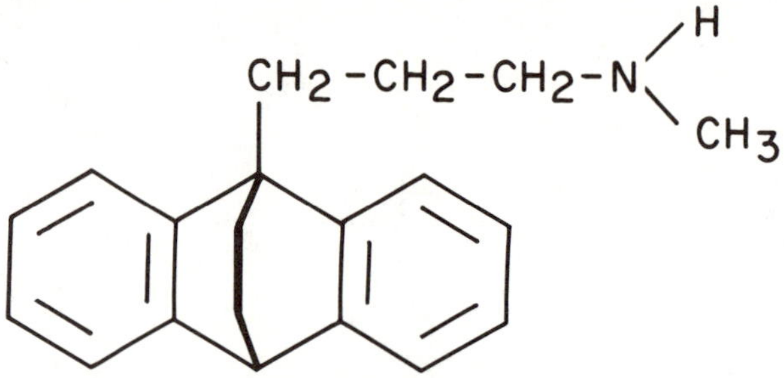

$$CH_2-CH_2-CH_2-N\begin{smallmatrix} H \\ \\ CH_3 \end{smallmatrix}$$

Figure 2E.6.   Chemical structure of maprotiline.

problematic with maprotiline than with the tricyclic antidepressants. Combining maprotiline in therapy with neuroleptics, a class of drugs with a reputation for stimulating epileptic activity, should be avoided.

Nortriptyline   This demethylated metabolite of amitriptyline has a lower degree of anticholinergic side effects and sedation, as compared with that of its precursor (Table 2E.2). The extent of this difference makes nortriptyline an acceptable antidepressant for some patients when amitriptyline is not. Nortriptyline has another advantage. It has the most established therapeutic plasma concentration range of all available cyclic antidepressants (11). Several studies have replicated a range of 50 to 150 ng/ml as optimal for treatment of endogenous depression. Steady-state plasma concentrations either below or above this range can be adjusted by means of dosage changes if clinical effects do not seem to be as robust as anticipated. However, as with all dose- or concentration-response relationships, some responders will be below and above the accepted target range which usually encompasses 20 to 80% of the responders. Overall, nortriptyline's monitoring parameters are similar to those of imipramine.

Nortriptyline may be the tricyclic antidepressant of choice for patients with significant problems with orthostatic hypotension (37). A pretreatment orthostatic systolic pressure drop of 10 mm Hg or greater may actually predict a favorable response to nortriptyline (38).

Protriptyline   As can be seen in Table 2E.3, protriptyline has the longest half-life of the available tricyclic antidepressants. In addition, its daily dose is less. This drug has gained the clinical reputation for being "activating" in occasional patients, rather than sedating, as is typical for other members of its drug class. It is similar to the remaining tricyclics in its indications and side effects.

Neurotransmitter Precursors

L-Tryptophan   Because a deficiency state or imbalance involving 5-hydroxytryptamine (5-HT) is suspected in the etiology of depression, L-tryptophan, as a precursor of 5-HT (see Chapter 1B), has been studied as an antidepressant. Generally, the results have been disappointing. There have been reports that it is better than placebo, is as effective as the tricyclics or electroconvulsive therapy, and may potentiate the tricyclics in combination therapy, but overall the results have largely been equivocal and have not confirmed the early excitement over L-tryptophan or 5-hydroxytryptophan as antidepressants (39, 40). The usual dose has been 6 to 9 gm/day. The most likely clinical situation involving L-tryptophan monitoring is combined therapy with lithium, a tricyclic, or a MAOI. Patients are likely to be more sedated than on monodrug therapy. Nausea and vomiting are problematic side effects.

REFERENCES

1. Malek-Ahmadi P, Williams JA: Rubidium in psychiatry: research implications. *Pharmacol Biochem Behav* 21(Suppl):49–50, 1984.
2. Prien RF, Caffey EM, Klett CJ: Prophylactic efficacy of lithium carbonate in manic-depressive illness. *Arch Gen Psychiatry* 28:337–341, 1973.
3. Fieve RR, Platman SR, Plutchik R: The use of lithium in affective disorders. I. Acute endogenous depression. *Am J Psychiatry* 125:487–491, 1968.
4. Hansen CJ, Retboll K, Schou M: Lithium in psychiatry. A review. *J Psychiatr Res* 6:67–95, 1968.
5. Post RM, Ballenger JC, Uhde TW, Bunney WE Jr: Efficacy of carbamazepine in manic-depressive illness: implications for underlying mechanisms. In: *Neurology of Mood Disorders*, Post RM, Ballenger JC (eds), Williams and Wilkins, Baltimore, 1984, pp 777–816.
6. Lambert P, Carraz G, Borselli S, et al: Dipropylacetamide in the treatment of manic-depressive psychosis. *Encephale* 1:25–31, 1975.
7. Jones BD, Chouinard G: Clonazepam in the treatment of recurrent symptoms of depression and anxiety in a patient with systemic lupus erythematosus. *Am J Psychiatry* 142:354–355, 1985.
8. Sulser F, Vetulani J, Mobley PL: Mode of action of antidepressants drugs. *Biochem Pharmacol* 27:257–261, 1978.
9. Hollister LE, Davis KL, Berger PA: Subtypes of depression based on excretion of MHPG and response to nortriptyline. *Arch Gen Psychiatry* 37:1107–1110, 1980.
10. Schildkraut JJ, Orsulak PJ, Schatzberg AF, et al: Toward a biochemical classification of depressive disorders. *Arch Gen Psychiatry* 35:1427–1433, 1978.
11. DeVane CL: Cyclic Antidepressants. In: *Applied Pharmacokinetics: Principles of Therapeutic Drug Monitoring*, Evans WE, Schentag JJ, Jusko WJ (eds), Applied Therapeutics, San Francisco, 1986, pp 852–907.
12. DeVane CL: Naming the cyclic antidepressants. *J Clin Psychopharmacol* 7:285–286, 1987.
13. Feighner JP: Clinical efficacy of the newer antidepressants. *J Clin Psychopharmacol* 1(Suppl):23S–26S, 1981.
14. Linnoila M, Karoum F, Potter WZ: Effect of low-dose clorgyline on 24-hour urinary monoamine excretion in patients with rapidly cycling bipolar affective disorder. *Arch Gen Psychiatry* 39:513–516, 1982.
15. Pickar D, Murphy DL, Cohen RM, et al: Selective and nonselective monoamine oxidase inhibitors: behavioral disturbances during their administration to depressed patients. *Arch Gen Psychiatry* 39:535–540, 1982.
16. Ballenger JC, Post RM: Carbamazepine in manic-depressive illness: a new treatment. *Am J Psychiatry* 137:782–790, 1980.
17. Post RM, Uhde TW, Ballenger JC, Squillace KM: Prophylactic efficacy of carbamazepine in manic-depressive illness. *Am J Psychiatry* 140:1602–1604, 1983.
18. Jann MW, Ereshefsky L, Saklad SR, et al: Effects of carbamazepine on plasma haloperidol levels. *J Clin Psychopharmacol* 5:106–109, 1985.
19. Chouinard G, Yong SN, Annable L: Antimanic effect of clonazepam. *Biol Psychiatry* 4:451–466, 1983.
20. Puzynski S, Klosiewicz L: Valproic acid amide in the treatment of affective and schizoaffective disorders. *J Affect Dis* 6:115–121, 1984.
21. McElroy SL, Keck PE Jr, Pope HG Jr: Sodium valproate: its use in primary psychiatric disorders. *J Clin Psychopharmacol* 7:16–24, 1987.
22. Sethy VH, Harris DW: Determination of biological activity of alprazolam, triazolam and their metabolites. *J Pharm Pharmacol* 34:115–116, 1982.
23. Pyke RE, Cohn JB, Feighner JP, Smith WT: Open-label studies of adinazolam in severe depression. *Psychopharmacol Bull* 19:96–98, 1983.
24. Feighner JP, Aden GC, Febre LF, et al: Comparison of alprazolam, imipramine and placebo in the treatment of depression. *JAMA* 249:3056–3064, 1983.
25. Goldberg SC, Ettigi P, Schulz PM, et al: Alprazolam versus imipramine in depressed outpatients with neurovegatative signs. *J Affect Dis* 11:139–145, 1986.

26. Preskorn SH, Simpson S: Tricyclic antidepressant-induced delirium and plasma drug concentration. *Am J Psychiatry* 139:822–823, 1982.
27. Lydiard RB, Genenberg AJ: Amoxapine—an antidepressant with some neuroleptic properties: a review of its chemistry, animal pharmacology and toxicology, human pharmacology, and clinical efficacy. *Pharmacotherapy* 1:163–175, 1981.
28. Tarsy D: Neuroleptic-induced extrapyramidal reactions: classification, description, and diagnosis. *Clin Neuropharmacol* 6(Suppl):9–26, 1983.
29. Zung WWK. Review of placebo-controlled trials with bupropion. *J Clin Psychiatry* 44[sec 2]:104–114, 1983.
30. Van Wych Fleet, Manberg PJ, Miller LL, et al: Overview of clinically significant adverse reactions to bupropion. *J Clin Psychiatry* 44[sec 2]:191–196, 1983.
31. Laizure SC, DeVane CL, Stewart JT, et al: Pharamacokinetics of bupropion and its major basic metabolites in normal subjects after a single dose. *Clin Pharmacol Ther* 38:586–589, 1985.
32. Golden RN, DeVane CL, Laizure SC, et al: Bupropion in depression: The role of metabolites in clinical outcome. *Arch Gen Psychiatry*, 45:145–149, 1988.
33. Golden RN, James SP, Sherer MA, et al: Psychoses associated with bupropion treatment. *Am J Psychiatry*, 142:1459–1462, 1985.
34. Thoren P, Asberg M, Cronholm B, et al: Clomipramine treatment of obsessive-compulsive disorder. *Arch Gen Psychiatry* 37:1281–1285, 1980.
35. Cohn JP, Wilcom C: A comparison of fluoxetine, imipramine, and placebo in patients with major depressive disorder. *J Clin Psychiatry* 46(3, sec 2):26–31, 1985.
36. Wells BG, Gelenberg AJ: Chemistry, pharmacology, pharmacokinetics, adverse effects, and efficacy of the antidepressant maprotiline. *Pharmacotherapy* 1:121–139, 1981.
37. Glassman AH, Bigger JT: Cardiovascular effects of therapeutic doses of tricyclic antidepressants. *Arch Gen Psychiatry* 38:815–820, 1981.
38. Stack JA, Reynolds CF III, Perel JM, et al: Pretreatment systolic orthostatic blood pressure and treatment response in elderly depressed inpatients. *J Clin Psychopharmacol* 8:116–120, 1988.
39. D'Elia G, Hansson L, Raotma H: L-trytophan and 5-hydroxytryptophan in the treatment of depression. A review. *Acta Psychiatr Scand* 27:239–252, 1978.
40. Byerley WF, and Risch SC: Depression and serotonin metabolism: rationale for neurotransmitter precursor treatment. *J Clin Psychopharmacol* 5:191–206, 1985.

3

Drug Therapy for Psychoses

Psychosis is a general term describing the severity of a behavioral disturbance that is characterized by an impaired sense of reality, impaired ability to communicate, and loss of emotional awareness and control and/or cognitive abilities. This leads to an inability to maintain personal relations and to compromised daily functioning. Behavior may be of psychotic proportions in several mental disorders, including mania, severe depression, organic brain syndrome, and schizophrenic disorders. The antipsychotic drugs are used to calm disturbed patients, whatever the cause, but their greatest use is for treatment of schizophrenia.

The schizophrenic disorders, described in Chapter 1F, are the major indications for the antipsychotic drugs. The incidence rate of schizophrenia is estimated at greater than 1 per 2000 individuals. The disorder makes its appearance usually before age 45 and most commonly in adolescence or early adult life. Men are usually affected earlier in life than women. Most patients experience an impairment of daily functioning and the illness runs a chronic course. Only about 15% of patients will fully recover. Another 50 to 70%, especially when untreated, will have intermittent psychotic episodes or continuous low level symptoms.

The antipsychotics are the most effective management for acute psychoses, particularly schizophrenia and acute mania. The decision whether to treat is relatively clear. The response to treatment of psychotic conditions is frequently good in the early stages of therapy. The target symptoms that can be expected to respond to antipsychotic medication include combativeness; hyperactivity; tension; hostility; hallucinations; negativism; poor sleep, dress, and appetite; acute delusions; and sociability. Some symptoms less likely to respond include insight, judgment, and memory. This incomplete reduction of symptoms is a major inadequacy of the currently available medications. About 15% of patients will experience chronic severe impairment and will require permanent nursing care in a hospital or will live in abandonment with life-threatening circumstances. About 25% of all hospital beds in the U.S. are occupied by schizophrenic patients.

As with the treatment of affective disorders, there will be long periods of drug administration to relatively symptom-free patients. This practice may appear as unnecessary medication, but the risk of relapse is great after an acute illness. Less clear is the need to continue indefinite treatment. The permanent neurological disability from tardive dyskinesia can have a tragic effect on the quality of a patient's life. Minimizing this risk requires vigilance in monitoring for early appearance of drug-related side effects.

In the following sections, databases are presented for two prototype antipsychotic drugs, chlorpromazine and haloperidol, a low and high potency antipsychotic, respectively. These are the most widely used antipsychotics and they reflect many characteristics of all of the medications in this class. With the possible exception of clozapine, all available antipsychotics produce neurological side effects. The antiparkinson drugs are often requisite adjuncts to the use of antipsychotic medication but have no intrinsic therapeutic benefit. A database for benztropine, a prototype antiparkinson drug, is presented because a knowledge of the clinical pharmacology of at least one of these drugs is necessary for antipsychotic drug monitoring.

A

Chlorpromazine Database

FORMULATIONS

Chlorpromazine hydrochloride tablets: 10 mg, 25 mg, 50 mg, 100 mg, 200 mg
Chlorpromazine hydrochloride capsules: 30 mg, 75 mg, 150 mg, 200 mg, 300 mg
Chlorpromazine hydrochloride syrup: 10 mg/5 ml; concentrate, 30 mg/5 ml
Chlorpromazine suppositories: 25 mg, 100 mg
Chlorpromazine hydrochloride injection: 25 mg/ml
Brand names: Thorazine (SKF); Prompar (Parke-Davis); various generic brands

BASIC PHARMACOLOGY

Chlorpromazine (Fig. 3A.1) has a myriad of pharmacological effects (1). As it represents the prototype phenothiazine and antipsychotic drug, its pharmacological properties are outlined in Table 3A.1. Despite an extensive knowledge about chlorpromazine's pharmacology, the actions underlying its therapeutic effects in psychotic states remain uncertain. The ability to block postsynaptic dopamine receptors in the brain has received the most research attention. Chlorpromazine also has α-adrenergic blocking effects and depresses the release of hypothalamic and pituitary hormones. The mechanism of action for the drug's antiemetic effects is believed to be an inhibition of the medullary chemoreceptor trigger zone. Chlorpromazine's sedative effects may result from an indirect reduction of stimuli in the brainstem. Its antiemetic, antimuscarinic, and sedative properties are shared by most drugs that are useful as antipsychotics; however, these properties for chlorpromazine are generally stronger by comparison.

Chlorpromazine frequently produces sedation when taken orally. A decrease in blood pressure is accompanied by resultant tachycardia. There is usually a slowing of psychomotor activity and an overall calming effect. In excited, agitated, or psychotic patients, this affective blunting can be very desirable. Experimental volunteers who are not actively psychotic frequently find the psychophysiological and behavioral effects of chlorpromazine to be very uncomfortable. Table 3A.2 lists the physiological effects from chlorpromazine therapy that may be easily monitored.

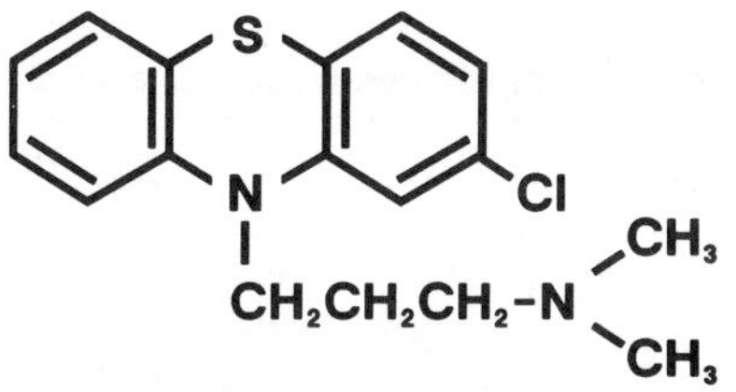

Figure 3A.1.   Chemical structure of chlorpromazine.

Table 3A.1.
Pharmacological Properties of Chlorpromazine

Property	Potential Effects
Inhibit the reuptake of norepinephrine and 5-HT[a] in cerebral cortex	Alter behavior mediated by these neurotransmitters in diffuse areas of the brain
Slowing of the EEG[a] with an increase in theta waves; lowering of convulsive threshold	Drug-induced seizures in susceptible patients
Blockade of dopamine receptors and increase of the turnover rate in corpus striatum	Therapeutic effects?
Inhibition of the release of growth hormone	Growth alterations in children?
Enhanced release of prolactin	Galactorrhea, gynecomastia, amenorrhea
Inhibition of apomorphine-induced emesis in hypothalamus	Therapeutic uses
Local anesthetic effects	
Peripheral α-adrenergic blocking actions	Orthostatic hypotension
Antihistaminic effects	Sedation
Cholinergic blocking effects	Decreased sweating and salivation
Decreased platelet adhesiveness	Beneficial effects in vascular disease?
Decreased sperm motility	Impaired fertility?

[a]5-HT, 5-hydroxytryptamine; EEG, electroencephalogram.

PHARMACOKINETIC PROPERTIES

Chlorpromazine undergoes rapid absorption when taken orally or when administered by intramuscular injection. In the gastrointestinal tract, it undergoes presystemic metabolism, including biotransformation in both the gut wall and the liver (2). Major metabolic pathways include sulfoxidation, demethylation, and hydroxylation. Chlorpromazine has several other potential metabolic pathways and has been hypothesized to have more than 100 metabolites; however, less than 20 have been specifically measured in human plasma.

Three of chlorpromazine's metabolites may substantially contribute to its pharmacological effects in humans. These are the 7-hydroxy, monodesmethyl, and N-oxide metabolites. The concentration of these metabolites in plasma is usually less than 20% of that of chlorpromazine. However, a lesser degree of

Table 3A.2.
Expected Physiological Effects from Chlorpromazine Therapy for Monitoring[a]

Parameter	Drug Effect
Cardiovascular status	
Heart rate	Frequent slight tachycardia
ECG	Prolongation of Q-T interval, S-T segment depression
Blood pressure	Orthostatic hypotension is common; fall in blood pressure
Respiratory function	Slight decrease in respiratory rate
Renal function	
Serum creatinine and clearance, BUN	Normal values should not change in most adults; occasional apparent diuretic actions
Hepatic function	
SGOT, SGPT, alkaline phosphatase	Transient benign increases may occur during first month. Substantial increases accompanied by increases in bilirubin should prompt further assessment of liver function. Occasional hypersensitivity reaction and obstructive jaundice occurs, usually in 2nd to 4th week of therapy with high levels of alkaline phosphatase and bilirubin.
Triglyceride, cholesterol	Serum concentrations have been reported to show no changes or transient rises after initiation of therapy. High density lipoprotein cholesterol may decrease.
Hematology status	
CBC	Leukocytosis, leukopenia, and eosinophilia may occur. Agranulocytosis and thrombocytopenia are rare.
Neuroendocrine status	
Glucose tolerance	Acute doses may cause hyperglycemia and inhibit insulin secretion; little effect is due to chronic low doses.
Serum prolactin	Elevated in men and women throughout therapy; no tolerance develops.
Other tests	
Serum magnesium, serum calcium	Slight decreases during therapy have been noted with other phenothiazines.

[a]Abbreviations: BUN, blood urea nitrogen; SGOT, serum glutamic-oxaloacetic transaminase; SGPT, serum glutamic-pyruvic transaminase; CBC, complete blood count.

protein binding of these metabolites could result in relatively high concentrations in the cerebrospinal fluid (CSF). Sedvall (3) found 7-hydroxychlorpromazine in CSF in a similar concentration as chlorpromazine. The 7-hydroxy metabolite was administered directly to humans, the most rigorous test of metabolite activity, and was found to have antipsychotic effectiveness equal to chlorpromazine given in the same dose (4). The ring sulfoxide metabolite is inactive.

Peak plasma concentration of the parent compound after an oral dose occurs between 30 and 60 minutes (5). The extent of presystemic metabolism varies

Table 3A.3.
Pharmacokinetic Parameters of Chlorpromazine

Parameter	Range
Bioavailability	Nearly complete absorption; total bioavailability reduced from extensive presystemic elimination
Time of peak concentration after single dose	Between 30 minutes and 4 hours
Plasma protein binding	90% or above
Volume of distribution	10 to 35 liters/kg (mean of 20)
Total plasma clearance	IM: mean of 0.6 liter/min
	Oral: approaches or exceeds hepatic blood flow (1.5 liters/min)
Renal clearance	Negligible
Elimination half-life	Range of 6 to 118 hours; mean of 30
Active metabolites	7-Hydroxychlorpromazine
Therapeutic range	30 to 350 ng/ml for antipsychotic effects; greater than 750 ng/ml associated with frequent adverse effects.

greatly among patients and, thus, peak concentration from an administered dose shows wide variations.

Chlorpromazine is widely distributed into most body tissues and easily crosses into the central nervous system. The drug is 92 to 97% plasma protein-bound. Less than 1% of an oral dose is normally excreted unchanged in the urine. Table 3A.3 lists the pharmacokinetic properties of chlorpromazine.

Several reports have suggested that patients chronically treated with chlorpromazine have lower plasma concentrations than have acutely treated patients (6). The mechanism of this effect is unknown as there is little evidence that chlorpromazine either decreases its absorption over time or induces its own metabolism. However, the within-subject variability of chlorpromazine plasma concentrations over time may be one of several factors contributing to the need for more frequent dosage adjustments in therapy.

INDICATIONS

Given its diverse pharmacologic effects (Table 3A.1), chlorpromazine has many potential uses. The Food and Drug Administration (FDA)-approved uses in psychiatry include the management of psychotic disorders and of the manic state of bipolar affective disorders and the short-term treatment of severe agitation, hyperactivity, or aggressiveness in disturbed children. Nonpsychiatric uses include relief of intractable hiccups, acute intermittent porphyria, hyperthermia, and restlessness and apprehension before surgery and control of nausea and vomiting. Table 3A.4 is a list of disorders for which chlorpromazine has been tried.

The treatment of psychotic behavior is the primary indication for chlorpromazine. Numerous controlled trials have indicated its utility in reducing the delusions, hallucinations, and bizarre behavior that accompanies schizophrenia. Psychotic behavior may be manifested in a number of treatable psychiatric disorders (Table 3A.4).

Table 3A.4.
Conditions for Which Chlorpromazine May Have Beneficial Effects

Psychotic disorders, including acute and chronic schizophrenia
Organically induced psychoses (PCP, amphetamine abuse)
Nausea and vomiting
Intermittent porphyria
Intractable hiccups
Tetanus
Surgical restlessness/apprehension
Antihypertensive after open-heart surgery
Schizoaffective disorder
Premenstrual psychotic or dysphoric symptoms

DOSAGE REGIMEN DESIGN

The dosage of chlorpromazine should be carefully individualized as the effective range is broad, between 30 and 1000 mg/day. The effect of this drug on a patient is difficult to predict based on clinical characteristics (7, 8). For debilitated or elderly patients or those with multiple organ disease, attention should be directed to baseline physiological status (Table 3A.2) before beginning therapy. Adverse effects (see below) may occur anytime during therapy with chlorpromazine.

Like the mood stabilizers and cyclic antidepressants, the optimal beneficial effects of antipsychotic therapy do not appear immediately but may take days or months to be fully apparent. However, at the initiation of therapy, patients may become calmer and less agitated. The symptoms of schizophrenia, discussed in Chapter 1, that show the most rapid improvement are the positive symptoms (see Table 1F.6). These include delusions and hallucinations. Those symptoms slowest to improve have been termed the negative symptoms of schizophrenia. They include a lack of insight into the illness, poor judgment, limited social organization, and ineffective planning for the future.

For most psychotic patients who have positive symptoms along with some degree of anxiety and agitation, the usual initial adult oral dosage is 100 to 200 mg/day divided into two to four doses. Some symptomatic improvement can be expected within days. The total daily dose may be increased according to patient tolerance, usually by 25 to 50 mg/day. Optimal doses are determined empirically by patient response. It should be remembered that a lag time occurs between increasing the daily dose and the full therapeutic expression of the increase.

Intramuscular (IM) administration will be needed in some patients. As this route of administration avoids the first pass elimination of drug in the liver, plasma concentrations of parent drug will be much higher after each dose. Hypotensive effects in the newly treated patient may occur with the first dose or early in therapy. The acutely manic or agitated patient may require repeated IM injections over the first couple of days of therapy to control behavior. Doses should be given no more frequently than 1 hour apart and with increased dosage intervals as soon as possible. Conversion from IM to oral dosing can take place at any time. Frequently, a higher oral dose will be needed to produce the same clinical effects as from intramuscular dosing. Total daily doses of chlorpromazine for most patients may not need to exceed 400 mg, although a few patients may be treated with doses as high as 2 g/day. There is no firmly established upper dosage limit. In general, the lowest possible dose should be used to avoid side effects; however, optimal therapeutic benefit should not be compromised with too low a daily dose. Doses in the range of 150 to 300 mg/day will be too low for some patients, whereas doses much greater than 600 mg/day will be unnecessary for most patients.

Many schizophrenic patients will be treated with chlorpromazine for long periods, some for decades. In general, the resolution of a psychotic episode should be accompanied by a reduction in the need for antipsychotic treatment. Patients in the residual phase of schizophrenia may be treated for 6 months with gradual dosage tapering and discontinuance when possible. A general guideline for maintenance therapy is to continue treatment for 3 months after the initial episode of psychosis, for up to a year after the second episode, and longer after the third episode. Attempts to decrease dosage should be made whenever feasible. Dosage reduction should proceed slowly, with the dose gradually decreased by 25 to 50 mg every few days.

Only limited data exist about dose-response relationships with antipsychotics (9). When doses of 300 mg or more of chlorpromazine or an equivalent dosage with other antipsychotics have been compared with dosage in the range of 1000 mg or more, the higher doses did not seem to be more effective than lower doses. This suggests a plateau in the dose-response curve for chlorpromazine above 300 mg/day for maintenance therapy for many patients (see Fig. 1C.3).

THERAPEUTIC DRUG MONITORING

Several characteristics of chlorpromazine and of the phenothiazines in general have made it difficult to relate plasma concentrations in a usual manner to clinical response. These include pharmacokinetic characteristics of high hepatic clearance, formation of active metabolites, a lag time in response after the initial dose, and the difficulty in obtaining precise, reproducible measures of clinical response (10).

Although daily dose is not a good predictor of chlorpromazine plasma concentration, the range at which a good antipsychotic response is seen is broad. An additional complication is that side effects also seem to have little relationship to steady-state plasma concentration. Several studies have addressed the issue of a therapeutic range for chlorpromazine, but only a weak correlation between plasma levels and therapeutic effect has been found (11).

The most rigorous reports of chlorpromazine's purported therapeutic range suggest that many patients will achieve a desirable response with a concentration between 30 and 350 ng/ml. This range is as broad as the daily doses used in the treatment of schizophrenia and, thus, does not serve as a reliable guide to follow in adjusting therapy in nonresponding patients. Plasma concentrations above 750 ng/ml seem to be associated with toxicity and, when present in nonresponding patients, suggest the need to reconsider diagnosis or institute an alternative therapy.

In one study, patients who showed high levels of chlorpromazine metabolites after a single dose tended to have poor clinical improvement after 3 months of chlorpromazine therapy. Responders showed the opposite pattern. This outcome could reflect patients with a lower hepatic extraction of chlorpromazine who received greater amounts of active drug systemically and hence did better clinically. The place of plasma concentration monitoring of chlorpromazine is not fully established. Overall, it may be useful in occasional nonresponding patients to document that adequate doses have been used before switching to alternative pharmacotherapy.

CONTRAINDICATIONS—WARNINGS—PRECAUTIONS

The precautions to be considered when using chlorpromazine are numerous as adverse effects can involve most organ systems. Chlorpromazine should not be administered to patients who are comatose or in the presence of large amounts of central nervous system (CNS) depressants (alcohol, barbiturates). Chlorpromazine may impair cognitive ability, and patients may find some usual daily activities, such as safely driving an automobile, to be compromised.

Chlorpromazine can impair body temperature regulation through its actions in the hypothalamus and by suppression of sweating. The extreme result of this effect has been fatal hyperpyrexia. The possibility of heat stroke can be reduced by avoiding combination therapy with other anticholinergic drugs and excessive outdoor activities associated with high temperatures and humidity. Patients who swim may occasionally complain of chills after body exposure in cold water.

DRUG INTERACTIONS

Chlorpromazine can participate in numerous drug interactions. The most investigated mechanisms are pharmacokinetic, including inhibition of absorption by other drugs and induction or inhibition of hepatic enzymes by concurrent drug theray. Given the broad range of effective doses and plasma concentrations, many interactions may go unnoticed. A list of prominent interactions is given in Table 3A.5. One should always be alert to changes in clinical state when drugs are added or deleted from a regimen of chlorpromazine.

ADVERSE REACTIONS—OCCURRENCE AND MANAGEMENT

The possible adverse reactions from chlorpromazine therapy involve all organ systems. The most worrisome reactions involve the blood, liver, eyes, and cardiovascular and neurological systems. The expected side effects of chlorpromazine therapy are listed in Table 3A.6.

Usually the first side effect to be noticed is drowsiness, particularly during the first few weeks of therapy. Orthostatic hypotension may also be troublesome. Patients who are heavy smokers may be less bothered by this effect (12). This would presumably be due to an enhanced first-pass effect from cigarette-induced hepatic enzyme induction. Anticholinergic effects are especially common early in therapy. Avoidance of those drugs producing a high incidence of certain side effects forms one basis for selection of initial antipsychotic therapy (see Chapter 3D).

As chlorpromazine blocks dopamine receptors in the nigrostriatal tract, extrapyramidal symptoms (EPS) may emerge during therapy. Acute dystonic reactions include bizarre contractions of muscles, frequently in the neck and head but also involving the limbs. This reaction typically occurs during the first few days of therapy. Akathisia is a subjective effect of inner restlessness that results in a desire to be in constant motion. Patients experiencing this reaction will be unable to sit motionless or may pace constantly. Pseudoparkinsonism has a typical onset of several weeks to months after the initiation of therapy.

Table 3A.5.
Drug Interactions with Chlorpromazine

Interacting Drug	Effect
Aluminum salts; antacids	Aluminum-based antacids, kaolin, attapulgite may decrease the absorption of chlorpromazine.
Barbiturates	Hepatic enzyme induction results in decreased chlorpromazine plasma concentrations; additive CNS depression can occur.
Methadone, alcohol	Additive CNS depression can occur.
Propranolol	Pharmacological effects of both drugs may be increased through alterations in the drugs' first-pass metabolism in the liver.
Epinephrine	Hypotension and tachycardia can result. The α-receptor blocking effects of chlorpromazine leave the β-adrenergic agonist activity of epinephrine unopposed.
Guanethidine	Inhibition of neuronal uptake by chlorpromazine may decrease antihypertensive effectiveness.
Cimetidine	Uncertain: the absorption of chlorpromazine may be delayed and the metabolites inhibited, producing variability in plasma concentrations.
Anticholinergics	Additive anticholinergic effects; an unsubstantiated decrease in chlorpromazine effectiveness
Cyclic antidepressants	A mutual metabolic inhibition can raise plasma concentrations of either drug or both; additive anticholinergic effects.

The symptoms are similar to those in true Parkinson's disorder. The patient may show a mask-like facial expression and drool. A tremor is usually present at rest involving the upper extremities. When walking, the patient may shuffle or experience periods of akinesia when voluntary movements are difficult. These reactions require that dosage be kept as low as possible. When EPS appear, anticholinergic agents or diphenhydramine may be used as treatment. Further discussion of neurological side effects from antipsychotic therapy is found in the haloperidol and benztropine databases (Chapters 3B and 3E).

Corneal opacities in patients treated with chlorpromazine have been regularly reported since the early 1960s. Visual acuity is usually not impaired, and the opacities improve slowly after the drug is discontinued (13). Patients with ocular disorders should be examined periodically by an ophthalmologist, especially if high dose chlorpromazine therapy is given. Any of the following symptoms encountered during monitoring may suggest ocular complications of phenothiazine therapy: complaints of blurred vision or photophobia, difficulty in reading, poor adjustment in changing from dimly to brightly lit rooms, or dryness of the eyes.

Skin changes from chronic chlorpromazine therapy occur in some patients. Melanosis, a tanning effect, occurs more frequently in women than men and seems to be related to the duration of treatment. Treatment consists of limiting the chlorpromazine dose or duration of therapy or switching to another antipsychotic such as haloperidol.

Table 3A.6.
Expected Side Effects of Chlorpromazine Therapy

Effect	Rare	Less Common	More Common
Dry mouth			X
Blurred vision		X	
Constipation			X
Nausea		X	
Vomiting		X	
Drowsiness			X
Dizziness			X
Ataxia		X	
Fainting		X	
Disorientation		X	
Headache		X	
Muscle spasms			X
Restlessness			X
Shuffling walk			X
Tic-like movements of head, face		X	
Difficult urination			X
Skin rash		X	
Blood pressure decrease			X
Tachycardia			X
Jaundice	X		
Breast swelling	X		
Gynecomastia (males)		X	

Chlorpromazine and other antipsychotics produce a variety of cardiovascular effects. In addition to orthostatic hypotension and tachycardia, electrocardiogram (ECG) changes are common (Table 3A.2). Sudden unexpected deaths in patients on high dose phenothiazine therapy have been hypothesized to be due to drug-induced arrhythmias. Several factors predispose to ECG changes (14). These include hypokalemia, recent food intake, heavy exercise, and alcohol abuse. Cardiac status should be monitored closely during combination therapy with the tricyclic antidepressants and antiparkinsonian drugs because these agents also produce ECG changes. Serum potassium should be monitored along with ECG in patients with cardiac disease, given the importance of this ion in regulating cardiac function.

An adverse effect of chlorpromazine and other antipsychotic drugs being increasingly recognized is the neuroleptic malignant syndrome (NMS) (15–17). This is an acute and potentially lethal reaction manifested by fever, muscular rigidity, CNS abnormalities, and autonomic dysfunction. It may occur at any time during antipsychotic drug treatment, even after the drug has been recently discontinued. Laboratory abnormalities frequently accompanying NMS include leukocytosis, elevated creatine phosphokinase in serum, and elevated values of liver function tests. A proposed mechanism involves altered neurochemical transmission. The treatment consists of discontinuing the suspected drug and providing supportive treatment and pharmacotherapy. Anticholinergic drugs may act to restore the central balance of dopamine and acetylcholine. Either benztropine, 1 to 2 mg IM, or diphenhydramine, 25 to 50 mg IM, has been recommended. Dopamine agonists have also been used to restore neurotransmitter balance. Amantadine, 200 mg/day (18), or bromocriptine, 15 mg/day (19), have been used. Finally, dantrolene sodium, 100 to 300 mg/day (20), has been successful in relieving skeletal muscle stiffness. Treatment may need to be continued for 1 to 3 weeks.

Bone marrow suppression is an occasional side effect of antipsychotic therapy. Agranulocytosis and granulocytopenia are serious concerns. Lithium may be useful to stimulate leukocyte production but may require weeks of therapy to show effectiveness.

MANAGEMENT OF OVERDOSE

The toxicity of chlorpromazine in overdosage resembles an extension of its pharmacological effects. Anticholinergic effects are exaggerated. Sedation proceeds to coma, and the lowering of seizure threshold may result in generalized seizures. ECG and cardiac arrhythmias, hypothermia, and respiratory and/or cardiovascular collapse can proceed to death. As with the cyclic antidepressants, there is no specific therapy to reverse the drug's toxic manifestations broadly. The treatment of chlorpromazine overdosage involves symptomatic and supportive care.

Anticholinergic toxicity is manifested peripherally by fever, ileus, flushing, urinary retention, increased sweat retention, blurred vision, and mydriasis. Myoclonus, choreoathetosis, seizures, and coma reflect central toxicity. The cardiac effects, similar to those of quinidine, include increased QRS-, QT-, and U-waves; bundle branch block; and various arrhythmias.

Treatment with physostigmine, a tertiary amine that crosses the blood-brain barrier, has reversed the central anticholinergic syndrome as well as electrocardiographic abnormalities of phenothiazine poisoning (21). The rationale behind using physostigmine in this type of toxicity is to inhibit cholinesterase, thereby increasing the natural levels of acetylcholine (see Chapter 1B). The safety of this treatment may be questionable, as has been documented with overdosage of the tricyclic antidepressants. The indications to use physostigmine should be limited to central and/or peripheral anticholinergic effects plus one or more of the following: (a) ventricular arrhythmias, (b) seizures, (c) agitation or hallucinations, (d) hypertension, or (e) coma. As with the cyclic antidepressants, the high lipid solubility of chlorpromazine, with its extensive tissue distribution and binding, suggests that dialysis procedures would not be efficient in enhancing the total body clearance of the drug (see Chapter 1D). Drug clearance by the patient's liver will eventually lower the amount of chlorpromazine in the body to help reverse the competitive antagonism of acetylcholine by the drug. Dialysis measures remain as heroic, last attempt measures to prolong life.

USE IN RENAL AND/OR HEPATIC DISEASE

No specific dosage adjustments are recommended for chlorpromazine in renal disease (22). As chlorpromazine is nearly fully metabolized, liver disease could be expected to alter its disposition (23). Chlorpromazine can cause hepatic sensitivity reactions, including cholestatic jaundice resembling infectious hepatitis. This is a sufficient reason to avoid its use in patients with hepatic disease. The jaundice from chlorpromazine usually occurs within a month after initiation of therapy. The incidence is low, less than 1% of treated patients. Laboratory findings would include eosinophilia, bilirubin in the urine, and elevated hepatic enzymes. The drug should be discontinued if these occur, especially when accompaning a yellow appearance of the skin or eyes. Serum bilirubin determinations during the first weeks of therapy would provide a screen for this adverse drug reaction, but ordinarily this degree of monitoring is unnecessary (see Chapter 1G).

USE IN CHILDREN AND ADOLESCENTS

The indications for antipsychotics are less specific in children than in adults partly because of less extensive experience with psychoactive drug use in children, a past reluctance to use antipsychotics in this patient population, and a lack of drug efficacy data from controlled trials. The best established uses are for infantile autism (24), Tourette's disorder (25), and behavioral symptoms associated with mental retardation (26). Schizophrenic disorders are rare in prepubertal children, and little research has been done in this area.

Among the disadvantages of using antipsychotics in children is the high degree of sedation sometimes produced. This may interfere with cognitive performance and intellectual development (27). For this reason, chlorpromazine may be avoided. Antipsychotics may lower the seizure threshold, which could be particularly disadvantageous for mentally retarded children with epilepsy. Antipsychotics produce extrapyramidal side effects in children as in adults (28). Acute dystonic reactions have been commonly treated with diphenhydramine orally or intramuscularly. Behavioral toxicity may be present as cognitive impairment, a decrease in psychomotor activity and verbal production, or an aggravation of preexisting symptoms. Careful monitoring of target symptoms is needed to assess behavioral toxicity.

The dosage requirements of children are generally less than those of adults. The usual chlorpromazine oral dose range is between 10 and 200 mg/day. Initial doses should be low, even with the expectation of ineffective doses, to allow careful assessment of the effects on target symptoms while avoiding any interference with cognitive functioning.

USE IN ELDERLY

Geriatric patients are more prone to the hypotensive effects of chlorpromazine, and initial doses should be lower than for young adult patients. Chlorpromazine is a potent anticholinergic drug, and this property makes it unsuitable for a first choice antipsychotic in many elderly. The elderly are especially prone to anticholinergic delirium and peripheral toxicities. The elderly also have a diminished capacity for drug metabolism. This may explain observations that older patients have higher chlorpromazine and metabolite concentrations compared to younger patients.

USE IN PREGNANCY

Given the lipophilic nature of chlorpromazine, it probably crosses the placenta in substantial amounts. Its safety during pregnancy has not been established. There is a suspicion of association between phenothiazine exposure and cardiovascular malformations. Chlorpromazine can be expected to appear in breast milk, and nursing should not be undertaken by women receiving chlorpromazine.

PATIENT INFORMATION

Chlorpromazine can impair cognitive ability and alertness. Patients should be warned of these effects and also the expected cardiovascular changes. All patients in southern climates should be told to wear a sunscreen, as a few people receiving chlorpromazine may become more sensitive to sunlight than normal and experience phototoxicity. Extrapyramidal reactions can be frightening to both patients and family, and these should be explained in detail. It is widely accepted that before informed consent is given, especially for psychotic patients receiving maintenance therapy, a discussion about the risk of tardive dyskinesia should take place.

REFERENCES

1. Gilman AG, Goodman LS, Roll TW, Murad (eds): *The Pharmacological Basis of Therapeutics*, Macmillan, New York, 1985, pp 393–408.
2. Curry SH, D'Mello A, Mould GP: Destruction of chlorpromazine during absorption in the rat in vivo and in vitro. *Br J Pharmacol* 42:403–411, 1971.
3. Sedvall G: Neurological side effects and plasma and CSF levels. In: *Clinical Pharmacology in Psychiatry: Neuroleptic and Antidepressant Research*, Usdin E, Dahl SG, Gram LF, Lingjaerde O (eds), MacMillan, London, 1980, pp 359–368.
4. Kleinman JE, Bigelow LB, Rogol A, Weinberger DR, Nazrallah HA, Wyatt RJ, Gillin JC: A clinical trial of 7-hydroxychlorpromazine in chronic schizophrenia. In: *Phenothiazines and Structurally Related Drugs: Basic and Clinical Studies*, Usdin E, Eckert H, Forrest IS (eds), Elsevier/North Holland, Amsterdam, 1980, pp 275–278.
5. Dahl SG, Strandjord R: Pharmacokinetics of chlorpromazine after single and chronic dosage. *Clin Pharmacol Ther* 21:437–448, 1977.
6. Rivera-Calimlim L, Gift T, Nasrallah HA, Wyatt RJ, Lasagna L: Low plasma levels of chlorpromazine in patients chronically treated with neuroleptics. *Comm Psychopharmacol* 2:113–121, 1978.
7. Sakurai Y, Rakahashi R, Nakahara T, Ikenaga H: Prediction of response to and actual outcome of chlorpromazine treatment in schizophrenic patients. *Arch Gen Psychiatry* 37:1057–1062, 1980.
8. Goldberg SC, Frosh WA, Drossman AK, et al: Prediction of response to phenothiazine in schizophrenia: a crossvalidation study. *Arch Gen Psychiatry* 26:367–373, 1972.
9. Davis JM, Schaffer CB, Killian GA, Kinard C, Chan C: Important issues in the drug treatment of schizophrenia. *Schizophr Bull* 6:70–87, 1980.
10. May PRA, Van Putten R: Plasma levels of chlorpromazine in schizophrenia: a critical review of the literature. *Arch Gen Psychiatry* 35:1081–1087, 1978.
11. Rivera-Calimlim L, Nasrallah H, Strauss J, Lasagna L: Clinical response and plasma levels: effect of dose, dosage schedules, and drug interactions on plasma chlorpromazine levels. *Am J Psychiatry* 133:646–652, 1976.
12. Swett C, Cole JO, Hartz SC, Shapiro SM, Slone D: Hypotension due to chlorpromazine: relation to cigarette smoking, blood pressure, and dosage. *Arch Gen Psychiatry* 34:661–663, 1977.
13. Prien RF, DeLong SL, Cole JO, Levine J: Ocular changes occurring with prolonged high dose chlorpromazine therapy. *Arch Gen Psychiatry* 23:464–468, 1970.
14. Nasrallah HA: Factors influencing phenothiazine-induced ECG changes. *Am J Psychiatry* 135:118–119, 1978.
15. Lew TY, Tollefson G: Chlorpromazine-induced neuroleptic malignant syndrome and its response to diazepam. *Biol Psychiatry* 18:1441–1446, 1983.
16. Caroff SN: The neuroleptic malignant syndrome. *J Clin Psychiatry* 41:79–82, 1980.
17. Birkhimer LJ, DeVane CL: The neuroleptic malignant syndrome: presentation and treatment. *Drug Intell Clin Pharm* 18:462–465, 1984.
18. McCarron MM, Boettger ML, Peck JJ: A case of neuroleptic malignant syndrome successfully treated with amantadine. *J Clin Psych* 43:381–382, 1982.
19. Mueller PS, Vester JW, Fermaglich J: Neuroleptic malignant syndrome—successful treatment with bromocriptine. *JAMA* 249:386–388, 1983.

20. May DC, Morris SW, Stewart RM, Fenton BJ, Gaffney FA: Neuroleptic malignant syndrome: response to dantrolene sodium. *Ann Intern Med* 98:183–184, 1983.
21. Weisdorf D, Kramer J, Goldbarg A, Klawans HL: Physostigmine for cardiac and neurologic manifestations of phenothiazine poisoning. *Clin Pharmacol Ther* 24:633–667, 1978.
22. Bennett W, Aronoff G, Morrison G: Drug prescribing in renal failure: Dosing guidelines for adults. *Am J Kidney Dis* 3:155–193, 1983.
23. Read A: Effects of chlorpromazine in patients with hepatic disease. *Br Med J* 3:497–499, 1969.
24. Anderson LT, Cambell M, Grega DM, et al: Haloperidol in the treatment of infantile autism: effects on learning and behavioral symptoms. *Am J Psychiatry* 141:1195–1202, 1984.
25. Shapiro AK, Shapiro ES: The treatment and etiology of tics and Tourette syndrome. *Compr Psychiatry* 22:193–205, 1981.
26. Breuning SE, Ferguson DG, Davidson NA, Poling AD: Effects of thioridazine on the intellectual performance of mentally retarded drug responders and nonresponders. *Arch Gen Psychiatry* 40:309–313, 1983.
27. Campbell M, Adnerson LT, Meier M, Cohen IL, Small AM, Samit C, Sachar EJ: A comparison of haloperidol and behavior therapy and their interaction in autistic children. *J Am Acad Child Psychiatry* 17:640–655, 1978.
28. Gualtieri CT, Harnhill J, McGimsey J, SchellD: Tardive dyskinesia and other movement disorders in children treated with psychotropic drugs. *J Am Acad Child Psychiatry* 19:491–510, 1980.

■ B

Haloperidol Database

FORMULATIONS

Haloperidol tablets: 0.5 mg, 1 mg, 2 mg, 5 mg, 10 mg, 20 mg
Haloperidol concentrate: 2 mg/ml
Haloperidol injection: 5 mg/ml
Haloperidol decanoate injection: 50 mg/ml
Brand names: Haldol (McNeil); various generic brands

BASIC PHARMACOLOGY

Haloperidol (Fig. 3B.1) is the most successful of the butyrophenone class of antipsychotic compounds. Its major pharmacological effect is to antagonize the effects of dopamine in the basal ganglia and limbic portions of the brain (1) (see Chapter 1B). It is a potent antipsychotic having less cross-reactivity with other receptor sites compared to chlorpromazine. It has more specific antidopaminergic action and less anticholinergic and anti-α-adrenergic activity. Haloperidol is a cleaner drug compared to the low potency antipsychotics with respect to its side effect profile, exhibiting little anticholinergic, hypotensive, or sedative activity. Because of its greater potency on dopaminergic neurons, particularly in the basal ganglia where neurons control extrapyramidal movements, the neurological side effects of haloperidol tend to be more frequent than those

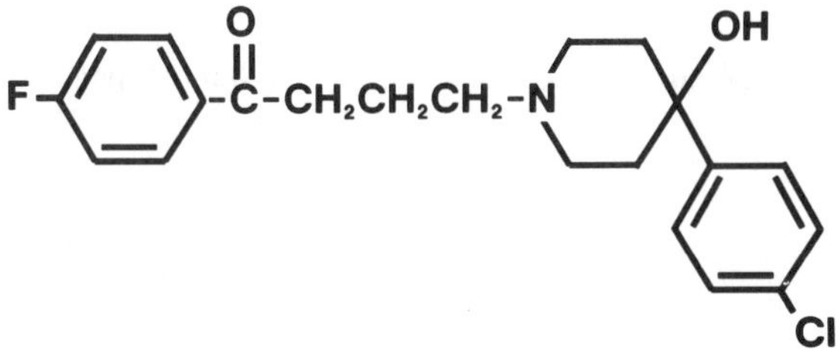

Figure 3B.1.   Chemical structure of haloperidol.

with some other antipsychotic drugs. The exact mechanism of the antipsychotic action of haloperidol is unknown.

As with chlorpromazine and other antipsychotics, haloperidol produces an uncomfortable feeling when taken by normal volunteers. Conversely, behaviorally disturbed patients experience a calming effect. Table 3B.1 lists objective physiological effects of haloperidol therapy that may be monitored.

PHARMACOKINETIC PROPERTIES

Haloperidol seems to be well absorbed when taken orally, with maximal blood levels reached in 2 to 6 hours after liquid and tablet dosage administration. The relative bioavailability compared to parenteral formulations is between 60 and 70% (2, 3). After intramuscular administration, maximal blood levels occur in approximately 30 minutes. Although not approved for intravenous use, haloperidol has been administered safely by this route. Nevertheless, sudden death has occurred after intravenous administration, which is not recommended.

Haloperidol has a volume of distribution of approximately 22 liters/kg. This value indicates that the drug is highly lipophilic and readily distributes outside the plasma into body tissues. In healthy volunteers, haloperidol had an elimination half-life of 13 to 35 hours. Table 3B.2 is a summary of the pharmacokinetic properties of haloperidol.

Haloperidol is highly metabolized by the liver. However, the elimination pathways for haloperidol are much less complex than those for any of the other antipsychotic drugs. A hydroxylated metabolite, reduced haloperidol, may have approximately 10% or more of the dopamine blocking activity of the parent drug (4). Indirect evidence for the importance of this metabolite includes its presence in the brain of postmortem schizophrenics previously treated with haloperidol, its measurable concentration in the CSF of patients, and plasma concentrations at times exceeding the concentration of haloperidol (5, 6). Reduced haloperidol's contribution to the therapeutic and toxic effects of haloperidol therapy are active research questions.

INDICATIONS

Haloperidol is a broadly useful drug in psychiatry. The FDA-approved indications are for use in management of the manifestations of psychotic disorders, for the control of tics and vocal utterances of Tourette's disorder in children and adults, and for the treatment of severe behavioral problems in children. Haloperidol is effective in the short-term treatment of hyperactive children who show excessive motor activity with accompanying conduct disorder. Unapproved uses of haloperidol include prevention and treatment of emesis due to

Table 3B.1.
Expected Physiological Effects from Haloperidol Therapy for Monitoring[a]

Parameter	Drug Effect and Time Course
Cardiovascular status	
Heart rate	Slight increase
ECG	Similar changes as with chlorpromazine; ST segment depression
Blood pressure	Slight decrease, occasional orthostatic response
Renal function	
Serum creatinine and clearance, BUN	Normal values should not change in most adults.
Hepatic function	
SGOT, SGPT, alkaline phosphatase	Transient benign increases may occur during 1st month. Substantial increases accompanied by increases in bilirubin should prompt further assessment of liver function.
Hematology status	
CBC	Mild and transient leukopenia or leukocytosis; minimal decrease in erythrocyte count. Thrombocytopenia occurs less often than with phenothiazines.
Neuroendocrine status	
Prolactin	Elevated concentrations throughout therapy

[a]For abbreviations, see Table 3A.2, footnote a.

Table 3B.2.
Pharmacokinetic Parameters of Haloperidol

Parameter	Range
Bioavailability	Nearly complete absorption; total bioavailability reduced from extensive presystemic elimination
Time of peak concentration after single dose	Oral: 0.5 to 4 hours IM: 0.3 hour IM decanoate: 4 to 11 days
Plasma protein binding	80 to 93% bound
Volume of distribution	13 to 25 liters/kg; mean of 22
Total plasma clearance	8 to 15 ml/kg/min; mean of 11
Renal clearance	Negligible
Elimination half-life	Mean of 18 ± 6 hours; 21 days from the decanoate formulation
Active metabolites	Reduced haloperidol
Steady-state metabolite to parent concentration ratio	Range of 0.2 to 2.0
Therapeutic range for antidepressant effect	5 to 15 ng/ml; toxicity range, 10 to 30 ng/ml

various causes, including cancer chemotherapy, irradiation, and gastrointestinal disorders and in postoperative patients (7). Haloperidol has shown promising effectiveness in the treatment of stuttering and in the treatment of autism in children (8).

DOSAGE REGIMEN DESIGN

Dosages are individualized according to the response of the patient and the desired therapeutic goals. Several dosage adjustments, upward or downward, may be necessary to obtain adequate symptom control. For oral administration in adults, moderate symptoms are treated with 1 to 6 mg a day in two or three divided doses. The severity of symptoms varies considerably among patients, and 20 to 80 mg/day may be necessary. Elderly patients should receive lower than usual initial doses, in the range of 0.5 to 2 mg/day. Some severely disturbed patients ultimately benefit from dosages of up to 100 mg/day. However, diagnosis of drug-induced delirium should be considered in all patients receiving drug doses of haloperidol or other psychoactive drugs at the upper extreme of clinically used doses.

IM doses of 2 to 10 mg may be used for the rapid control of a severely agitated patient. Peak concentrations occur earlier from IM than oral administration. Most patients can be managed on a 4- to 8-hour dosage schedule; however, particularly severe cases may require IM injections on an hourly basis to achieve control (9). This reflects a general clinical impression that, the more intense the initial dosing schedule, the faster the clinical response; however, much evidence exists to show that, above some minimal antipsychotic dose, acutely psychotic patients do not improve faster. A lag time exists for full antipsychotic response with haloperidol analogous to the clinical situation with cyclic antidepressants. Defining a minimal effective dose is a clinical challenge.

The injectable form should be switched to the oral form as soon as practical. For an initial approximation of the total daily dose, a dose at least equal to and up to twice the parenteral dose administered during the preceding 24 hours may be used. As bioavailability may vary considerably among patients, clinical signs and symptoms must be monitored carefully and used to guide further dosage adjustments.

Haloperidol decanoate is available for treatment of chronically psychotic patients who require prolonged therapy. The slow release of haloperidol from its decanoate ester formulation confers an effective elimination half-life of approximately 3 weeks. The recommended initial dose is 10 to 15 times the daily oral dose given at an interval of 4 weeks.

Upon achieving a satisfactory therapeutic response, dosage by either oral or intramuscular administration should be gradually reduced to the lowest effective maintenance level. After remission of a first acute psychotic episode, the dose of haloperidol should be gradually decreased and probably discontinued within 6 to 12 months. Suddenly stopping haloperidol is not recommended. This practice may result in tachycardia, restlessness, and abdominal distress. It has been postulated that a cholinergic rebound or a hyperdopaminergic state can occur, producing uncomfortable withdrawal symptoms.

THERAPEUTIC DRUG MONITORING

Dosage adjustments with haloperidol are generally guided by the control of psychotic symptoms and/or the appearance of side effects rather than by plasma level monitoring. The absence of multiple active metabolites makes haloperidol an appropriate drug to study the relationship between plasma concentration and clinical response and toxicity. The conclusion from several studies suggests that plasma concentrations between 5 and 15 ng/ml are positively correlated with therapeutic effects in adult psychotic patients (10–12). Recent evidence indicating significantly higher plasma concentrations of reduced haloperidol compared to haloperidol support the need to include this metabolite in future pharmacodynamic studies. This is a complex issue as haloperidol and reduced haloperidol may undergo interconversion, or reversible metabolism, in the body. Some evidence suggests that children with Tourette's syndrome may show improvement at a lower range of haloperidol concentrations, from 1 to 4 ng/ml. An increasing risk of neurological side effects can be expected as steady-state haloperidol concentrations exceed 15 ng/ml.

CONTRAINDICATIONS—WARNINGS—PRECAUTIONS

Haloperidol is contraindicated in severe CNS depression, in comatose states from any cause, and in individuals who have Parkinson's disease or who are hypersensitive to the drug. It may impair mental and/or physical abilities required for operating machinery or driving a car. The ambulatory patient should be warned accordingly. Alcohol should not be used with haloperidol because of the additive impairment of mental or physical functioning and the possibility of contributing to hypotension.

Although haloperidol has a relatively mild hypotensive effect, patients with severe cardiovascular disorders may experience transient hypotension and/or precipitation of anginal pain. If a vasopressor is required, norepinephrine or dopamine rather than epinephrine should be used as the latter leads to unopposed β-receptor stimulation and will possibly induce further hypotension.

Haloperidol may lower the seizure threshold, so anticonvulsant therapy should be monitored closely in patients with seizure disorders. When using antipsychotic drugs in patients with a seizure history, gradual dosage adjustment is recommended to avoid seizures.

DRUG INTERACTIONS

Concomitant haloperidol and lithium therapy resulted in symptoms of encephalopathy, confusion, extrapyramidal symptoms, and fever in several patients with mania (13). However, given the extensive use of this drug combination in the acute phase of mania, criticism has been made of the validity of these reports. Additional survey data do not support the hazard of this combination (14). A possible mechanism may be related to greater lithium distribution intracellularly in the presence of haloperidol or phenothiazines (15). This interaction may only become significant with high doses of one or both of the drugs. The risk of toxicity may be higher in acutely manic patients who have marked psychotic symptoms and intense anxiety (16). Table 3B.3 lists other interactions of haloperidol that may be clinically significant.

ADVERSE REACTIONS—OCCURRENCE AND MANAGEMENT

The principal adverse reactions of haloperidol involve the autonomic and extrapyramidal systems. Anticholinergic side effects with haloperidol are mild but may include dry mouth, blurred vision, urinary retention, and constipation

Table 3B.3.
Drug Interactions with Haloperidol

Interacting Drug	Effect
Lithium	Questions about enhanced neurotoxicity have not been fully resolved. Use of the combination should be closely monitored for neurological toxicity.
Phenytoin, barbiturates, carbamazepine, smoking	Hepatic enzyme induction results in decreased plasma concentrations.
Guanethidine	Due to inhibition of neuronal uptake of guanethidine by haloperidol, the antihypertensive effectiveness may be reduced.
Tricyclic antidepressants	A mutual metabolic inhibition may raise plasma concentrations of either drug. The pharmacodynamic consequences remain to be fully defined.

(Table 3B.4). The patient can be encouraged to increase fluid intake or suck on sugarless candy for dry mouth. A laxative or stool softener may be prescribed for constipation. Haloperidol rarely causes hypotension, with the exception of the overdose situation. Haloperidol is only mildly sedating; however, appropriate precautions should be given to the patient.

Extrapyramidal symptoms (EPS) occur frequently with haloperidol, often in the first 3 days of treatment. Symptoms include dystonias, akathisias, and parkinsonism (akinesia, tremor, rigidity). Dystonias readily respond to anticholinergic therapy with such agents as benztropine, trihexylphenidyl, or diphenhydramine. Even so, the potential consequences of EPS are grave. Antipsychotic drug-induced laryngeal and/or pharyngeal dystonia can precipitate cardiac arrhythmias, presumably through vagal reflexes. As young adults, especially men, seem to be at high risk for haloperidol-induced dystonias, it has been recommended to give prophylactic anticholinergic therapy during the first few days of treatment. The anticholinergic can be discontinued after 1 week, frequently without the appearance of EPS. The usual dosage to treat EPS is discussed in Chapters 3E and F.

Anticholinergics should be withdrawn after 1 to 2 weeks to determine their continued need. In patients refractory to or intolerant of anticholinergic drugs, amantadine may be tried. The usual dosage is 100 mg two times a day (see Chapter 3F).

Extrapyramidal effects are not consistently dose-related, and in some cases extrapyramidal effects from high dose therapy may be less severe than those occurring at moderate dose therapy. An apparent threshold is sometimes encountered in dosage, above which extrapyramidal symptoms seem less bothersome. An alternative explanation is that the drug's anticholinergic effects at increasing dosage could counteract the EPS (see Fig. 1C.5). Dystonias sometimes seem to be triggered by stress. Anxiety can increase the intensity of neuroleptic-induced EPS.

Tardive dyskinesia (TD) may occur with haloperidol therapy. TD generally appears with an insidious onset after at least 3 months of therapy. It may occur in approximately 15% of patients treated with antipsychotic drugs. Patients

Table 3B.4.
Expected Side Effects from Haloperidol Therapy

Effect	Rare	Less Common	More Common
Dry mouth		X	
Blurred vision	X		
Constipation		X	
Nausea		X	
Vomiting		X	
Drowsiness		X	
Dizziness		X	
Ataxia		X	
Fainting		X	
Disorientation		X	
Headache		X	
Muscle spasms			X
Restlessness			X
Shuffling walk			X
Tic-like movements of head, face			X
Difficult urination	X		
Skin rash	X		
Blood pressure decrease		X	
Tachycardia		X	
Jaundice	X		
Gynecomastia (males)		X	

above 50 years of age seem to have a greater risk of developing TD and have a poorer prognosis for remission. The incidence of TD seems to be higher in women.

Ideal treatment upon the appearance of TD is discontinuation of haloperidol or other offending antipsychotics (17). However, such a decision must be based on the severity of the patient's illness and the continued need for the medication. If the dyskinesia is mild, then low doses of a benzodiazepine (clonazepam or diazepam) or phenobarbital may be adequate treatment.

In patients with persistent, distressing, or disabling dyskinesia, it may be necessary to use dopamine-blocking agents for treatment. This carries the risk of aggravating the severity of TD and reducing the likelihood of remission. Low potency dopamine blockers such as thioridazine are often selected, although they have not been proven safe. Before resorting to a dopamine blocker, a trial of a presynaptic dopamine-depleting agent, such as reserpine, is recommended as it does not bind to postsynaptic dopamine receptor sites and has rarely been incriminated as causing tardive dyskinesia.

MANAGEMENT OF OVERDOSE

Haloperidol overdosage is treated by following general principles of overdose management, attempting to prevent further drug absorption, and providing symptomatic treatment. Unless the patient is comatose, is convulsing, or has lost the gag reflex, emesis can be initiated. If one of these contraindications is present, endotracheal intubation should precede gastric lavage. Activated charcoal is frequently administered in a dose of 60 to 100 gm for adults and 30 to 60 gm for children. A saline cathartic may also be used. The usual dose of magnesium sulfate is 30 gm for adults and 250 mg/kg for children.

Symptomatic treatment may be needed for seizures. They can be treated with intravenous (IV) diazepam. The adult dose is up to 10 mg slowly, repeated if necessary. For children the dose is 0.1 to 0.3 mg/kg slowly. Respiratory status should be monitored while diazepam is administered. If seizure activity is unresponsive, phenytoin in a dose of 15 mg/kg IV, given no faster than 0.5 mg/kg/min, is an alternative. Hypotension can occur in these circumstances. Hypotension is initially treated by administration of fluids and by placing the patient in the Trendelenburg position. Vasopressor drugs (dopamine or norepinephrine) may be necessary to prevent shock. Epinephrine should be avoided as this drug may worsen shock.

Phenytoin may be also administered in cases of cardiotoxicity to revert the depressed intraventricular conductivity of the myocardium associated with a prolonged Q-T interval. The recommended phenytoin loading dose for adults and children is 15 mg/kg up to 1 gm administered intravenously, not to exceed a rate of 0.5 mg/kg/min or 50 mg/min.

For dystonic reactions, diphenhydramine, 1 to 2 mg/kg up to 50 mg/dose IM or IV over 2 minutes, is effective. An alternative is to use benztropine mesylate, 1 to 2 mg parenterally, followed with maintenance oral therapy for 2 days.

USE IN RENAL AND/OR HEPATIC DISEASE

As haloperidol is extensively metabolized by the liver, no dosage adjustment is usually required for the presence of renal impairment. In addition, due to its high lipid solubility, no dosage adjustment is specifically indicated for patients undergoing hemodialysis.

USE IN CHILDREN AND ADOLESCENTS

Psychotic disorders in children are treated with 0.05 to 2.0 mg/kg/day. Doses for nonpsychotic behavioral disorders and Tourette's disorder are 0.05 to 0.075 mg/kg/day. There is little evidence to indicate that behavioral improvement is enhanced in dosages beyond 6 mg/day. No controlled studies have been performed for the safe use of IM administration to children.

Haloperidol has been reported to be highly effective in treating schizophrenic children ages 6 to 12 (18). In most controlled trials, reported side effects are low and the drug is well tolerated. In patients with infantile autism, children as young as 3 have shown clinical improvement (19). Haloperidol causes children to become calmer and also frequently improves their response to other nonpharmacological therapies (20). School instruction is facilitated for some patients. The drug is not recommended in children less than 3 years of age.

Little is known of the pharmacokinetics of haloperidol in children. It is suspected that the drug is more highly plasma protein-bound than in adults. Steady-state plasma concentrations show a large variability from usual doses, as occurs in adults. In Tourette's syndrome, the plasma concentration associated with clinical improvement appears frequently in the range of 1 to 4 ng/ml (21). Haloperidol may show favorable response in up to 90% of patients with this disorder.

USE IN ELDERLY

Haloperidol is one of the most popular antipsychotic drugs used in the elderly. The elderly can be very sensitive to the usual doses of haloperidol and should be monitored closely for adverse reactions. The elimination half-life of haloperidol can be expected to be prolonged from what would be typical in a younger adult.

USE IN PREGNANCY

Although there are isolated cases of teratogenicity associated with haloperidol, no cause and effect relationship has been established. It is suggested that haloperidol use be limited to psychotic patients requiring long-term therapy. Two cases of limb malformations have been reported in infants whose mothers received haloperidol plus other drugs between the 25th and 37th days of gestation (22). Although normal infants have been born after mothers took this drug during the first trimester, the existing evidence indicates that haloperidol should be avoided by pregnant women during the first trimester, the critical period for limb development. Complete avoidance is recommended.

Haloperidol seems to be only minimally excreted into breast milk. Although adverse effects in nursing infants are not frequently reported, the effect on infants of small concentrations of haloperidol in breast milk is unknown. Thus, careful consideration of the need for antipsychotic therapy should be given when patients are mothers nursing their infants.

PATIENT INFORMATION

Outpatients should be told that the drug may cause drowsiness and that they should exercise caution while driving a car or operating machinery. Dry mouth may occur with this medication, and sucking on sugarless candy or ice chips may help lessen this side effect. Dizziness may occur. The patient should be told to avoid alcoholic medications or drugs that may cause drowsiness (antihistamines, nonprescription sleep aids) as additive sedation may occur. The possibility of tardive dyskinesia appearing with long-term therapy should be discussed in terms of risks and benefits.

REFERENCES

1. Gilman AG, Goodman LS, Gilman A: *The Pharmacological Basis of Therapeutics*, ed 6, MacMillan, New York, 1980.
2. Forsman A, Ohman R: Pharmacokinetic studies on haloperidol in man. *Curr Ther Res* 20:319–336, 1976.
3. Holley FO, Magliozzo JR, Stanske DR, et al: Haloperidol kinetics after oral and intravenous doses. *Clin Pharmacol Ther* 33:477–484, 1983.
4. Forsman A, Larsson M: Metabolism of haloperidol. *Curr Ther Res* 24:567–568, 1978.
5. Korpi ER, Wyatt RJ: Reduced haloperidol: effects on striatal dopamine metabolism and conversion to haloperidol in the rat. *Psychopharmacology* 83:34–37, 1984.
6. Ereshefsky L, Davis CM, Harrington CA, et al: Haloperidol and reduced haloperidol plasma levels in selected schizophrenic patients. *J Clin Psychopharmacol* 4:138–142, 1984.
7. Plotkin DA, Plotkin D, Okun R: Haloperidol for treatment of nausea and vomiting due to cytotoxic drug administration. *Curr Ther Res* 15:599–602, 1973.
8. Cohen IL, Campbell M, Posner D, et al: A study of haloperidol in young autistic children. *Psychopharm Bull* 16:63–65, 1980.
9. Donlon PT, Hopkin J, Tupin JP: Overview: efficacy and safety of the rapid neuroleptization method with injectable haloperidol. *Am J Psychiatry* 136:273–278, 1979.
10. Magliozzi JR, Hollister LE, Arnold KV, et al: Relationship of haloperidol levels to clinical response in schizophrenic patients. *Am J Psychiatry* 138:365–367, 1981.
11. Morselli PL, Bianchetti G, Dugas M: Haloperidol plasma level monitoring in neuropsychiatric patients. *Ther Drug Monit* 4:51–58, 1982.
12. Itoh H, Fujii Y, Ichikawa K: Blood level studies of haloperidol. *Adv Hum Psychopharmacol* 3:29–88, 1984.

13. Cohen WJ, Cohen NH: Lithium carbonate, haloperidol and irreversible brain damage. *JAMA* 230:1283–1287, 1974.
14. Baastrup PC, Hollnagel P, Sorensen R, Schou M: Adverse reactions in treatment with lithium carbonate and haloperidol. *JAMA* 236:2645–2646, 1976.
15. Pandey GN, Goel I, Davis JM: Effect of neuroleptic drugs on lithium uptake by the human erythrocyte. *Clin Pharmacol Ther* 26:96–102, 1979.
16. West AP, Meltzer HY: Paradoxical lithium neurotoxicity: a report of five cases and a hypothesis about risk for neurotoxicity. *Am J Psychiatry* 136:963–966, 1979.
17. Tarsy D: Tardive dyskinesia. *Ann Rev Med* 35:605–623, 1975.
18. Engelhardt DM, Polizos P, Waizer J, Hoffman SP: A double-blind comparison of fluphenazine and haloperidol in outpatient schizophrenic children. *J Autism Child Schizophrenia* 3:128–137, 1973.
19. Anderson LT, Campbell M, Grega DM, et al: Haloperidol in the treatment of infantile autism: effects on learning and behavioral symptoms. *Am J Psychiatry* 141:1195–1202, 1984.
20. Campbell M, Anderson LT, Meier M, et al: A comparison of haloperidol and behavior therapy and their interaction in autistic children. *J Am Acad Child Psychiatry* 17:640–655, 1978.
21. Morselli PL, Bianchetti G, Durand G, et al: Haloperidol plasma level monitoring in pediatric patients. *Ther Drug Monit* 1:35–46, 1979.
22. Kopelman AE, McCullar FW, Heggeness L: Limb malformations following maternal use of haloperidol. *JAMA* 231:62–64, 1975.

C

Clozapine Database

FORMULATIONS

Clozapine tablets: 25 and 100 mg
Brand names: Clozaril; Leponex (Sandoz)

BASIC PHARMACOLOGY

Clozapine (Fig. 3C.1) is the most recently available antipsychotic medication. It is a tricyclic dibenzodiazepine derivative that is similar in structure to loxapine. However, it differs in pharmacological properties from the classical neuroleptic agents (Chapters 3A and 3B). It was registered in many European, Asian, and African countries for marketing in the 1970s but, because of an unacceptably high incidence of fatal agranulocytosis, it was withdrawn from the Finnish and subsequently other markets (1). Recently completed clinical trials in the United States have shown that it is superior to both chlorpromazine and haloperidol in selected patients refractory to these drugs (2–4). An overall risk versus benefit assessment concluded that clozapine is an important drug that can provide superior therapy for some groups of schizophrenic patients but requires close monitoring to avoid its potentially dangerous bone marrow suppression (5).

Clozapine's pharmacological properties that are relevant to therapeutics are outlined in Table 3C.1 (6). Of primary interest is its ability to inhibit dopamine-sensitive adenylate cyclase (7) (see Chapter 1B). This effect suggests an appar-

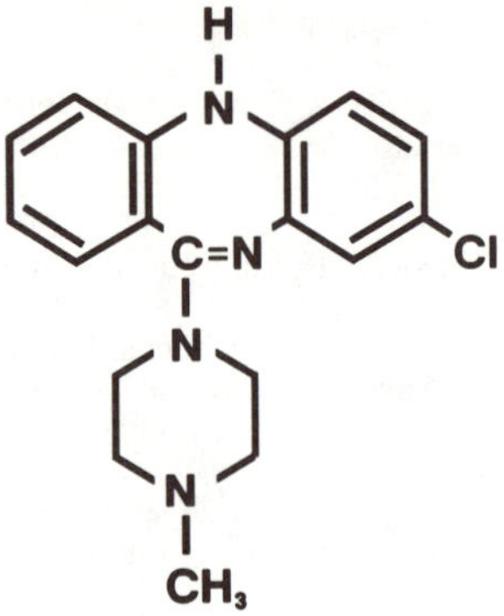

Figure 3C.1. Structure of clozapine.

Table 3C.1.
Pharmacological Properties of Clozapine

Property	Potential Effects
Inhibition of dopamine (D-1)-sensitive adenylate cyclase	Antipsychotic effects
Blockade of serotonergic (S2) receptors	Antipsychotic effects (?)
Slight, transient elevations of prolactin	Low propensity for galactorrhea
α_1-Adrenergic blocking actions	Orthostatic hypotension
Antihistaminic (H1) effects	Sedation
Anticholinergic (muscarinic) blockade	Reduced incidence of EPS, anticholinergic side effects
Increase in REM sleep; decrease in REM latency	Improvement in sleep; intensification in dreams

ently greater selectivity toward D-1 rather than D-2 receptors. This selectivity is in contrast to the classical antipsychotics like haloperidol. Interactions in the CNS with dopamine may also occur more prominently in the limbic rather than in the striatal system. Together, these effects confer antipsychotic activity with only a low propensity to cause extrapyramidal side effects. In addition, tardive dyskinesia has not yet been reported with clozapine despite many years of clinical use abroad. There is cautious optimism that clozapine may even benefit some patients with abnormal movement disorders (8, 9). The effectiveness of clozapine without the disabling extrapyramidal side effects of the classical neuroleptics gives new hope that other neuroleptics can be developed for psychotic conditions with an even greater margin of safety. The expected physiological effects for monitoring are outlined in Table 3C.2.

PHARMACOKINETIC PROPERTIES

Clozapine's pharmacokinetic properties have been studied with gas chromatographic and radioimmunoassay methods (10–12). The drug is nearly completely absorbed when taken orally, following a lag time of approximately 30 minutes. Its peak concentration in plasma occurs between 1 and 4 hours. Because of presystemic elimination, the effective bioavailability is reduced to approximately 70%. The drug is completely metabolized with negligible renal clearance. Metabolites include demethylated and other oxidized products. The

Table 3C.2.
Expected Physiological Effects from Clozapine Therapy for Monitoring[a]

Parameter	Drug Effect
Cardiovascular status	
Heart rate	Sinus tachycardia, up to 120 beats/minute
ECG	Occasional flattening of T-wave, shortening of P-Q interval
Blood pressure	Orthostatic hypotension can occur, sometimes severe.
Renal function	
Serum creatinine and clearance, BUN	Normal values should not change in most adults. Occasional apparent diuretic actions.
Hepatic function	
AST (SGOT), ALT (SGPT), alkaline phosphatase	Transient increases may occur during first few weeks of therapy unaccompanied by physical symptoms. Increases in bilirubin should prompt further assessment of liver function.
Hematology status	
CBC	Leukocytosis, leukopenia, and eosinophilia may occur. Reversible granulocytopenia can occur. CBC is recommended weekly for the duration of therapy. If WBC is below 3500, then it should be rechecked bi-weekly. WBC below 3000 or granulocyte count below 1500 is an indication for discontinuing therapy.
Neuroendocrine status	
Body temperature	Hyperthermia is common in 10% or more of patients, but is usually mild and self-limited.

[a]Abbreviations: BUN, blood urea nitrogen; AST, aspartate aminotransferase; SGOT, serum glutamic-oxaloacetic transaminase; ALT, alanine aminotransferase; SGPT, serum glutamic-pyruvic transaminase; WBC, white blood cell count.

distribution of clozapine in the body, as determined from animal studies, is extensive. The drug is present in most major organs. Plasma protein binding is high, greater than 90%. Tissue binding is presumably also extensive.

Clozapine seems to follow linear disposition kinetics with doses between 75 and 300 mg/day, the usual range of daily doses during therapy. The elimination half-life averages 16 hours. Clozapine can be classified as a high clearance drug with values in some patients approaching hepatic blood flow.

Expected steady-state clozapine concentrations in patients taking 150 mg a day are in the range of 100 to 300 ng/ml (10). There is a severalfold variability in the steady-state concentrations achieved among patients receiving the same daily dose. This variability is expected with drugs highly cleared by hepatic metabolism (see Chapter 1D). Clozapine's pharmacokinetic parameters in healthy adults are summarized in Table 3C.3.

INDICATIONS

Clozapine is indicated for use in the management of acute and chronic psychotic disorders in three types of patients. The first group is those patients who are refractory to treatment with conventional neuroleptics. In clinical trials these patients have shown inadequate clinical response to at least two different antipsychotic drugs and have been treated for an adequate duration of time.

Table 3C.3.
Pharmacokinetic Parameters of Clozapine

Parameter	Range
Bioavailability	Nearly complete absorption; total bioavailability reduced to approximately 70% from presystemic elimination
Time of peak concentration after single dose	Between 1 and 4 hours
Plasma protein binding	90% or above
Volume of distribution	1 to 10 liters/kg (mean of 4.6)
Total plasma clearance	Oral: 11 to 105 liters/hr (mean of 45 liters/hr)
Renal clearance	Negligible
Elimination half-life	Range of 6 to 33 hours; mean of 16
Active metabolites	Uncertain; demethylated metabolites could have some activity.
Therapeutic range	Not established; no correlation has been found in limited studies between plasma concentration and either efficacy or adverse effects. Usual doses produce plasma concentrations with a range of 100 to 600 ng/ml.

Many of these patients will have a history of multiple hospital admissions. Typically, florid psychotic symptoms are present despite doses of antipsychotics at the upper range of recommended doses. In controlled trials, clozapine proved superior to chlorpromazine for this type of patient (2–4). Many patients had also shown unsatisfactory response to haloperidol. During the largest multicenter trial (2), clozapine proved superior to chlorpromazine for improving positive symptoms of schizophrenia during the entire 6-week active treatment period and proved superior for treatment of negative symptoms from weeks 2 to 6.

A second group of patients are those who cannot receive adequate doses of typical antipsychotics to control their symptoms because of intolerable extrapyramidal side effects. As discussed later (see Chapter 3E) some patients do not respond to antiparkinson drugs and are difficult to treat. The low incidence of extrapyramidal symptoms with clozapine makes it an apppropriate choice in many of these patients.

Finally, a third group of schizophrenic patients with tardive dyskinesia must continue to be treated because of psychotic symptoms, yet are drug-intolerant. These patients either develop a worsening of dyskinetic movements with continued antipsychotic treatment or are dysfunctional because of their tardive dyskinesia. Some patients' symptoms of tardive dyskinesia were suppressed during treatment with clozapine. However, low doses, less than 250 mg/day, do not seem effective. Guidelines for treating these patients are needed from further clinical research.

Clozapine has been tried as a treatment for abnormal involuntary movement disorders (13, 14). The results have been equivocal. Two patients with Huntington's disease showed a marked decrease in movements, but other patients with Tourette's syndrome showed no improvement. Some patients with tardive dyskinesia had a suppression of their symptoms of tardive dyskinesia while taking clozapine (14). This is not unexpected, as typical antipsychotics will suppress tardive dyskinesia, although eventually breakthrough symptoms occur as the illness progresses (15). However, in one case of clozapine treatment of tardive dyskinesia, no breakthrough symptoms were described during therapy for 15 months (9). This is an encouraging therapeutic prospect for other patients. Clozapine is not specifically indicated as a treatment for tardive dyskinesia but may eventually find a role in its management.

DOSAGE REGIMEN DESIGN

Dosage must be individualized according to patient response. An intramuscular dosage form, marketed in Europe, is not yet available in the United States; only oral tablets are available at present. The recommended dose for initial treatment is 25 to 50 mg/day and should be no higher than 75 mg/day. The usual dosage schedule is to administer clozapine three times daily, at intervals of 4 to 6 hours. It can be given less frequently. As clozapine produces a high degree of sedation, the bulk of the daily dose can be given in the evening.

Increases should be made on the basis of response to target symptoms (see Chapter 1F). It may be necessary to titrate the dose very slowly during the 1st week as hypotension, tachycardia, and sedation may be profound during this period. The average dose to manage most patients is 150 to 450 mg/day. A maximum of 900 mg/day should not be exceeded. A minimal effective dose should be sought in all patients once symptoms are stabilized.

Schizophrenic patients who respond to clozapine usually begin to show improvement by the end of 2 weeks. It is recommended to evaluate efficacy at 6 weeks to determine the potential benefits of continuing therapy (5). Patients who have shown no improvement at this time may wish to reconsider going forward because they would be at increased risk of agranulocytosis with continued therapy (discussed below). A maximal rate of improvement should be achieved by the end of the 3rd month of treatment, but many patients seem to continue to improve for many months longer. In addition to improving positive symptoms of schizophrenia (delusions, hallucinations), many patients will show improvement in social functioning, tension, anxiety, and blunted affect.

There are no specific guidelines for maintenance therapy. Some patients have been on continued therapy for as long as 12 years.

THERAPEUTIC DRUG MONITORING

At present, plasma concentration monitoring would be of limited value in clozapine therapy. Very little data address the issue of whether a plasma concentration range of clozapine is associated with therapeutic effect. There could be some utility of monitoring as a check of compliance once dosage is stabilized and concentrations during assured therapy have been established.

Only minimal concentration data relate to clozapine toxicity. One case in which a generalized seizure occurred revealed a plasma concentration of over 2000 ng/ml at the time of the seizure (11). This was above the expected steady-state concentrations of patients taking the usual daily dose, which is generally less than 600 ng/ml (10). In some circumstances, for example, when daily doses are at the upper level of recommended doses, concentration monitoring might reveal unusually rapid metabolism; however, the analytical methods for clozapine monitoring are not yet widely available and additional studies are needed to demonstrate their value.

CONTRAINDICATIONS—WARNINGS—PRECAUTIONS

Agranulocytosis has occurred in patients receiving clozapine (see "Adverse Reactions," below). This drug reaction, reversible upon early detection, is apparently an unpredictable, possibly immunological phenomenon unrelated to dosage. The risk is as high as 1 to 2% of patients treated for a year. Fatalities have occurred but only in patients identified after the onset of symptoms of infection (1). This risk must be balanced against the very poor prognosis for some chronic refractory schizophrenics. State hospitals contain many psychotic patients whose quality of life is dismal and whose prospects for useful interactions with society are limited to custodial care.

The incidence of bone marrow suppression with clozapine is no greater than exists with many chemotherapeutic agents and some other widely prescribed drugs (16). For example, estimates of the frequency of neutropenia associated with sustained-release procainamide is 0.55 to 4.4% (17). However, clozapine's estimated incidence of bone marrow suppression is higher than that of other antipsychotic agents.

Routine frequent monitoring of blood cell counts is the best possible approach to detection of drug-induced hematological abnormalities. However, this is not a fail-safe practice as occasionally granulocytopenia can occur rapidly. Attention should be paid to any symptoms that suggest infection, and appropriate investigation and treatment should be initiated when indicated. Patient fatalities from agranulocytosis usually result from secondary infections.

Clozapine should not be used in combination with other drugs known to depress bone marrow function, including other antipsychotics, or in patients with a history of myeloproliferative disorders.

Unless toxicity requires rapid discontinuation of clozapine, it should be withdrawn gradually. Two patients developed pronounced psychotic symptoms within 48 hours when clozapine was abruptly discontinued (18). Ordinarily, patients do not relapse for 2 weeks or longer after discontinuing antipsychotic therapy, although many patients will relapse within 6 months. These two cases of rapid clinical deterioration suggest that a clozapine-induced supersensitivity psychosis may have occurred.

Like most antipsychotics, clozapine can lower the seizure threshold. Seizures have been reported with clozapine. At doses of 600 mg/day and higher, the risk seems to be greater than with other antipsychotics (11). Generally, there seems to be a relationship between the dose of antipsychotic given and the incidence of seizures. This suggests that patients with a history of seizure disorder should be given the lowest possible dose of all antipsychotics. Anticonvulsant medication should be continued in patients receiving clozapine, but attention should be paid to the possibility that adding clozapine to an existing anticonvulsant regimen may result in a drug interaction. Plasma concentrations of anticonvulsants should be monitored if toxicity is suggested or seizure frequency increases.

DRUG INTERACTIONS

Specific drug interactions with clozapine have not been reported. However, some interactions can be predicted based on the drug's similarity to loxapine and its known pharmacological properties. These are listed in Table 3C.4. As clozapine is very sedating, it is likely that, in combination with other CNS depressants (benzodiazepines, barbiturates, alcohol), additive sedative effects

Table 3C.4.
Predicted Drug Interactions with Clozapine

Interacting Drug	Effect
Alcohol, barbiturates, benzodiazepines	Enhanced sedative effects
Epinephrine	Hypotension and tachycardia can result. The α-receptor blocking effects of clozapine leave the β-adrenergic agonist activity of epinephrine unopposed.
Anticholinergics	Additive anticholinergic effects; delirium could occur.
Cyclic antidepressants	Have been successfully coadministered, but highly anticholinergic drugs could lead to delirium.
Enzyme inhibitors (cimetidine, disulfiram, isoniazid)	Could interfere with the metabolism and elimination of clozapine
Enzyme inducers (rifampin, cigarette smoking)	Could hasten the elimination of clozapine and lower its steady-state concentrations

would occur along with psychomotor deterioration. An analogous situation exists when clozapine is combined with other anticholinergic drugs. The possibility of delirium would be increased. There should be no need to add an antiparkinson drug to a regimen of clozapine, and highly anticholinergic antidepressants, like amitriptyline, should be avoided.

As clozapine is highly extracted and metabolized by the liver, it could compete for drug-metabolizing enzymes with other drugs. The most likely candidates are other antipsychotic compounds, the cyclic antidepressants, and β-adrenergic blockers. The well-known enzyme inhibitors, cimetidine and disulfiram, are likely to interfere with the metabolism of clozapine. Similiarly, enzyme inducers such as rifampin and polycyclic hydrocarbons contained in cigarette smoke are likely to enhance the elimination rate of clozapine (see Chapter 1D, Table 1D.5). Although none of these interactions have specifically been reported to result in patient problems, potential interactions should be kept in mind when monitoring therapy.

ADVERSE REACTIONS—OCCURRENCE AND MANAGEMENT

There are six major adverse reactions of which all clinicians should be aware. The best known is reversible bone marrow suppression (see "Contraindications—Warnings—Precautions," above). Other significant reactions are hyperthermia, hypersalivation, drowsiness, seizures, and cardiovascular effects, especially hypotension and tachycardia.

The most serious reaction is agranulocytosis, which can be fatal. The estimated incidence is between 1 and 2% for patients treated a year or longer, about 10 times as high as with the traditional neuroleptics. This reaction seems to have a definite time-dependent component. Most cases of bone marrow suppression occur between 6 weeks and 6 months after therapy begins. For this reason, patient progress should be assessed at 6 weeks (see "Dosage Regimen design," above) to justify continued treatment as the risk of agranulocytosis will increase

Respiratory depression: 1/2000 → 1/1000
. ≥ ↑ dose on beginning tx
· P̄ c̄ recent BZP usage
· resp arrest possible

after this time. A weekly complete blood count (CBC) (see Chapter 1G) is recommended for the duration of therapy. Prodromal signs of bone marrow suppression are those associated with infection. These include sore throat, low grade fever, or flu-like symptoms. If significant blood cell production is suppressed (see Table 3C.2), the drug should be discontinued. Preventive measures against infection may be necessary, including reverse isolation and antibiotic therapy. Recovery is likely to occur over a 2- to 3-week period, during which time a CBC should be monitored frequently. Antipsychotic therapy can be reinstituted, but it is recommended that an alternative to clozapine be given. A small number of patients restarted on clozapine after bone marrow suppression have had a recurrence of the same reaction.

As many as 20% of patients will experience temperature elevations of 1 to 2°F or more. The peak incidence of this effect is between the 10th and 20th days of therapy. Ordinarily, the fever will remit spontaneously; however, signs of infection should be sought and the CBC monitored. Temperature spikes are transient and should return to normal within 4 to 7 days. This is not an indication for discontinuing the drug unless bone marrow suppression is present. There seems to be no relationship between this hyperthermic reaction and other laboratory test deviations. It is not expected to recur with continued treatment.

Neuroleptic malignant syndrome (NMS) is associated with hyperthermia, and this possibility should be kept in mind when observing a temperature spike during clozapine therapy. The other cardinal symptoms of NMS are muscular rigidity, CNS abnormalities, and autonomic dysfunction. NMS is not reported with clozapine alone but has occurred rarely in combination with lithium. If NMS is suspected, clozapine should be discontinued and appropriate therapy instituted (19).

Hypersalivation occurs in a high percentage of patients treated with clozapine. One-third or more of patients will experience this effect. It is not a sufficient reason to discontinue therapy unless patient management is severely compromised.

Cardiac effects may occur with clozapine. Hypotension and sinus tachycardia are the most common. An increase in heart rate of up to 25 beats/minute can occur. These effects are most prominent during the early phase of therapy.

Sedation may also be prominent. If this reaction compromises daytime functioning, the majority of the daily dose could be given in the evening. Other, less common adverse reactions are outlined in Table 3C.5. Clozapine does not elevate prolactin levels and thus does not share with other antipsychotics the propensity for galactorrhea, amenorrhea, and impotence.

MANAGEMENT OF OVERDOSE

Symptoms of overdosage include those related to CNS depression, including drowsiness, lethargy, and decreased reflexes. Seizure is likely, and coma can occur in severe cases. Cardiac symptoms include tachycardia, hypotension, and arrhythmias. Hypersalivation is likely to be present along with mydriasis and blurred vision. No specific antidote is available for acute overdosage. General measures of treatment are recommended. This would include hospitalization and continuous cardiac and respiratory monitoring. Electrolyte balance should be maintained.

As with overdosage from other antipsychotics with α-adrenergic blocking properties, epinephrine is best avoided when hypotension is present. β-Adren-

Table 3C.5.
Expected Side Effects of Clozapine Therapy

Effect	Rare	Less Common	More Common
Hypersalivation			X
Drowsiness, sedation			X
Nasal stuffiness			X
Blood pressure decrease			X
Tachycardia			X
Hyperthermia			X
Bone marrow suppression		X	
Leukopenia		X	
Dry mouth		X	
Blurred vision		X	
Constipation		X	
Nausea		X	
Vomiting		X	
Headache		X	
Akathisia		X	
Tremor		X	
Rigidity		X	
Skin rash		X	
Weight gain		X	
Jaundice	X		
Difficult urination	X		

ergic stimulation from epinephrine would be left unopposed, which could lead to further decreases in blood pressure.

USE IN RENAL AND/OR HEPATIC DISEASE

Renal or hepatic disease is not a specific contraindication to the use of clozapine. As clozapine is a highly metabolized drug, liver disease would likely interfere with its disposition and prolong its elimination. Starting doses are recommended to be smaller than usual. The same precaution can be given for renal disease.

USE IN CHILDREN AND ADOLESCENTS

Safety and efficacy in children have not been established. Although some experience with clozapine therapy in children has been obtained in Europe, the drug is not approved for this age group in the United States and should be avoided. There is an attractiveness to a drug with a low degree of extrapyramidal side effects for use in children, but this is an area for further clinical research before recommendations can be made.

USE IN ELDERLY

The effect of hypotension and tachycardia on cardiac status in the elderly should be kept in mind. Patients who have limited cardiac reserve would be at higher risk for untoward events. Dosage in the elderly should be substantially reduced.

USE IN PREGNANCY

Animal studies have not revealed adverse effects on pregnancy. Clozapine is classified in pregnancy category B. There are no adequate studies in pregnant women to suggest its safety, and it should be avoided, if possible, in pregnancy. Animal studies suggest that clozapine may be excreted in breast milk. Therefore, nursing should not be performed by mothers taking this drug.

PATIENT INFORMATION

The common side effects of clozapine therapy should be explained to patients, and they should be willing participants in their therapy. These side effects include sedation, hypersalivation, body temperature changes, hypotension, tachycardia, and bone marrow suppression.

As drowsiness can be a profound side effect of clozapine, patients should be informed of the possibility that complete mental alertness may be impaired during the early days of therapy. Patients should be alerted to the signs of infection that would suggest a decrease in white blood cell production. These include a sore throat, flu-like symptoms, and a fever. The importance of weekly blood sampling to determine blood count should be explained.

REFERENCES

1. de la Chapelle A, Kari C, Nurminen M, Hernberg S: Clozapine-induced agranulocytosis: a genetic and epidemiologic study. *Hum Genet* 37:183–194, 1977.
2. Kane J, Honigfeld G, Singer J, Meltzer H, et al: Clozapine for the treatment-resistant schizophrenic. *Arch Gen Psychiatry* 45:789–796, 1988.
3. Claghorn J, Honigfeld G, Abuzzahab FS, et al: The risks and benefits of clozapine versus chlorpromazine. *J Clin Psychopharmacol* 7:377–384, 1987.
4. Shopsin B, Klein H, Aaronsom M, Collora M: Clozapine, chlorpromazine and placebo in newly hospitalized, acutely schizophrenic patients. *Arch Gen Psychiatry* 36:657–664, 1979.
5. Marder SR, Van Putten T: Who should receive clozapine? *Arch Gen Psychiatry* 45:865–867, 1988.
6. Sayers AC, Amsler HA: Clozapine. In: *Pharmacological and Biochemical Properties of Drug Substances*, Goldberg ME (ed), American Pharmaceutical Association, Washington, 1977, pp 1–31.
7. Karobath M, Leitich H: Antipsychotic drugs and dopamine-stimulated adenylate cyclase prepared from corpus striatum of rat brain. *Proc Natl Acad Sci USA* 71:2915–2918, 1974.
8. Small JG, Milstein V, Marhenke JD, Hall DD, Kellams JJ: Treatment outcome with clozapine in tardive dyskinesia, neuroleptic sensitivity, and treatment-resistant psychosis. *J Clin Psychiatry* 48:263–287, 1984.
9. Meltzer HY, Luchins DJ: Effect of clozapine in severe tardive dyskinesia: a case report. *J Clin Psychopharmacol* 4:286–287, 1984.
10. Choc MG, Lehr RG, Hsuan F, et al: Multiple-dose pharmacokinetics of clozapine in patients. *Pharm Res* 4:402–405, 1987.
11. Simpson GM, Cooper TA: Clozapine plasma levels and convulsions. *Am J Psychiatry* 135:99–100, 1978.
12. Kane JM, Cooper TB, Sachar EJ, Halpern FS, Bailine S: Clozapine: plasma levels and prolactin response. *Psychopharmacology* 73:184–187, 1981.
13. Caine ED, Polinsky RJ, Kartzinel R, Ebert MH: The trial use of clozapine for abnormal involuntary movement disorders. *Am J Psychiatry* 136:317–320, 1979.
14. Simpson GM, Lee JH, Shrivastara RK: Clozapine in tardive dyskinesia. *Psychopharmacology* 56:75–80, 1978.
15. Jeste DV, Wyatt RJ: Clozapine and tardive dyskinesia. *Arch Gen Psychiatry* 40:347–348, 1983.
16. Pisciotta V: Drug-induced agranulocytosis. *Drugs* 15:132–143, 1978.

17. Meyers DG, Gonzalez ER, Peters LL, et al: Severe neutropenia associated with procainamide: comparison of sustained release and conventional preparations. *Am Heart J* 109:1393–1394, 1985.
18. Ekblom B, Eriksson K, Lindstrom LH: Supersensitivity psychosis in schizophrenic patients after sudden clozapine withdrawal. *Psychopharmacology* 83:293–294, 1984.
19. Birkhimer LJ, DeVane CL: The neuroleptic malignant syndrome. *Drug Intell Clin Pharm* 18:462–465, 1984.

D

Intraclass Comparisons of Antipsychotics

The drugs useful as antipsychotics come from several chemical classes. Those most widely used in the United States are listed in Table 3D.1. A suggested approach to the use and monitoring of antipsychotic medications is to learn first the differences between a high and a low potency drug. The databases for chlorpromazine and haloperidol, presented in Chapters 3A and 3B, will aid in this understanding. The relatively minor pharmacological differences among the major antipsychotics in various classes will then become evident. Clozapine represents a unique antipsychotic, and clinicians who monitor therapy of chronic schizophrenics will want to become familiar with its clinical pharmacology (Chapter 3C).

The phenothiazine derivatives are the oldest and most popular antipsychotics (see Chapter 1A and Table 3D.1). These drugs block the actions of dopamine in at least two distinct anatomical regions of the brain: the nigrostriatal and mesolimbic tracts (1). Drug actions in these areas are thought to produce the extrapyramidal and antipsychotic effects, respectively, of the phenothiazines.

Distinction is made between three chemical subgroups of phenothiazines. The aliphatic side-chain group, represented by the prototype chlorpromazine, is relatively low in antipsychotic potency and high in sedative effects. The piperidine side-chain group is represented by thioridazine and its metabolite, mesoridazine. The prototype piperazine antipsychotic is trifluoperazine. Members of this subclass of phenothiazines are more potent in antipsychotic effect than either the aliphatic or piperidine drugs. They also cause less sedation. However, the piperazine group is more likely to produce extrapyramidal reactions at equivalent therapeutic doses.

Chemically similar to the phenothiazines are the thioxanthenes, the most prominent being chlorprothixene and thiothixene, although the latter drug is used more often in practice. Loxapine and molindone are from chemical classes unrelated to the phenothiazines, but their pharmacological profile is similar to the piperazine subgroup.

Haloperidol (Chapter 3B) is the most important member of the butyrophenone class. Droperidol is useful as an adjunct to anesthesia but not as an antipsychotic.

Table 3D.1.
Classification of Antipsychotics and Usual Daily Doses

Chemical Class & Generic Name	Approximate Equivalent Dose (mg)	Usual Daily Dose Range (mg/day)	
		Outpatient	Inpatient
PHENOTHIAZINES:			
Aliphatic			
Chlorpromazine	100	50–400	200–1600
Piperidine			
Thioridazine	100	50–400	200–800
Mesoridazine	50	25–200	100–400
Piperazine			
Perphenazine	10	8–24	12–64
Butaperazine	10	10–30	10–100
Trifluoperazine	5	4–10	10–60
Fluphenazine	2–3	1–5	2–60
THIOXANTHENE:			
Thiothixene	5	6–30	10–120
DIBENZOXAZEPINE:			
Loxapine	10	15–40	40–160
INDOLE:			
Molindone	10	15–60	40–225
BUTYROPHENONE:			
Haloperidol	2–3	2–6	4–100
DIBENZAZEPINE:			
Clozapine	50	50–400	50–800

Haloperidol is best considered having actions like a piperazine phenothiazine, i.e., high potency relative to other drugs and minimal sedative actions. Extrapyramidal side effects are high, particularly acute dystonic reactions.

Clozapine, previously available for a brief time in Europe, is the newest antipsychotic available in the United States and possesses a different side effect profile from the other drugs. This drug, discussed in Chapter 3C, should become an important alternative in the future to the phenothiazines for patients refractory to usual therapy.

All antipsychotics are therapeutically equivalent when used in equipotent doses (2). Differences in potency should not be confused with differences in efficacy (see Chapter 1C), which seem to be minimal. However, intersubject variation in response exists and some individuals show better response with one antipsychotic than another. Unfortunately, this response is not reliably predictable on the basis of presenting symptoms. Therefore, drug selection is usually based on the patient's previous response to an antipsychotic and the side effect profile of the available drugs with consideration of the individual patient's characteristics.

If a medication history is unavailable from the patient, an initial antipsychotic can be chosen on the basis of differences in potential side effects and toxicity of the various drugs (3, 4). The major side effects of some prominent antipsychotic drugs are compared in Table 3D.2. For example, if a high degree of psychomotor agitation is present, then sedation may be useful. The most sedative drugs are chlorpromazine and thioridazine. If sedation is undesirable, a piperazine

Table 3D.2.
Pharmacological Comparison and Relative Side Effect Profile of Some Prominent
Antipsychotics

Drug or Drug Class	Sedation Potential	Muscarinic Blockade	Orthostatic Hypotension	EPS Potential
Phenothiazines:				
Aliphatic	strong	moderate	strong	moderate
Piperidine	moderate	strong	moderate	moderate
Piperazine	weak	weak	weak	strong
Thiothixene	strong	moderate	strong	moderate
Loxapine	moderate	moderate	moderate	moderate
Haloperidol	weak	weak	weak	strong
Molindone	weak	weak	weak	moderate
Clozapine	strong	strong	moderate	weak

phenothiazine or haloperidol is an appropriate choice. Sedative effects generally decrease as one goes down the list in Table 3D.2. α-Adrenergic blocking
properties, which result in cardiovascular effects, including orthostatic hypotension and tachycardia, also generally decrease in this manner. When
extrapyramidal effects are to be particularly avoided in a patient, thioridazine
would be a reasonable choice. The high anticholinergic nature of this drug may
partly offset its disturbance of dopamine and acetylcholine balance in the
nigrostriatal pathway and minimize extrapyramidal side effects (EPS).
Clozapine, which possesses the lowest potential to produce EPS, is not indicated as initial antipsychotic therapy.

Generally, the anticholinergic actions of the antipsychotic drugs minimize
their propensity to cause extrapyramidal side effects. The neurological side
effects of these drugs seem to be inversely proportional to their affinity for
central muscarinic receptors (5). Thus, the drugs with the least anticholinergic
effects seem to cause a greater degree of neurological side effects.

When high dose, long-term therapy is necessary, the more potent pipera-
zines and haloperidol may avoid the skin pigmentation and retinopathy associated with chronic high dose therapy with aliphatic and piperidine
phenothiazines.

All antipsychotic drugs alter susceptibility to seizures, although the overall
rate of seizure induction is low. Occasionally, there is a need to choose a drug
to minimize this effect (6). A rough preference exists for using haloperidol
before trifluoperazine and either of these high potency drugs over thioridazine.
Experience suggests that chlorpromazine should be avoided in patients considered to be at risk for seizures. Seizures are more likely to be a problem in
psychiatric patients with a history of a seizure disorder, mental retardation, or
organic brain disease or in patients in whom drug dosage is rapidly escalated
(7).

The side effect profile of high and low potency antipsychotics (Table 3D.2) is
usually upheld in formal comparisons. Branchey et al (8) compared thioridazine
and fluphenazine in elderly psychiatric patients. The high potency phenothiazine caused more extrapyramidal effects but less sedation, anticholinergic
effects, and cardiovascular effects than thioridazine. Thioridazine caused more
weight gain in elderly patients than fluphenazine but less rigidity. In this and

Table 3D.3.
Pharmacokinetic Parameters of Antipsychotics

Drug	Oral Availability	Volume of Distribution (liters/kg)	Elimination Half-life (hours)	Active Metabolites
Chlorpromazine	0.25–0.75	10–35	mean of 30	7-hydroxy
Clozapine	0.9	2.2–10	6 to 33	
Haloperidol	0.25–0.75	13–25	mean of 18	reduced haloperidol
Thioridazine	0.4–0.9	10–20	9-10	mesoridazine

similar studies, psychiatric evaluations seemed equal regardless of the drug's potency.

The rate at which symptoms improve can vary widely among patients. Some psychotic patients improve within a few days of treatment; however, most of the therapeutic gain occurs during the first 6 weeks of therapy. The duration of treatment is based on the history of the disorder in the individual and his life situation. The chance of another occurrence of an acute illness is lessened if prophylactic treatment is continued for 6 months to a year after remission of a psychotic episode (9). In most situations, maintenance therapy will be continued with the same drug used to treat the acute episode. Combining two antipsychotics for chronic use cannot be justified. It may be occasionally necessary to start a new antipsychotic briefly while tapering the existing drug when switching agents because of unacceptable side effects or inefficacy.

The major pharmacokinetic properties for several antipsychotics are listed in Table 3D.3. Overall, the antipsychotics have properties similar to those of the tricyclic antidepressants. They demonstrate high hepatic and low renal clearance, extensive plasma protein and tissue binding, and high volumes of distribution. These drugs all seem to be well absorbed when taken orally but are extensively metabolized during their first pass through the liver and possibly in the gut wall. Their hepatic extraction ratios are high, in the range of 0.5 to 0.9. These drug characteristics result in the production of numerous metabolites, some of which are pharmacologically active (10). Because the antipsychotic drugs have large volumes of distribution, most of the body burden of drug resides outside the circulation. Thus, plasma concentrations of these drugs are low relative to tissue concentrations. Unfortunately, this characteristic predicts that hemodialysis, peritoneal dialysis, and other means of extracorporeal drug removal are poorly effective as aids in treating overdosage.

Only the most sensitive analytical methods can accurately measure plasma concentrations of antipsychotics, which often circulate in the nanogram per milliliter range (11). Thin-layer, gas, and liquid chromatography, radioimmunoassay, and more recently, the radioreceptor assay have been used to measure blood and plasma concentrations of antipsychotic drugs (see Chapter 1G). The use of plasma concentrations for monitoring antipsychotic therapy has been controversial (11–13). When used with discretion for longitudinal monitoring, compliance may be improved and toxic and therapeutic thresholds may be identified (13). However, broad application of proposed therapeutic ranges for antipsychotic drugs, with the possible exception of haloperidol (see Chapter 3B), cannot be recommended for routine clinical practice.

Evidence continues to accumulate that monitoring the plasma concentration of haloperidol, of all the antipsychotics, is most likely to be of benefit. Overall, therapeutic drug monitoring of other antipsychotics has thus far contributed little to improved patient care for psychotic patients. Some authorities suggest that plasma concentration monitoring, if applied on a more widespread basis, could be clinically useful; however, problems remain, including technically difficult analytical methods, uncertainty about the role of active metabolites, and questions regarding patient diagnosis and clinical evaluation of improvement.

INDIVIDUAL AGENTS

Acetophenazine

This piperazine phenothiazine is less potent than chlorpromazine as an anticholinergic drug and can be expected to cause slightly more extrapyramidal side effects. It is similar in action to the other drugs in its class, including perphenazine, fluphenazine, and trifluoperazine.

Chlorpromazine

The first phenothiazine available for clinical use, chlorpromazine (Chapter 3A), revolutionized psychiatric care in the 1950s and 1960s. Its degree of antipsychotic efficacy has not been surpassed by subsequently marketed drugs, with the possible exception of clozapine in refractory patients (Chapter 3C). Chlorpromazine remains an extremely useful drug, available in a variety of dosage forms.

Chlorprothixene

This drug is a thioxanthene derivative, similar to thiothixene but not as potent a dopamine antagonist. As it is available in an intramuscular form, it has been suggested for use as a rapid tranquilizing agent (14) but offers no advantages over haloperidol for this purpose. It can be considered to have similar pharmacological actions to chlorpromazine.

Clozapine

This antipsychotic interacts more specifically with dopamine D-1 receptors than other available antipsychotics. Some evidence suggests that D-1 receptors are primarily involved with antipsychotic efficacy, while D-2 receptor interactions are responsible for both efficacy and extrapyramidal side effects. This specificity of clozapine's actions on dopamine receptor subtypes could explain the drug's apparent lack of EPS in contrast to standard agents like haloperidol, which interact preferentially with D-2 receptors, while still retaining potent antipsychotic effects (15). Clozapine has provided symptom relief for some patients who are refractory to both chlorpromazine and haloperidol (16, 17). However, a major drawback is clozapine's hematopoietic toxicity (18). Because clozapine can depress white blood cell production and has caused agranulocytosis, monitoring of its therapy should include weekly blood cell counts. Clozapine is also highly anticholinergic. Physiological monitoring parameters are listed in Table 3C.1.

Fluphenazine

Fluphenazine is a high potency piperazine phenothiazine available in oral tablets, in solution, and for parenteral injection. The oral form in standard daily doses (up to 30 mg/day) generally causes a good to excellent clinical response. Megadoses (1000 mg/day or more) have been tried in treatment-resistant schizophrenics but have not been shown to be consistently better than low dosage (19). The drug causes a significant number of extrapyramidal side effects in usual daily doses.

The introduction of fluphenazine enanthate and decanoate in the 1960s made it possible to treat many psychiatric patients who were noncompliant with oral therapy by allowing injectable drug administration at weekly, biweekly, or monthly intervals (20). These depot antipsychotics are synthesized by esterfication of the active drug with a long-chain fatty acid and then dissolved in a vegetable oil for intramuscular injection. This formulation process results in slow release of the drug into the systemic circulation, which markedly prolongs the apparent elimination rate of the drug from the body (21). Therapy can be initiated with the depot drugs, but this practice is not advisable. Therapy with an oral dosage form should first be initiated to test both efficacy and tolerance of the patient to the drug.

Fluphenazine has been marketed as both decanoate and enanthate esters, both dissolved in sesame oil. The latter formulation was more painful on injection than the decanoate, and questions about its efficacy and side effects compared to the decanoat ester resulted in a lack of acceptance (22).

The dosage of fluphenazine decanoate should be individualized. The manufacturer's information for fluphenazine states that, once antipsychotic therapy is stabilized, a rough equivalent dosage is 12.5 mg of decanoate every 3 weeks for each 10 mg of fluphenazine hydrochloride administered daily. Clinical practice may deviate considerably from this recommendation (23), with usual doses ranging between 12.5 and 100 mg/dose with a frequency of every 2, 3, or 4 weeks. The persistence of fluphenazine in plasma for as long as 3 months after stopping therapy with the decanoate formulation suggests that the dosage interval may be increased as therapy continues (24).

There is no precise conversion factor between oral antipsychotics and long-acting drugs. Fluphenazine decanoate should be dosed as if it were a separate drug from its hydrochloride counterparts. A recent review (21) of the depot antipsychotics stated the following mean conversion ratio: 1.6 times the oral daily dose of fluphenazine in milligrams per day = fluphenazine decanoate intramuscular dose in milligrams per week. Another recommendation (25) is to calculate one-fourth of the biweekly oral fluphenazine dose, reduce this further by 25%, and administer an injection every 2 weeks. Whatever the calculated depot dose, most authorities agree that some supplementary therapy with oral medication may be necessary for the first few days after the beginning of parenteral dosing. No precise guidelines can be given for oral dosage during this transition period.

Haloperidol

Over 25 years of experience has shown haloperidol (Chapter 3B) to be an extremely versatile agent. Recently, haloperidol decanoate became available for clinical use. Its recommended dosage schedule is once monthly, which is less frequent than the fluphenazine products. The longer half-life of haloperidol in this slow release formulation results in effective concentrations persisting for as long as a month (26).

Loxapine

Loxapine is a dibenzoxazepine derivative with low anticholinergic activity compared to the phenothiazines and a similar or slightly smaller propensity to cause extrapyramidal side effects compared to haloperidol. The patterns of its clinical use seem to relegate it to a second line choice of antipsychotic. Loxapine, like all available antipsychotics, is thought to be clinically equivalent in effectiveness and is probably underutilized. The incidence of seizures may be particularly high when loxapine is taken in acute overdosage.

Mesoridazine

This drug is the side-chain sulfoxide metabolite of thioridazine. Its lesser degree of plasma protein binding compared to thioridazine may account for its approximate twofold greater potency (Table 3D.1). It has similar clinical characteristics as the piperidine phenothiazines and a side effect profile similar to or slightly better than that of thioridazine.

Molindone

Weight gain in chronically treated psychotic patients is an unfortunate drug-related side effect. Retrospective reviews have suggested that loxapine and molindone are the least likely to cause this effect among the available antipsychotics, but published reports are conflicting. Like loxapine, molindone may be underutilized.

Perphenazine

Perphenazine is a piperazine phenothiazine with all of the characteristics of this subgroup, including a moderate propensity to cause neurological side effects.

Thioridazine

Thioridazine is available in many different dosage forms, which gives it useful dosing flexibility, but it is not available for intramuscular administration. It has been widely used at both extremes of age. It has a low propensity to cause EPS or photosensitivity. A ceiling dose of 800 mg/day has been established to minimize the possibility of pigmentary retinopathy. Thioridazine is notable for a high frequency of cardiac effects (27). It has caused hypotension, premature ventricular contractions, and torsades des pointes arrhythmia accompaning QT prolongation, even at moderate doses in occasional individuals. Interestingly, thioridazine has been found to be a potent calcium channel blocker, which may partly explain its cardiac effects. Overall, thioridazine is a broadly useful drug with an extensive history of clinical experience.

Thiothixene

This drug is the prototype thioxanthene derivative. It represents an alternative to the phenothiazines for difficult patients but offers no particular therapeutic advantage over the other available drugs. Some treatment-resistant schizophrenics have responded to megadoses, but this type of pharmacotherapy should be reserved for unusual cases because some patients may experience an exacerbation of schizophrenic symptoms at high doses of antipsychotics.

Therapeutic plasma concentration ranges have been proposed for thiothixene, but the evidence for a curvilinear range is meager. Most patients will respond at plasma concentrations of less than 10 ng/ml.

In a clinical comparison (28), thiothixene seemed to be equal in efficacy to chlorpromazine when used in acute mania, both in rate and degree of improvement. This confirms the general impression of equal efficacy among most antipsychotics; however, expected side effects were typical of the high potency drugs.

Trifluoperazine

As a piperazine phenothiazine, trifluoperazine possesses all of the characteristics of a high potency antipsychotic, including low anticholinergic and high extrapyramidal effects.

REFERENCES

1. Hokfelt T, Ljungdahl A, Fuxe K, Johansson O: Dopamine nerve terminals in the rat limbic cortex: aspects of the dopamine hypothesis of schizophrenia. *Science* 184:177–179, 1974.
2. Seeman P, Lee T, Chau-Wong M, Wong K: Antipsychotic drug doses and neuroleptic/dopamine receptors. *Nature* 261:717–719, 1976.
3. Hollister LE: Choice of antipsychotic drugs. In: *Drugs in Psychiatry, Vol. 3: Antipsychotics*, Burrows GD, Norman TR, Davies B (eds), Elsevier Science Publishers, Amsterdam, 1985, pp 141–145.
4. Van Putten T, May PRA, Marder SR: Prediction of response to antipsychotic drugs. In: *Drugs in Psychiatry, Vol. 3: Antipsychotics*, Burrows GD, Normal TR, Davies B (eds), Elsevier Science Publishers, Amsterdam, 1985, pp 47–54, 1985.
5. Snyder S, Greenberg D, Yamamura HI: Antischizophrenic drugs and brain cholinergic receptors: affinity for muscarinic sites predicts extrapyramidal effects. *Arch Gen Psychiatry* 31:58–61, 1974.
6. Remick PA, Fine SH: Antipsychotic drugs and seizures. *J Clin Psychiatry* 40:78–80, 1979.
7. Jabbari B, Bryan GE: Incidence of seizures with tricyclic and tetracyclic antidepressants. *Arch Neurol* 42:480–481, 1985.
8. Branchey MH, Lee JH, Amin R, Simpson GM: High- and low-potency neuroleptics in elderly psychiatric patients. *JAMA* 239:1860–1862, 1978.
9. Davis JM: Overview: maintenance therapy in psychiatry. I: schizophrenia. *Am J Psychiatry* 132:1237–1245, 1975.
10. Dahl SG: Active metabolites of neuroleptic drugs: possible contribution to therapeutic and toxic effects. *Ther Drug Monit* 4:33–40, 1982.
11. Cooper TB: Plasma level monitoring of antipsychotic drugs. *Clin Pharmacokinet* 3:14–38, 1978.
12. Curry SH: Commentary: the strategy and value of neuroleptic drug monitoring. *J Clin Psychopharmacol* 5:263–271, 1985.
13. Morselli PL: Clinical significance of neuroleptic plasma level monitoring. In: *Clinical Pharmacology in Psychiatry, Neuroleptic and Antidepressant Research*, Usdin E, Dahl SG, Gram LF, Lingjaerde O (eds), MacMillan, London, 1981, pp 199–209.
14. Nilson JA: Immediate treatment expedites hospital release. *Hosp Community Psychiatry* 20:36–38, 1969.
15. Creese I, Leff SE: Dopamine receptors: a classification. *J Clin Psychopharmacol* 2:329–335, 1982.
16. Matz R, Rick W, OH D, Thompson H, Gershon S: Clozapine: a potential antipsychotic agent without extrapyramidal manifestations. *Curr Ther Res* 16:687–695, 1974.
17. Shopsin B, Klein H, Aaronsom M, Collora M: Clozapine, chlorpromazine, and placebo in newly hospitalized, acutely schizophrenic patients. *Arch Gen Psychiatry* 36:657–664, 1979.
18. de la Chapelle A, Dari C, Nurminen M, Hernberg S: Clozapine-induced agranulocytosis. *Hum Genet* 37:183–194, 1977.

19. Quitkin F, Rifkin A, Klein DF: Very high dosage vs. standard dosage fluphenazine in schizophrenia—a double-blind study of nonchronic treatment-refractory patients. *Arch Gen Psychiatry* 32:1276–1281, 1975.
20. Groves JE, Mandel MR: The long-acting phenothiazines. *Arch Gen Psychiatry* 32:893–900, 1975.
21. Jann MW, Ereshefsky L, Saklad SR: Clinical pharmacokinetics of the depot antipsychotics. *Clin Pharmacokinet* 10:315–333, 1985.
22. Van Praag HM, Dols LCW: Fluphenazine enanthate and decanoate: a comparison of their duration of action and motor side effects. *Am J Psychiatry* 130:801–804, 1973.
23. Johnson DAW: Observations on the dose regime of fluphenazine decanote in maintenance therapy of schizophrenia. *Br J Psychiatry* 126:457–461, 1975.
24. Gitlin MJ, Midha KK, Fogelson D, Nuechterlein K: Persistence of fluphenazine in plasma after decanoate withdrawal. *J Clin Psychopharmacol* 8:53–56, 1988.
25. Hollister LE: *Clinical Pharmacology of Psychotherapeutic Drugs*, Churchill Livingstone, New York, 1978, p 165.
26. Deberdt R, Elens P, Berghams W, et al: Intramuscular haloperidol decanoate for neuroleptic maintenance therapy, efficacy, dosage schedule and plasma levels. *Acta Psychiatr Scand* 62:356–363, 1980.
27. Risch SC, Groom GP, Janowsky DS: The effects of psychotropic drugs on the cardiovascular system. *J Clin Psychiatry* 43:16–32, 1982.
28. Janicak PG, Brwesnahan DB, Sharma R, et al: A comparison of thiothixene with chlorpromazine in the treatment of acute mania. *J Clin Psychopharmacol* 8:33–37, 1988.

▬ E ▬

Benztropine Database

FORMULATIONS

Benztropine mesylate tablets: 0.5 mg, 1.0 mg, 2.0 mg
Benztropine mesylate injection: 1 mg/ml in 2-ml ampules
Brand name: Cogentin (Merck)

BASIC AND PRECLINICAL PHARMACOLOGY

Benztropine (Fig. 3E.1) is a synthetic tertiary amine that is closely related chemically to atropine. The drug resembles both atropine and diphenhydramine in structure and can produce anticholinergic, antihistaminic, and local anesthetic effects (1). At high doses, it blocks dopamine uptake in animal preparations (2). Only the anticholinergic properties have been established as therapeutically significant in the management of Parkinson's disease. This drug is referred to as antimuscarinic because at normal doses it blocks cholinergic stimuli at muscarinic receptors. It has no effect on cholinergic stimuli at the nicotinic receptors at normal doses. Being an antimuscarinic, benztropine competitively binds to postsynaptic receptors and inhibits the stimulus produced by acetylcholine or other cholinergic stimuli (see Chapter 1B).

Healthy adults experience noticeable anticholinergic effects from benztropine similar to the effects felt from single doses of nonsedating tricyclic antidepres-

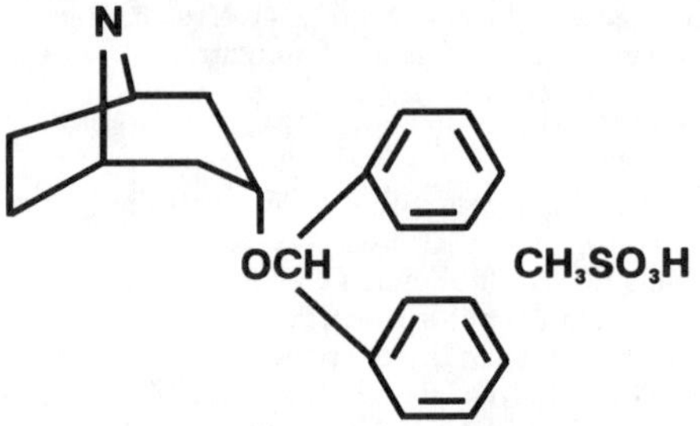

Figure 3E.1. Chemical structure of benztropine mesylate.

sants. The expected effects on standard physiological parameters are given in Table 3E.1.

PHARMACOKINETIC PROPERTIES

The pharmacokinetics of benztropine have not been well elucidated, and only general information is available (3). Being a tertiary amine, benztropine is readily absorbed from the gastrointestinal tract when taken orally; however, the presence of food may decrease the absorption efficiency. Atropine reaches a peak concentration in 15 to 50 minutes after intramuscular administration. Benztropine, being similar in structure, may have similar absorption characteristics.

The distribution of most antimuscarinics has not been well studied. Benztropine is rapidly distributed in body tissues, including the central nervous system. It is not known whether it crosses the placenta or whether it is present in breast milk. Benztropine is excreted in the urine approximately 30 to 50% as unchanged drug. A comparison of the daily oral dose of benztropine with serum concentrations, measured as atropine equivalents using a radioreceptor assay (see Chapter 1G), revealed an 8- to 10-fold variability in effective steady-state concentrations (4).

INDICATIONS

Benztropine is used as an adjunct in the therapy of all forms of Parkinson's disease. It is also used in the control of extrapyramidal side effects caused by antipsychotic drugs (5). It is not used for the treatment of tardive dyskinesia.

DOSAGE REGIMEN DESIGN

The dosage must be individualized. Therapy is begun with a low dose that is gradually increased if needed. For drug-induced extrapyramidal disorders, 1 to 4 mg once or twice daily is administered. Cumulative effects occur over the first several doses, and therapy may be increased in increments of 0.5 mg gradually at 5- or 6-day intervals. The maximal daily dose is 6 mg.

For acute dystonic reactions, 1 to 2 mg intramuscularly (IM) or intravenously (IV) usually relieves the condition quickly. The onset of effects from IM administration is rapid so the IV route is seldom needed. After initial therapy, 1 to 2 mg orally, 2 times daily, usually prevents recurrence. Many extrapyramidal disorders occurring soon after the initiation of antipsychotic therapy may be transient. Therefore, after 1 or 2 weeks of benztropine therapy, the drug should be gradually withdrawn to determine the need for continued use.

Table 3E.1.
Expected Physiological Effects from Benztropine Therapy for Monitoring[a]

Parameter	Drug Effect
Cardiovascular status	
Heart rate	Effects similar to those of atropine. Low dose: transient decrease (4 to 8 beats/minute) due to central vagal stimulation; high dose: increasing tachycardia by blocking vagal effects on the S-A nodal pacemaker. Heart rate increases by as much as 35 to 40 beats/minute after IM administration.
ECG	Atrial arrhythmias and atrioventricular dissociation possible with high doses
Blood pressure	Normally expect little change.
Renal function	
Serum creatinine and clearance, BUN	Normal values should not change in most adults.
Hepatic function	
SGOT, SGPT, alkaline phosphatase	Normal values should not change in most adults.
Hematology status	
CBC	Normal values should not change in most adults.
Neuroendocrine status	
DST, plasma cortisol	Not reported

[a]For abbreviations, see Table 3C.2, footnote a. DST, dexamethasone suppression test.

Many patients may be successfully withdrawn from benztropine or other antiparkinson drugs without a return of their antipsychotic-related side effects (6, 7). This forms an argument for using these medications for as short a time as possible. However, clinical benefits may accrue from reducing subtle side effects (8). The current trend is toward prophylactic and maintenance therapy with antiparkinson drugs for many patients. This is a controversial area in clinical psychopharmacology, and each patient's therapy should be carefully evaluated at periodic intervals.

THERAPEUTIC DRUG MONITORING

At present, benztropine therapy is monitored by treatment response. However, receptor binding assay studies for anticholinergic drugs have identified the inadequacy of standard dosage regimens in some individuals (4). The assay methods exist to determine the plasma concentration of most antiparkinsonian medications, but few studies have determined the value, if any, of plasma concentration monitoring (3). As the therapeutic endpoints in treating extrapyramidal side effects are readily apparent, plasma concentration monitoring would seem to be of limited utility.

CONTRAINDICATIONS—WARNINGS—PRECAUTIONS

Benztropine is contraindicated in children under 3 years of age. It should only be used cautiously in older children. Hypersensitivity to benztropine is a rare contraindication.

Benztropine may decrease sweating because of its similarity to atropine. Therefore, it should be administered cautiously during hot weather, especially when given with other anticholinergic drugs to the chronically ill, those with central nervous system disease, and those who do manual labor in a hot environment. Hyperthermia is a possible consequence of anhidrosis, and fatalities have occurred.

Benztropine should not be used in people with glaucoma, particularly angle-closure glaucoma; pyloric or duodenal obstruction; stenosing peptic ulcers; prostatic hypertrophy or bladder neck obstructions; or mysasthenia gravis. Patients taking benztropine who report gastrointestinal complaints should be promptly questioned about the cause and further investigation started, if necessary. Paralytic ileus, sometimes fatal, has been reported in patients taking anticholinergic-type antiparkinson drugs in combination with phenothiazines and/or tricyclic antidepressants.

The subjective effects of antiparkinsonian medications have been perceived as pleasurable by some individuals. This has led to benztropine and similar drugs becoming substances of abuse (9, 10). Trihexylphenidate (see Chapter 3F) seems to be the preferred drug. Single doses of only 2 to 4 times the usual daily dose may produce the disorientation and visual hallucinations typical of anticholinergic delirium. However, a steep dose-response curve (see Chapter 1C) between mild euphoria and toxicity has prevented widespread popularity of this form of substance abuse. Clinicians should take a careful drug history to uncover antiparkinsonian drug abuse. It may be difficult to distinguish between psychopathology and the behavioral effects from mild intoxication.

DRUG INTERACTIONS

Additive anticholinergic effects may result when antiparkinsonian drugs are administered concomitantly with phenothiazines, tricyclic antidepressants, or some antihistamines. Therapy with benztropine and any of these drugs may represent an increased risk for developing adverse anticholinergic effects.

It has long been suspected, but unproven, that antiparkinsonian drugs adversely interact with the antipsychotics (11). When antiparkinsonian drugs are withdrawn from patient's antipsychotic drug regimens, an increase can occur in the plasma concentration of the antipsychotic (12). This result suggests that a pharmacokinetic interaction occurs when antiparkinsonian drugs are used to treat extrapyramidal side effects. The reduction in neurological side effects could be due to an anticholinergic-induced decrease in gastrointestinal absorption of the antipsychotic. If this hypothesis were true, then a simple dose reduction of the antipsychotic would be preferable to giving an antiparkinsonian drug. However, a widespread opinion is that pharmacokinetic interactions between these drugs do occur but account for only a negligible impact on therapeutic outcome. Antiparkinsonian medications counteract the effects of antipsychotics on striatal cholinergic neurons apart from their effect on drug absorption. Other antiparkinsonian interactions are summarized in Table 3E.2.

ADVERSE REACTIONS—OCCURRENCE AND MANAGEMENT

Adverse effects may be anticholinergic or antihistaminic in nature. Dry mouth, blurred vision, nausea, vomiting, urinary retention, disorientation, drowsiness, irritability, tachycardia, and impotence may occur. If dry mouth is severe to the point of difficulty in swallowing or speaking, the dosage should be reduced or discontinued temporarily. Nausea unaccompanied by vomiting can

Table 3E.2.
Drug Interactions with Benztropine

Interacting Drug	Effect
Acetaminophen Cimetidine Levodopa	Reduced effect of interacting drug. Benztropine as an anticholinergic can theoretically alter the absorption of drugs by slowing gastrointestinal transit time. Many of these reports are suspect and unsubstantiated.
Atenolol Digoxin, thiazide diuretics	Enhanced effects of these interacting drugs from increased absorption
Haloperidol, other antipsychotics	Suspected reversal of antipsychotic effects; see text for discussion
Piperidine phenothiazines, tricyclic antidepressants, many antihistamines	The additive anticholinergic effects may predispose to anticholinergic side effects and delirium.

usually be disregarded. However, a slight reduction in dosage may control the nausea and still give sufficient relief of symptoms. Vomiting should be controlled by temporarily discontinuing therapy. Other adverse reactions include constipation, numbness in the fingers, and listlessness. Occasionally, an allergic reaction develops and a skin rash may appear.

MANAGEMENT OF OVERDOSE

Severe overdosage with benztropine can be expected to resemble atropine poisoning. Severe toxicity can include circulatory collapse, cardiac arrest, respiratory depression or arrest, and central nervous system depression preceded or followed by stimulation, shock, coma, or stupor. Seizures may occur or patients may appear ataxic, incoherent, and combative. Hyperpyrexia is frequent, accompanied by hot, dry skin. Dry mucous membranes are common, and dilated and slowly reactive pupils may appear.

Treatment of overdose can be both symptomatic and specific. The general approach is to establish respiration with the creation of an artifical airway, if necessary. Unless the patient is comatose or seizing, prevention of absorption may be attempted by initiating emesis. If contraindications are present, endotracheal intubation should precede gastric lavage with a large-bore tube.

Physostigmine salicylate, a cholinesterase inhibitor, has been reported to reverse most cardiovascular and neurological effects of anticholinergic overdosage, although treatment failures may occur (13, 14). For adults, the dose is 1 to 3 mg given intramuscularly or intravenously slowly over 3 minutes. Because physostigmine has a short duration of action, additional doses may be needed at 30- to 60-minute intervals (15). Although some neurological symptoms will respond within 30 minutes, mental status may deteriorate again in 1 to 2 hours. This treatment should be used cautiously as physostigmine can precipitate seizures, cholinergic crisis, bradyarrhythmias and asystole. Stimulants such as pentylenetetrazol should be avoided because of their convulsant effects. A local miotic for mydriasis and cycloplegia may be helpful. Ice bags or other cold applications and alcohol sponges are used for hyperpyrexia. A dark room may be helpful when photophobia is a problem. Urinary retention may require catheterization.

USE IN RENAL AND/OR HEPATIC DISEASE

No special dosage adjustments are recommended for renal or hepatic disease; however, caution should be used in these types of patients as they are frequently more sensitive to usual doses of a variety of drugs.

USE IN CHILDREN AND ADOLESCENTS

Benztropine is contraindicated in children under 3 years of age; safety and efficacy for use in older children has not been established.

USE IN ELDERLY

Geriatric patients frequently display an unusual sensitivity to anticholinergic drugs. Occasionally, mental confusion and disorientation may occur from drug administration. Other symptoms of an anticholinergic syndrome include agitation, hallucinations, and psychotic-like delusions (16). Older patients are less likely to tolerate larger doses, which may be needed in younger patients. It has been a common finding in anticholinergic-induced delirium for patients to be receiving three anticholinergic medicines. Close monitoring of medication intake is advised to avoid polypharmacy, which can lead to behavioral toxicity.

USE IN PREGNANCY

The safe use of benztropine has not been established in pregnancy. It should only be used when clearly needed and when the potential benefits outweigh the unknown hazard to the fetus. Breast feeding is inadvisable. Infants are sensitive to anticholinergic effects, and some benztropine probably crosses through breast milk. An anticholinergic-induced inhibitory effect on lactation is also possible.

PATIENT INFORMATION

Patients should be told that the drug may cause drowsiness and to be cautious when driving a car or operating dangerous machinery. Benztropine may cause drowsiness, dizziness, or blurred vision. The patient should notify the physician if rapid or pounding heartbeat, confusion, eye pain, or rash occurs. This medication should be used cautiously in hot weather as it may increase the susceptibility to heat stroke.

REFERENCES

1. Gilman AG, Goodman LS, Gilman A: *The Pharmacological Basis of Therapeutics*, ed 6, MacMillan, New York, 1980.
2. Church WH, Justice JB Jr, Byrd LD: Extracellular dopamine in rat striatum following uptake inhibition by cocaine, nomifensine and benztropine. *Eur J Pharmacol* 139:345–348, 1987.
3. Cedarbaum JM: Clinical pharmacokinetics of anti-parkinson drugs. *Clin Pharmacokinet* 13:141–178, 1987.
4. Tune L, Coyle JT: Serum levels of anticholinergic drugs in treatment of acute extrapyramidal side effects. *Arch Gen Psychiatry* 37:293–297, 1980.
5. Chouinard G, Annable L, Ross-Chouinard A, Kropsky ML: Ethopropazine and benztropine in neuroleptic-induced parkinsonism. *J Clin Psychiatry* 40:147–152, 1979.
6. Perenyi A, Gardos G, Samu I, et al: Changes in extrapyramidal symptoms following anticholinergic drug withdrawal. *Clin Neuropharmacol* 6:55–61, 1983.
7. Orlov P, Kasparian G, DiMascio A, Cole JO: Withdrawal of antiparkinson drugs. *Arch Gen Psychiatry* 25:410–412, 1971.
8. Rifkin A, Quitkin F, Klein DF: Akinesia—a poorly recognized drug-induced extrapyramidal behavior disorder. *Arch Gen Psychiatry* 35:483–489, 1975.

9. Crawshaw JA, Mullen PE: A study of benzhexol abuse. *Br J Psychiatry* 145:300–303, 1984.
10. McInnis M, Petursson H: Trihexyphenidyl dependence. *Acta Psychiatr Scand* 69:538–542, 1984.
11. Singh MM, Smith JM: Reversal of some therapeutic effects of an antipsychotic agent by an antiparkinson drug. *J Nerv Ment Dis* 157:50–58, 1973.
12. Gautier J, Jus A, Villeneuve A, Jus K, Pires P, Villeneuve R: Influence of the antiparkinsonian drugs on the plasma level of neuroleptics. *Biol Psychiatry* 12:389–399, 1977.
13. Duvoison RC, Katz R: Reversal of central anticholinergic syndrome in man by physostigmine. *JAMA* 206:1963–1965, 1968.
14. Granacher RP, Baldessarini RJ: Physostigmine—its use in acute anticholinergic syndrome with antidepressant and antiparkinsonian drugs. *Arch Gen Psychiatry* 32:375–380, 1975.
15. El-Yousef MK, Janowsky DS, Davis JM, Sekerke HJ: Reversal of antiparkinsonian drug toxicity by physostigmine: a controlled study. *Am J Psychiatry* 130:141–145, 1973.
16. Hall RCW, Fox J, Stickney SK, et al: Anticholinergic delirium: etiology, presentation, diagnosis and management. *J Psychedelic Drugs* 10:237–241, 1978.

F

Intraclass Comparisons of Antiparkinson Drugs

Parkinson's disease is a neurological disorder characterized by tremor, rigidity, akinesia, and difficulties in maintaining posture and equilibrium. Several causes are recognized. The pathophysiological basis is complex but partly involves a deficiency of dopamine in the basal ganglia area of the brain (Chapter 1B). This results in an imbalance between acetylcholine and dopamine. Some of the drugs that are effective in reversing the symptoms of parkinsonism either increase neurotransmission by acting as dopamine agonists (L-DOPA, amantadine, bromocriptine) or decrease cholinergic neurotransmission by acting as muscarinic antagonists.

Symptoms of parkinsonism may be drug-induced. All of the effective antipsychotic drugs, with the possible exception of clozapine, can produce pseudoparkinsonism and other neurological side effects (1–3). These are collectively known as extrapyramidal symptoms (EPS). The most common are dystonias and akathisia. A comparison is shown in Table 3F.1. The presence of these side effects can seriously undermine the therapeutic goals of antipsychotic drug therapy, prolong hospitalization, and contribute to the patient's inactivity. Some dystonias (e.g., oculogyric crises) can present as serious medical conditions. Akathisia can be distressing and result in maladaptive reactions, even contributing to suicidal behavior. The anticholinergic drugs can reverse or prevent most antipsychotic-induced EPS. L-DOPA, the immediate precursor of dopamine, has not been systematically studied for the treatment of antipsychotic-induced EPS.

Table 3F.1.
Neurological Side Effects of Antipsychotic Drugs

Reaction	Features	Usual Time of Appearance during Therapy	Treatment
Acute dystonia	Spasm of muscles of tongue, face, neck	1 to 5 days	Antiparkinson agents (IM or IV, then oral)
Pseudoparkinsonism	Bradykinesia, rigidity, variable tremor, mask facies, shuffling gait	5 to 30 days	Antiparkinson agents (oral)
Akathisia	Motor restlessness	5 to 60 days	Reduce dose or change drug; antiparkinson drugs usually help
Tardive akathisia	Motor restlessness	weeks after withdrawal of antipsychotic	Antiparkinson agents (oral)
Tardive dyskinesia	Oral-facial dyskinesia; choreoathetosis	months to years	No adequate therapy; antiparkinson drugs are not recommended

Most of the medications available for use as anticholinergic drugs are similar in structure to the atropine-like alkaloids. Diphenhydramine, an antihistamine, is also useful. Amantadine is the only indirect dopamine agonist that is useful in treating EPS. Unfortunately, there is no well-defined basis for choosing among these drugs. Trihexylphenidyl and benztropine are the most popular. Trihexylphenidyl is available generically, and benztropine has the advantage of availability in a parenteral form. Additionally, the dosage intervals for benztropine are longer, every 12 or 24 hours, compared to every 6 or 8 hours for the other available anticholinergics. There is no systematic evidence that one antiparkinson drug is consistently superior to another for treatment of EPS. Table 3F.2 compares the usual doses for the most widely used drugs.

The antiparkinson drugs have also been used to treat psychoactive drug withdrawal symptoms (4). Specifically, benztropine and atropine have been used to reverse gastrointestinal symptoms and insomnia in patients who had recently been withdrawn from cyclic antidepressants. It is hypothesized that the etiology of psychoactive drug withdrawal symptoms is from central cholinergic rebound after long-term therapy with highly potent anticholinergic drugs. The tricyclic antidepressants frequently produce these symptoms, in both adults and children (5, 6).

The ability of the antiparkinson drugs to produce adverse reactions has long been recognized (7, 8). They appear as extensions of the drug's pharmacological effects. Minor side effects include blurred vision as a result of paralysis of accommodation, dry mouth, slurred speech, tachycardia as a result of vagal

Table 3F.2.
Usual Dosages of Antiparkinson Drugs for EPS

Drug	Brand Name	Dose Range (mg/day)	Equivalent Dose (mg)
Benztropine	Cogentin	0.5–8	2
Trihexyphenidyl	Artane	2–20	5
Procyclidine	Kemadrin	5–20	5
Biperiden	Akineton	4–8	4
Diphenhydramine	Benadryl	25–200	50
Amantadine	Symmetrel	100–300	100

blockade, constipation, and difficulty in urination. Combining therapy with antidepressants and antipsychotics, as discussed in Chapters 2 and 3, may result in additive anticholinergic effects. Mydriasis, facial flushing, and decreased sweating are additional problems that can occur. Occasionally, a sense of euphoria occurs.

The manifestations of anticholinergic toxicity are summarized in Table 3F.3. This syndrome can occur from use of any anticholinergic drug, including the tricyclic antidepressants, or when drugs from different classes of psychoactive drugs with anticholinergic properties are combined. Many outpatients will be self-medicating with over-the-counter sedatives, which are frequently anticholinergic antihistamines. This emphasizes the importance of obtaining an accurate medication history (Chapter 1E). The onset of symptoms can be insidious, occurring over a 1- to 3-week period.

Physostigmine may occasionally be useful in diagnosing and treating an acute anticholinergic syndrome (9). This drug is a reversible cholinesterase inhibitor that results in enhanced central and peripheral cholinergic actions. A dose of 1 mg, intramuscularly, should reverse the mental confusion and peripheral anticholinergic toxicity from benztropine and other anticholinergic agents. Before administering this drug, vital signs should be observed and pupil size noted. Cardiac monitoring is recommended as anticholinergic drugs may produce arrhythmias. Physostigmine can also be administered slowly intravenously; however, atropine should be available if misdiagnosis results in a physostigmine-induced hypercholinergic state. This would be suggested by bradycardia and miosis. Appropriate treatment would be 0.5 mg of atropine for each 1.0 mg of physostigmine administered.

Anticholinergic psychosis may occur in patients who are drug abusers. Occasional patients may feign extrapyramidal symptoms to obtain benztropine or trihexyphenidyl to achieve a euphoria (10). Tales abound of prison inmates who use benztropine as a kind of currency to obtain favors. Two cases have been reported that suggest concern for a dependence lability of trihexyphenidyl (11), the anticholinergic drug most frequently associated with abuse (12).

Monitoring of antiparkinson therapy is usually by pharmacological response. However, the radioreceptor assay has allowed assessment of plasma anticholinergic activity through serum measurements of atropine equivalents (13). Studies have suggested that the dose-response curve for eliminating EPS is close to that adversely affecting memory (14) (see Chapter 1C). The measurement instrument in this study was a verbal recall test administered to reflect encoding of recent memories. This finding suggests that antiparkinson drugs should be used at their lowest dose. Some experimentation may be necessary to find the

Table 3F.3.
Medical and Psychiatric Manifestations of Anticholinergic Toxicity

Peripheral
  Tachycardia
  Dry mucous membranes
  Urinary retention
  Blurred vision
  Constipation
Central
  Delirium
  Disorientation
  Ataxia
  Reduced ability to concentrate
  Euphoria
  Seizures in severe cases
  Confusion
  Recent memory difficulties
  Hallucinations, visual or auditory
  Delusions
  Irritability
Predisposing factors
  High (greater than 450 ng/ml) plasma concentrations of tricyclics
  Polypharmacy (two or more drugs with anticholinergic properties)
  Advanced age
  Concurrent CNS disease

minimal effective dose. Frequently, dosage can be lowered after 1 or 2 weeks of continuous therapy. The benefits of therapy can be followed objectively with rating scales for abnormal movements (15).

The pharmacokinetics of the antiparkinson drugs have received less study than other psychoactive drug classes (16). Their basic properties are outlined in Table 3F.4 (17–19). In most studies, a lack of correlation was found between serum drug concentration and relief of EPS.

INDIVIDUAL MEDICATIONS
Diphenhydramine

Parenteral diphenhydramine in a dose of 12.5 to 25 mg is very effective in counteracting acute dystonic reactions such as torticollis or oculogyric crises. Another use of diphenhydramine is oral administration at bedtime as a sedative. It is less often used compared with other oral anticholinergic drugs for the treatment of EPS. Diphenhydramine is biotransformed to a demethylated metabolite that has a half-life averaging 7 to 9 hours, similar to that of unchanged diphenhydramine (20).

Trihexylphenidyl

Trihexylphenidyl is useful for all forms of parkinsonism. For EPS, the usual dose is 1 mg orally two or three times daily and may be increased to a total of 20 mg daily. The usual dose is between 5 and 15 mg/day. For many patients, the dosage regimen will require administration three times daily. Clinical pharmacokinetic studies have found that serum levels are unrelated to response in the

Table 3F.4.
Comparative Pharmacokinetics of Antiparkinson Drugs

Drug	Percent of Dose Absorbed	Peak Concentration (hr)	Volume of Distribution (liters/kg)	Clearance (liters/hr)	Half-life (hr)
Diphenhydramine	0.5–0.8	1–2	4–12	28–140	4–15
Trihexylphenidyl	0.95	1–2		26	5–15
Orphenadrine	0.95	2–4			13–20
Procyclidine	0.5–0.9	1–2		4	12
Biperidine		1–1.5			18
Amantadine		1–4	5–10	6–18	10–30

treatment of EPS; therefore, dosage must be individualized (21) according to clinical response. A reduction in dosage after a few days when EPS symptoms are under control should be attempted.

Biperidine

Biperidine has not been extensively used in the United States. Despite a long half-life, averaging 18 hours, it must be given two or three times a day. Pharmacokinetic evaluations have shown that its anticholinergic effects are not mirrored by serum concentrations (22).

Orphenadrine

Orphenadrine is the *o*-methyl analog of diphenhydramine. It has been used as a skeletal muscle relaxant, but early studies of its efficacy to control fluphenazine-induced EPS found it to be no better than placebo (23). Another drug with proven efficacy should be used in its place.

Procyclidine

Procyclidine is an effective agent for EPS although not very popular. This may be due to its availability in only oral dosage forms. Dosage for EPS is 2.5 mg three times daily, increased as necessary to 20 mg daily.

Amantadine

Amantadine is not an anticholinergic compound; rather, it posesses antiparkinsonian effects through dopamine receptor agonist activity (24). It has comparable efficacy to benztropine and possibly fewer side effects (25, 26). However, an occasional patient will experience disturbances in memory and orientation or a worsening of positive symptoms of schizophrenia. Other side effects are insomnia, nightmares, and mood disturbances, both mood elevations and depression. Some patients who were successfully treated for akathisia with amantadine later developed tolerance to its therapeutic effects. As amantadine is renally excreted, caution must be exercised in patients with renal dysfunction (27). It has potential usefulness in the treatment of some neuroleptic side effects such as gynecomastia and galactorrhea, which are mediated by increases in prolactin secretion. Amantadine, as a dopamine agonist, should have the ability to reverse these endocrine effects of antipsychotics.

REFERENCES
1. Swett C Jr, Cole JO, Shapiro S, Stone D: Extrapyramidal side effects in chlorpromazine recipients. *Arch Gen Psychiatry* 34:942–943, 1977.

2. Goetz CG, Klawans HL: Drug-induced extrapyramidal disorders—a neuropsychiatric interface. *J Clin Psychopharmacol* 1:297–303, 1981.
3. Rifkin A, Quitkin F, Klein DF: Akinesia: a poorly recognized drug-induced extrapyramidal behavioral disorder. *Arch Gen Psychiatry* 32:672–673, 1975.
4. Dilsaver SC, Feinberg M, Greden JF: Antidepressant withdrawal symptoms treated with anticholinergic agents. *Am J Psychiatry* 140:249–251, 1983.
5. Kramer JC, Dlein DF, Fink M: Withdrawal symptoms following discontinuation of imipramine therapy. *Am J Psychiatry* 118:549–550, 1961.
6. Law W III, Petti TA, Kazdin AE: Withdrawal symptoms after graduated cessation of imipramine in children. *Am J Psychiatry* 138:647–650, 1981.
7. Woody GE, O'Brien CP: Anticholinergic toxic psychosis in drug abusers treated with benztropine. *Compr Psychiatry* 15:439–442, 1974.
8. Stephens DA: Psychotoxic effects of benzhexol hydrochloride (Artane). *Br J Psychiatry* 113:213–218, 1967.
9. Granacher RP, Baldessarini RJ: Physostigmine: its use in acute anticholinergic syndrome with antidepressant and antiparkinson drugs. *Arch Gen Psychiatry* 32:375–380, 1975.
10. Rubinstein JS: Abuse of antiparkinsonism drugs. *JAMA* 239:2365–2366, 1978.
11. McInnis M, Petursson H: Trihexyphenidyl dependence. *Acta Psychiatr Scand* 69:538–542, 1984.
12. Smith JM: Abuse of antiparkinson drugs: a review of the literature. *J Clin Psychiatry* 41:351–354, 1980.
13. Creese I, Snyder SH: A simple and sensitive radioreceptor assay for antischizophrenic drugs in blood. *Nature* 270:180–182, 1977.
14. Tune LE, Strauss ME, Lew MK, Breitlinger E, Coyle JT: Serum levels of anticholinergic drugs and impaired recent memory in chronic schizophrenic patients. *Am J Psychiatry* 139:1460–1462, 1982.
15. Simpson GM, Angus JWS: A rating scale for extrapyramidal effects. *Acta Psychiatr Scand* 212(suppl):11–19, 1970.
16. Cedarbaum JM: Clinical pharmacokinetics of anti-parkinsonian drugs. *Clin Pharmacokinet* 13:141–178, 1987.
17. Whiteman PD, Fowle ASE, Hamilton MJ, Peck AW, Bye A, Dean K, Webster A: Pharmacokinetics and pharmacodynamics of procyclidine in man. *Eur J Clin Pharmacol* 38:73–78, 1985.
18. Nation RL, Triggs EJ, Vine J: Metabolism and urinary excretion of benzhexol in humans. *Xenobiotica* 3:165–169, 1978.
19. Pacifici GM, Nardine M, Ferrari P, Latini R, Fieschi C, Morselli PL: Effect of amantadine on drug-induced parkinsonism: relationship between plasma levels and effect. *Br J Clin Pharmacol* 3:883–889, 1976.
20. Blyden GT, Greenblatt DJ, Scavone JM, Shader RI: Pharmacokinetics of diphenhydramine and a demethylated metabolite following intravenous and oral administration. *J Clin Pharmacol* 26:529–533, 1986.
21. Burke RE, Fahn S: Serum trihexyphenidyl levels in the treatment of torsion dystonia. *Neurology* 35:1066–1069, 1985.
22. Hollmann M, Brode E, Greger G, Muller-Peltzer H, Wetzelsberger N: Biperiden effects and plasma levels in volunteers. *Eur J Clin Pharmacol* 27:619–621, 1984.
23. Mindham RHS, Gaind R, Anstee BH, Rimmer L: Comparison of amantadine, orphenadrine, and placebo in the control of phenothiazine-induced parkinsonism. *Psychol Med* 2:406–413, 1972.
24. Aoki FY, Sitar DS: Clinical pharmacokinetics of amantadine hydrochloride. *Clin Pharmacokinet* 14:35–51, 1988.
25. DiMascio A, Bernardo DL, Greenblatt DJ, Marder JE: A controlled trial of amantadine in drug-induced extrapyramidal disorders. *Arch Gen Psychiatry* 33:599–602, 1976.
26. Greenblatt DJ, Dimascio A, Harmatz JS, et al: Pharmacokinetics and clinical effects of amantadine in drug-induced extrapyramidal symptoms. *J Clin Pharmacol* 17:704–708, 1977.
27. Horadam VW, Sharp JG, Smilack JD, et al: Pharmacokinetics of amantadine hydrochloride in subjects with normal and impaired renal function. *Ann Intern Med* 94:454–458, 1981.

4
Drug Therapy for Anxiety and Insomnia

Anxiety and insomnia are ubiquitous complaints in Western culture. This is reflected partly by the high emphasis given to these problems in the lay press. The popularity of treatments, including excessive self-medication with alcohol, also attests to this fact. Although anxiety serves a physiological function by inducing arousal and aiding performance, excess anxiety can undermine coping skills and reduce the ability to function appropriately. Accurate diagnosis and appropriate treatment can minimize the impact of anxiety disorders on the quality of life.

Pathological anxiety can occur in all age groups. As discussed in Chapter 1F, anxiety is no longer thought to represent a continuum between enhanced arousal and a pathological state. Discrete heterogenous disorders are proposed to exist. This concept has received validation from pharmacological research. Clinical trials have demonstrated that specific drugs are better for certain anxiety disorders. For example, clomipramine seems to be superior in its treatment outcome for obsessive-compulsive disorder compared with the benzodiazepines. In provocation studies, lactate infusions will generally not precipitate a panic attack in patients with generalized anxiety disorder as typified in patients with panic disorder. The response of posttraumatic stress disorder to monoamine oxidase inhibitors is frequently more rewarding than to benzodiazepines. These observations suggest that the pathogenesis differs according to the specific anxiety disorder. As many medical conditions can be accompanied by symptoms of anxiety, these must always be ruled out or documented and appropriately treated before initiating antianxiety treatment. Thus, careful consideration must be given to the source of anxiety in deciding upon treatment and to the expected outcome from using antianxiety drugs.

The first modern therapies for anxiety and insomnia were the barbiturates. These drugs are essentially broad central nervous system (CNS) depressants. The difference between their anxiolytic effects and further CNS depression proceeding to anesthesia, coma, and death is only a matter of dosage. The barbiturates and nonbarbiturate sedative-hypnotics (methylprylon, gluthethimide, methaqualone) have been extensively prescribed despite recognition of their severe lethality in overdosage. Fortunately, these drugs can be abandoned with the availability of safer, more specific medicines.

An ideal antianxiety agent should reduce anxiety without causing excessive sedation. The benzodiazepines have generally met this characteristic, but they have the drawbacks of producing dependence and withdrawal symptoms in a small proportion of users. When taken alone in overdoses, death is not expected to occur. The benzodiazepines continue to be some of the most widely prescribed drugs in the world because of their safety and efficacy.

In the first database that follows, diazepam, the prototype benzodiazepine, is discussed. It has been the most widely prescribed drug in its class. By considering the pharmacokinetic properties of the benzodiazepines, discussed in Chapter 4C, a basis is provided for selecting these drugs for individual patients. Buspirone deserves attention as the first of a new class of nonbenzodiazepine anxiolytics (Chapter 4B). Although the benzodiazepines all share similar pharmacological properties, three have been marketed specifically as sedatives. Flurazepam (Chapter 4D), the first to become available, is described in detail. Finally, triazolam, temazepam, and other alternative sedatives are discussed within the context of drug therapy for insomnia (Chapter 4E).

A

Diazepam Database

FORMULATIONS

Diazepam tablets: 2 mg, 5 mg, 10 mg
Diazepam capsules: 15 mg sustained release
Diazepam oral solution: 5 mg/ml
Diazepam injection: 5 mg/ml
Brand names: Valium (Roche); various generic brands

BASIC PHARMACOLOGY

Diazepam is the prototype 1,4-benzodiazepine (Fig. 4A.1). Historically, chlordiazepoxide was synthesized first, but diazepam was subsequently found to have stronger sedative, muscle-relaxant, anticonvulsant, and taming properties in animals. Since its marketing, it has frequently headed the list of the most widely prescribed drugs in the United States. Millions of people worldwide take diazepam daily for one or more of its numerous indications.

The benzodiazepines have been widely accepted in clinical practice to treat a variety of specific anxiety disorders. These medications have replaced the barbiturates and meprobamate for several reasons (1). They are more specific and effective for anxiety symptoms, producing more than simple CNS depression, and they produce fewer side effects and are safer in overdosage. Diazepam produces marginal enzyme induction or inhibition, and its dependence and addictive properties are less severe compared to the barbiturates. Although newer, nonbenzodiazepine anxiolytics, in addition to buspirone (Chapter 4B), are expected to be marketed in the 1990s, the benzodiazepines are likely to remain the most extensively prescribed psychoactive drugs.

In 1977, specific recognition sites for the benzodiazepines were identified in mammalian brain (2, 3). These receptors are located in high concentrations in limbic structures including the amygdala, hippocampus, and frontal cortex (see Chaper 1B). These findings renewed interest in the field of anxiolytic pharmacology (4). Subsequently, it was shown that benzodiazepines enhanced the actions of γ-aminobutyric acid (GABA), the major inhibitory neurotransmitter

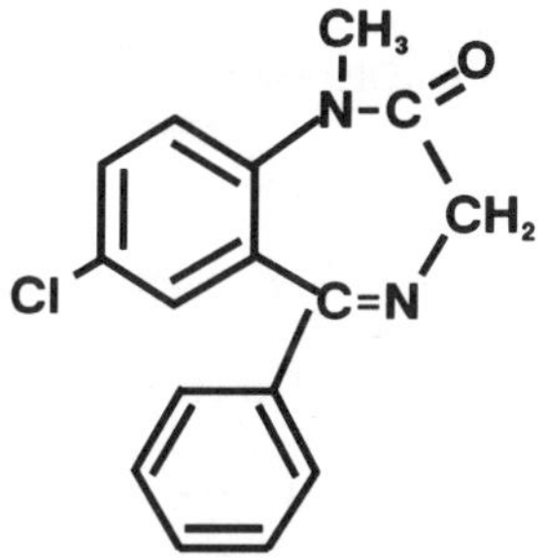

Figure 4A.1.   Structure of diazepam.

in various regions of the brain and spinal cord (see Chapter 1B). Currently, the benzodiazepine receptor is viewed as a modulatory site that is functionally coupled on the same molecule to GABA receptors that regulate chloride ion channels (5). The binding of benzodiazepines to their receptor sites seems to parallel their antianxiety potencies in vivo.

Just as the discovery of the opiate receptors for morphine resulted in the isolation and identification of their endogenous ligands, the enkephalins, the existance of benzodiazepine receptors suggests that endogenous substrates must exist that mediate stress (6). Inappropriate responses to stress are eventually manifested as pathological anxiety. The benzodiazepines ameliorate this response. The search to discover the endogenous substrates of anxiety is a major area of current research.

Diazepam illustrates several classical benzodiazepine actions. It is an effective skeletal muscle relaxant acting by inhibiting spinal cord afferent pathways at high doses; however, these effects are not prominent at usual doses. It may also directly depress motor nerve function. The benzodiazepines do not extinguish an abnormal seizure focus but suppress the spread of seizure activity and are thus effective anticonvulsants.

In usual doses, the benzodiazepines have little effect on cardiovascular, autonomic, and respiratory function. Diazepam in doses exceeding 20 mg/day may lower cortisol levels (7). This effect could potentially falsely normalize the dexamethasone suppression test (see Chapter 1G). Diazepam's expected effects on physiological status and various laboratory tests are outlined in Table 4A.1.

PHARMACOKINETIC PROPERTIES

Diazepam's pharmacokinetic properties are summarized in Table 4A.2. Diazepam has been extensively investigated as it can be considered a model compound for various physiological factors that influence drug disposition (8). It is almost entirely metabolized, with less than one % of a dose being excreted in the urine in an unchanged form. The major metabolic pathways are demethylation to desmethyldiazepam and hydroxylation to N-methyloxazepam. These metabolites are further converted to oxazepam, conjugated with glucuronide, and excreted in the urine.

After oral administration, diazepam is rapidly and nearly completely absorbed and achieves peak plasma concentrations within 30 to 90 minutes. The high lipid solubility of diazepam allows it to diffuse rapidly to active brain sites. Volunteers experience a variety of mental effects shortly after taking diazepam. Depending on the experience and expectations of patients and volunteers,

Table 4A.1.
Expected Physiological Effects from Diazepam Therapy for Monitoring[a]

Parameter	Drug Effect
Cardiovascular status	
Heart rate	No effect or slight increase in patients with lung disease
ECG	No expected effects
Blood pressure	Modest reduction in systolic pressure after IV administration
Renal function	
Serum creatinine and clearance, BUN	Normal values should not change
Hepatic function	
AST (SGOT), ALT (SGPT), alkaline phosphatase	Rare elevation of AST and ALT; jaundice has been reported.
Hematology status	
CBC	Rare leukopenia and eosinophilia
Neuroendocrine status	
Cortisol	No change or decrease in plasma cortisol; potential interference with DST during chronic, high dose therapy
Thyroid indices	These may be altered, but the patient remains euthyroid.
Growth hormone	No change or increase
ACTH	No change or decrease

[a]Abbreviations: ECG, electrocardiogram; BUN, blood urea nitrogen; AST, aspartate aminotransferase; SGOT, serum glutamic-oxaloacetic transaminase; ALT, alanine aminotransferase; SGPT, serum glutamic-pyruvic transaminase; CBC, complete blood count; ACTH, adrenocorticotropic hormone; DST, dexamethasone suppression test.

these effects range from a feeling of inner calm and relaxation to deterioration of mental function, loss of coordination, or feelings of dysphoria.

Diazepam shows a pronounced distribution phase of rapidly falling concentrations after the occurrence of its peak concentration in plasma. This pattern of concentration changes over time is consistent with the classical two-compartment pharmacokinetic model. The distribution phase is followed by a slower terminal phase of drug elimination. The rapid fall in plasma concentration from a peak, with distribution to other tissue sites, is probably accompanied by rapidly falling brain concentration. This would explain the diminution in the initially perceived mental effects. For some dependence-prone patients, this deterioration in early effects serves as a reinforcement for frequent drug intake. After multiple doses, diazepam accumulates to higher plasma concentrations because of the slower elimination phase and its inherent metabolic clearance rate. This accumulation to steady state extends the duration of action of antianxiety effects.

Diazepam is extensively plasma protein-bound, in the range of 90 to 98%, mostly to albumin. Not surprisingly, diazepam is stored in body fat, in addition to its distribution to lipid-rich areas such as brain tissue. It is present in breast milk and readily passes the placenta to the fetus.

Table 4A.2.
Pharmacokinetic Parameters of Diazepam

Parameter	Range
Bioavailability	Oral: nearly complete
Time of peak concentration after single dose	Oral: 30 to 90 minutes IM: erratic
Plasma protein binding	Greater than 95%
Volume of distribution	1 to 2 liters/kg
Total plasma clearance	0.3 to 1.0 ml/min/kg
Renal clearance	Negligible
Elimination half-life	Young adults: Mean of 20 hours Elderly: Range 30 to 70 hours with mean of 40 hours
Active metabolites	Desmethyldiazepam
Steady-state metabolite to parent concentration ratio	Greater than 1.0
Therapeutic range for antianxiety effect	Not established; usual plasma steady-state concentrations are in the range of 100 to 600 ng/ml.

The elimination half-life of diazepam is dependent upon the patient's age (9). In young healthy adults, the average half-life is 20 hours; this rises dramatically in the elderly. Patients older than 65 require 30 to 100 hours to eliminate half of the drug. The mean half-life in the elderly is approximately 40 hours. Diazepam is a low extraction drug, and clearance is in the range of 0.3 to 1.0 ml/min/kg. In general, men show an earlier deterioration than women in the ability to oxidize many drugs. Diazepam clearance is reduced in elderly men more prominently than in elderly women, although a prolonged half-life exists in both sexes compared to young adults.

The demethylation of diazepam produces desmethyldiazepam, an active metabolite common to several benzodiazepines (see Chapter 4C). This metabolite is slowly eliminated with a half-life of 36 to over 96 hours (10). Its clearance is slower than that of diazepam and it accumulates to a plasma concentration at steady state in excess of diazepam. Thus, upon chronic dosing of diazepam, steady-state concentrations of drug and metabolite may not be reached for up to 10 days or longer.

INDICATIONS

Diazepam is effective for the management of anxiety disorders or for the short-term relief of the symptoms of anxiety. This Food and Drug Administration (FDA)-approved labeling statement implies efficacy in specific anxiety disorders as well as anxiety associated with medical conditions. The various anxiety disorders were outlined in Chapter 1F. Table 4A.3 lists various medical conditions that may be accompanied with anxiety symptoms amenable to benzodiazepine therapy. The benzodiazepines are the drugs of choice for most anxiety states, but they are not superior to the monoamine oxidase inhibitors or tricyclic antidepressants for treatment of panic disorder and agoraphobia (11).

Diazepam is useful in states of acute alcohol withdrawal (12). It reduces the agitation and associated symptoms of impending delirium tremens. Although

Table 4A.3.
Conditions for Which Diazepam or Benzodiazepines May Have Beneficial Effects

Medical conditions with accompaning anxiety
    Angina pectoris
    Alcohol withdrawal states
    Chronic obstructive pulmonary disease
    Mitral valve prolapse
    Myocardial infarction
    Organic brain syndromes
    Pain
    Pheochromocytoma
    Thyrotoxicosis
    Trauma
Anesthetic therapy
    Tracheal intubation
    Adaptation to ventilator rhythm
    Psychomotor agitation
    Eclampsia
    Decerebrate fits
    Tetanus
Neurology
    Postherpetic neuralgias
    Spasticity
    Tetanus
    Status epilepticus

chlordiazepoxide has been promoted for this use, it has no inherent advantages over diazepam.

Diazepam has been commonly used as a premedication for numerous surgical conditions. As a preoperative, it is used parenterally before cardioversion and as an adjunct before endoscopic procedures.

Diazepam is used orally as a skeletal muscle relaxant. It decreases the severity of muscle contractions in stiff-man syndrome, a condition characterized by severe spasm of somatic musculature (trunk and abdominal wall) that may last for a few hours or up to a few days. Early studies with cats demonstrated that diazepam had high potency for inhibition of the linguomandibular reflex. It was better in this model of muscle relaxation than either N-desmethyldiazepam or oxazepam. This potency difference may account for diazepam's greater popularity as a muscle relaxant than other benzodiazepines. Diazepam is also used parenterally in the treatment of tetanus.

Diazepam administered 5 to 10 mg intravenously is useful in status epilepticus and recurrent convulsive seizures (13). It is also used to treat myoclonic and akinetic seizures and infantile spasms. It may be added to other anticonvulsant regimens in patients with generalized tonic-clonic seizures whose seizures are precipitated by tension and anxiety.

There is some evidence that diazepam may be an effective alternative to anticholinergics for the treatment of akathisia (14). Although this therapy is usually not considered until anticholinergic medications have failed, some evidence exists for successful use of diazepam in dystonic reactions that are otherwise unresponsive (15).

DOSAGE REGIMEN DESIGN

Dosage is individualized on the basis of subjective symptoms associated with anxiety (see Chapter 1F). For the management of most anxiety states, a starting dosage of 2 mg administered two to four times a day, orally, is recommended. Dosage should always begin low and be increased only if needed. When titrating dosage to target symptom endpoints, up to 40 mg/day may be necessary for some patients to maintain control; however, the lowest effective dose should be sought. Many patients can be managed with a total of 20 mg/day or less.

There seems to be little rationale for using the sustained release formulation of diazepam. A rare patient who feels dysphoric during the rapid absorption phase of orally administered tablets or some geriatric or debilitated patients may benefit from this dosage form. An occasional patient may prefer to take the entire day's dosage at one time. Cumulative effects occur upon multiple dosing. The inherent prolonged activity of N-desmethyldiazepam seems to argue against the need for a sustained release preparation. It is far more expensive than generic diazepam.

When diazepam is used in the treatment of status epilepticus, a dose of 10 mg given intravenously usually stops the seizures (13); however, the effect may last less than 30 minutes. The rate of administration should be 5 mg/min or slower. Caution should be exercised in repeated administrations because of the possibility of causing hypotension and respiratory depression (16).

THERAPEUTIC DRUG MONITORING

Several studies have addressed the relationship between plasma diazepam concentrations and clinical effects (17, 18). The most widely quoted study is that of Dasberg et al (18), in which patients with acute anxiety were found to do best when their diazepam concentrations were near 400 ng/ml. Other results have indicated a lack of a relationship between plasma concentration and subjective clinical effects (17). Overall, no satisfactory relationship has been found, in part because of the difficulty in objective measurement of clinical response in patients with anxiety.

When analytical support is available, some patients may be monitored for treatment compliance. Plasma concentration monitoring may be of value in identifying patients who have escalated their dosage. Plasma concentrations in these patients will be elevated without concomitant sedative effects because of the development of tolerance. However, such an assessment should include a previous steady-state concentration measurement, as plasma concentration during multiple dosing can vary severalfold among different patients. Steady-state concentrations are usually in the range of 100 to 600 ng/ml. Careful observation of clinical response remains the best approach to monitoring diazepam therapy.

CONTRAINDICATIONS—WARNINGS—PRECAUTIONS

Unwanted CNS depression can be expected to be worse in patients given diazepam for anxiety who have low serum albumin concentrations, less than 3.0 gm/100 ml (19). This adverse consequence of therapy may be a result of reduced plasma protein binding and increased free drug concentration. The elderly, patients with burns, or those with trauma may be at risk for greater side effects from usual doses due to decreased protein binding.

Table 4A.4.
Drug Interactions with Diazepam

Interacting Drug	Effect
Magnesium-aluminum antacids	Delays rate and possibly extent of absorption
Rifampin	Increases clearance
Isoniazid	Decreases clearance and prolongs elimination half-life
Disulfiram, cimetidine, oral contraceptives	Inhibits clearance
Nicotine	Cigarette smoking increases clearance and decreases clinical effects.
Phenytoin	Diazepam possibly interferes with phenytoin metabolism.
Alcohol	Additive depressant effects

Diazepam is water-insoluble and is marketed for injection dissolved in propylene glycol and ethanol. It precipitates if diluted for intravenous injection and causes phlebitis at the site of injection relatively frequently. It should not be mixed with other drugs or diluted but should be injected slowly, no faster than 5 mg (1 ml)/min. Diazepam adsorbs to plastic intravenous tubing and, therefore, the delivered dose may be less than that calculated. If patients are to receive diazepam intravenously, equipment for respiratory or cardiovascular assistance should be readily available as rare episodes of apnea have occurred.

Psychological and physical dependence is a risk associated with the chronic use of all benzodiazepines. These problems are more likely to occur with diazepam when therapy is prolonged and doses are excessive. Nevertheless, dependence from normal doses can occur.

When discontinuing therapy, a tapering schedule should be used. This will minimize the possibility of withdrawal symptoms. These are usually mild in character, consisting of flu-like symptoms mimicking cholinergic rebound. However, severe symptoms consisting of tremor and convulsions can occur. Propranolol has been used to attenuate the severity of benzodiazepine withdrawal symptoms, but its use cannot be expected to reduce the incidence of withdrawal symptoms.

DRUG INTERACTIONS

Diazepam's effects may be altered from a number of pharmacokinetic drug interactions. These are summarized in Table 4A.4. Magnesium-aluminum hydroxide antacids have been found to reduce the rate and/or extent of absorption of benzodiazepines (20, 21). Greenblatt et al (20) found a blunted response to single doses of chlordiazepoxide when taken concurrently with antacid. Although it is a common practice to administer benzodiazepines and other psychoactive drugs with antacids, this practice alters benzodiazepine bioavailability. This interaction would have less clinical significance with multiple-dose diazepam administration. During multiple dosing, this interaction would contribute to dose-to-dose variability in absorption, but the clinical effects of diazepam are cumulative and less dependent upon any single dose administration.

Antituberculous drugs interact with diazepam. Ochs et al (22) found that isoniazid prolonged diazepam's elimination half-life from 34 to an average of 45 hours in healthy volunteers. Other data suggested that rifampin, a recognized enzyme inducer (see Table 1D.5, Chapter 1D), enhanced the clearance of diazepam. The clinical implication is that adding antituberculous drugs to a dosage regimen of diazepam may result in altered clinical or enhanced adverse effects. Therefore, a dosage adjustment may be necessary when combining these drugs.

Cimetidine inhibits the metabolism of diazepam (23). The effect is pronounced, substantially increasing the diazepam plasma concentration and prolonging its elimination half-life within a day of beginning cimetidine therapy. The effects persist throughout therapy with cimetidine. Elderly patients or those with liver disease may want to avoid cimetidine in favor of ranitidine, which does not impair the hepatic elimination of diazepam (24). This interaction is pharmacokinetically significant, but it may have little clinical consequence for most patients.

Probably the most important diazepam interaction and that most thoroughly studied is with alcohol. Sellers et al (25) administered diazepam intraveously on two occasions, with and without a preceding dose of alcohol. Pharmacokinetic data indicated an inhibition by alcohol of the hepatic clearance of diazepam. Using several psychometric tests, it was observed that alcohol enhanced the mental impairment caused by diazepam. Several other studies confirmed that coadministration of alcohol enhances diazepam's effects (26, 27). Thus, the clinical adage of advising against using alcohol during treatment with antianxiety drugs is well substantiated. The concomitant ingestion of benzodiazepines with ethanol seems to result in greater impairment of psychomotor skills than that produced by either agent alone. This makes driving a car especially dangerous, and patients should be accordingly warned.

Disulfiram is a general metabolic inhibitor (see Chapter 6A). It inhibits not only aldehyde dehydrogenase, the enzyme responsible for metabolizing ethanol, but also a number of other hepatic enzymes. Disulfiram will decrease the clearance of diazepam. Therefore, smaller doses of diazepam should be used if these drugs must be combined in therapy (28).

Limited data suggest that diazepam may elevate phenytoin concentrations (29). When these drugs are combined, phenytoin plasma concentrations should be followed closely to avoid insipient toxicity. Given the nonlinear disposition of phentyoin (see Chapter 1D), even a relatively small inhibitory effect by diazepam could have greater than expected results on phenytoin serum concentration and clinical effect.

Fortunately, diazepam seems not to interact with tricyclic antidepressants (30). These drugs are sometimes used together in patients with agitated depression who have a high degree of psychomotor activity.

ADVERSE REACTIONS—OCCURRENCE AND MANAGEMENT

The most frequent adverse effects from diazepam therapy are extensions of its pharmacological effects. These include fatigue, weakness, dizziness, and confusion. Tolerance to these effects frequently occurs during therapy but may necessitate a reduction in dosage. Tolerance to diazepam's antianxiety effects is not expected to occur. Other adverse effects are listed in Table 4A.5.

Occasional fatal complications can occur from intravenous diazepam administration for cardioversion and endoscopy or as a supplement to anesthesia.

Table 4A.5.
Expected Side Effects from Diazepam Therapy

Effect	Rare	Less Common	More Common
Dry mouth		X	
Blurred vision		X	
Gastrointestinal disorders		X	
Nausea		X	
Vomiting	X		
Drowsiness			X
Dizziness			X
Ataxia		X	
Fainting	X		
Disorientation		X	
Headache		X	
Restlessness	X		
Excitement	X		
Skin rash	X		
Blood pressure decrease		X	
Tachycardia		X	
Jaundice	X		

Apnea is an idiosyncratic response and should be especially anticipated in elderly or debilitated patients (31). In patients with chronic obstructive pulmonary disease, diazepam may have a negative effect on alveolar ventilation (16).

Benzodiazepines have long been thought to interfere with the memory consolidation process. No tolerance develops to this effect. Diazepam seems to slightly impair performance on learning and memory tasks. Retrieval of previously learned information seems to be unaffected (32). This effect of benzodiazepines is an advantage when used as an adjunct to anesthesia, but suspicion of an adverse effect should be considered in patients who complain of forgetfulness.

MANAGEMENT OF OVERDOSE

Diazepam is one of the safest drugs used in medical practice. Deaths from overdosage are extremely rare; most occur when ingested in combination with alcohol or other drugs. Patients have recovered from acute ingestions as high as 2 gm (33, 34). Coma may occur, and there is morbidity associated with coma for any reason. Ingestions of less than 400 mg, 10 times the upper level of recommended daily dosage, usually do not result in coma or in the need for assisted ventilation; however, when taken with alcohol or other drugs, profound CNS depression may result (33).

Treatment of acute overdosage consists of general supportive therapy. Respiration, pulse, and blood pressure should be monitored. If necessary, pharmacotherapy for profound hypotension may consist of intravenous (IV) norepinephrine or metaraminol. IV fluids should be administered and care taken to prevent aspiration. If the overdose is recent, activated charcoal or gastric lavage may be used to retard further drug absorption. Dialysis is of limited value. Most patients recover rapidly after overdosage with diazepam alone.

USE IN RENAL AND/OR HEPATIC DISEASE

As would be expected of a highly metabolized drug, diazepam demonstrates impaired clearance in liver disease (35, 36). Viral hepatitis has produced a two-fold increase in elimination half-life whereas cirrhosis has produced up to a fivefold increase. The impaired disposition in cirrhotic patients was associated with increased sedation (36). Unfortunately, there seems to be no relationship between the impairment in drug disposition and the elevation of various liver function tests. Patients with liver disease should receive reduced doses of diazepam to avoid excessive effects. A 50% reduction in initial dosage is recommended.

Renal disease should not have a profound effect on diazepam disposition. However, the possibility should be kept in mind that hypoalbuminemia associated with renal impairment could alter plasma protein binding and possibly lead to exaggerated clinical effects.

USE IN CHILDREN AND ADOLESCENTS

Diazepam is used in children mostly for its anticonvulsant actions and less for antianxiety or muscle-relaxant effects. The pharmacokinetics of benzodiazepines have been reviewed in children (37). Prescribing patterns in adolescents are similar to those in adults.

USE IN ELDERLY

Diazepam elimination half-life is prolonged and metabolic clearance is reduced in the elderly (Table 4A.2). These effects have clinical implications when diazepam is used chronically. The elderly are more sensitive than the young to benzodiazepines (38, 39). Sedation is more profound for the same dosage rate. Salzman et al (9) demonstrated that diazepam accumulation in healthy volunteers aged 60 years and older was extensive, washout was slow, and desmethyldiazepam was measurable in plasma for 2 weeks after the last dose, during which time sedative effects persisted. Overall, these data argue for greatly reduced dosage of diazepam when used in the elderly and for the use of benzodiazepines with kinetic properties less influenced by advanced age (see Chapter 4C).

USE IN PREGNANCY

There are equivocal data that use of diazepam in pregnancy results in birth defects (40). The possibility exists that first trimester use increases oral clefts, and patients with a positive family history should avoid benzodiazepines during pregnancy.

The administration of diazepam to mothers in labor lowers Apgar scores at birth, causes reluctance to feed, and can produce apneic spells. Diazepam was detectable in infants for up to eight days after maternal administration (41). The transfer of diazepam to the fetus is apparently rapid.

Diazepam is secreted into breast milk. Drowsiness in neonates may be attributed to diazepam and desmethyldiazepam. Infants metabolize these compounds more slowly than adults, and an accumulation of them is possible (42). Breast feeding mothers given diazepam should be alerted to this possibility.

PATIENT INFORMATION

As with all psychoactive drugs, side effects should be explained to patients. The fear of requiring antianxiety therapy to cope with the stresses of daily living should be allayed. Some patients will be apprehensive about beginning therapy because of ignorance about the dependence potential of benzodiazepines.

Laboratory test skills that measure tasks presumably reflecting driving skills are impaired by diazepam in a dose-dependent fashion. This suggests that diazepam plus alcohol could further impair driving ability. Patients should be warned that diazepam may impair their ability to drive a car or perform complicated psychomotor tasks.

Because of the possibility of withdrawal symptoms from rapid discontinuation of benzodiazepines, patients should be told not to stop taking diazepam abruptly.

REFERENCES

1. Greenblatt DJ, Shader RI: *Benzodiazepines in Clinical Practice*, Raven Press, New York, 1973.
2. Squires RF, Braestrup C: Benzodiazepine receptors in rat brain. *Nature* 266:732–734, 1977.
3. Mohler H, Okada T: Benzodiazepine receptor: demonstration in the central nervous system. *Science* 198:849–851, 1977.
4. Tallman JF, Paul SM, Skolnick P, Gallager DW: Receptors for the age of anxiety: pharmacology of the benzodiazepines. *Science* 207:274–281, 1980.
5. Skolnick P, Paul SM: Benzodiazepine receptors in the central nervous system. *Int Rev Neurobiol* 23:103–140, 1982.
6. Guidotti A, Forchetti CM, Corda MG, Kondel D, Bennet CD, Costa E: Isolation, characterization and purification of an endogenous polypeptide putative with agonistic action on benzodiazepine receptors. *Proc Natl Acad Sci USA* 80:3531–3535, 1983.
7. Gram LF, Christensen P: Benzodiazepine suppression of cortisol secretion: a measure of anxiolytic activity? *Pharmacopsychiatry* 19:19–22, 1986.
8. Greenblatt DJ, Shader RI, Divoll M, Harmatz JS: Benzodiazepines: a summary of pharmacokinetic properties. *Br J Clin Pharmacol* 11(suppl):11–16, 1981.
9. Salzman C, Shader RI, Greenblatt DJ, Harmatz JS: Long v short half-life benzodiazepines in the elderly: kinetics and clinical effects of diazepam and oxazepam. *Arch Gen Psychiatry* 40:294–297, 1983.
10. Shader RI, Greenblatt DJ, Ciraulo DA, Divoll M, Harmatz JS, Georgotas A: Effect of age and sex on disposition of desmethyldiazepam formed from its precursor clorazepate. *Psychopharmacology* 75:193–197, 1981.
11. Zitrin CM, Klein DF, Woerner MG: Treatment of agoraphobia with group exposure in vivo and imipramine. *Arch Gen Psychiatry* 37:63–72, 1980.
12. Sellers EM, Jaranjo CA, Harrison M, Devenyi P, Roach C: Simplifying treatment of alcohol withdrawal: diazepam loading. *Clin Pharmacol Ther* 31:268, 1982 (abstr).
13. Delgado-Escueta AV, Wasterlain C, Treiman DM, Porter RJ: Management of status epilepticus. *N Engl J Med* 306:1337–1340, 1982.
14. Director KL, Muniz CE: Diazepam in the treatment of extrapyramidal symptoms: a case report. *J Clin Psychiatry* 43:160–161, 1982.
15. Gagrat D, Hamilton J, Belmaker R: Intravenous diazepam in the treatment of neuroleptic-induced acute dystonia and akathisia. *Am J Psychiatry* 135:1232–1233, 1978.
16. Rao S, Sherbaniuk RW, Prasad K, et al: Cardiopulmonary effects of diazepam. *Clin Pharmacol Ther* 14:182–189, 1972.
17. Mandelli M, Tognoni G, Garattini S: Clinical pharmacokinetics of diazepam. *Clin Pharmacokinet* 3:72–91, 1978.
18. Dasberg HH, van der Kleign E, Guelen P, van Praag H: Plasma concentration of diazepam and of its metabolite N-desmethyldiazepam in relation to anxiolytic effect. *Clin Pharmacol Ther* 15:473–483, 1974.

19. Greenblatt DJ, Koch-Weser J: Clinical toxicity of chlordiazepoxide and diazepam in relation to serum albumin concentration: a report from the Boston Collaborative Drug Surveillance Program. *Eur J Clin Pharmacol* 7:259–262, 1974.

20. Greenblatt DJ, Shader RI, Harmatz JS, Franke KS, Koch-Weser J: Absorption rate, blood concentrations, and early response to oral chlordiazepoxide. *Am J Psychiatry* 134:559–562, 1977.

21. Shader RI, Georgotas A, Greenblatt DJ, Harmatz JS, Allen MD: Impaired absorption of desmethyldiazepam from clorazepate by magnesium aluminum hydroxide. *Clin Pharmacol Ther* 24:308–315, 1978.

22. Ochs HR, Greenblatt DJ, Roberts GM, Dengler HJ: Diazepam interaction with antituberculous drugs. *Clin Pharmacol Ther* 29:671–678, 1981.

23. Klotz U, Reimann I: Delayed clearance of diazepam due to cimetidine. *N Engl J Med* 302:1012–1014, 1980.

24. Klotz U, Reimann IW, Ohnhaus EE: Effect of ranitidine on the steady-state pharmacokinetics of diazepam. *Eur J Clin Pharmacol* 24:357–360, 1983.

25. Sellers EM, Naranjo CA, Giles HG, Frecker RC, Beeching M: Intravenous diazepam and oral ethanol interaction. *Clin Pharmacol Ther* 28:638–645, 1980.

26. Linnoila M, Mattila MJ: Drug interaction on psychomotor skills related to driving: diazepam and alcohol. *Eur J Clin Pharmacol* 7:337–342, 1973.

27. Laisi U, Linnoila M, Seppala T, Himberg JJ, Mattila MJ: Pharmacokinetic and pharmacodynamic interactions of diazepam with different alcoholic beverages. *Eur J Clin Pharmacol* 16:263–270, 1979.

28. MacLeod SM, Sellers EM, Giles HG, Billings BJ, Martin PR, Greenblatt DJ, Marshman JA: Interaction of disulfiram with benzodiazepines. *Clin Pharmacol Ther* 24:583–589, 1978.

29. Vajda FJE, Prineas RJ, Lovell RRH: Interaction between phenytoin and the benzodiazepines. *Br Med J* 1:346, 1971 (letter).

30. Gram LF, Overo KF, Kirk L: Influence of neuroleptics and benzodiazepines on metabolism of tricyclic antidepressants in man. *Am J Psychiatry* 131:863–866, 1974.

31. Hall SC, Ovassapian A: Apnea after intravenous diazepam therapy. *JAMA* 238:1052, 1977.

32. Petersen R, Ghoneim M: Diazepam and human memory: influence on acquisition, retrieval and state-dependent learning. *Prog Neuropsychopharmacol* 4:81–89, 1980.

33. Greenblatt DF, Allen MD, Noel BJ, Shader RI: Acute overdosage with benzodiazepine derivatives. *Clin Pharmacol Ther* 21:497–514, 1977.

34. Greenblatt DJ, Woo E, Allen MD, Orsulak PJ, Shader RI: Rapid recovery from massive diazepam overdose. *JAMA* 240:1872–1874, 1978.

35. Klotz U, Avant GR, Hoyumpa A, Schenker S, Wilkinson GR: The effects of age and liver disease on the disposition and elimination of diazepam in adult man. *J Clin Invest* 55:347–359, 1975.

36. Ochs HR, Greenblatt DJ, Eckardt B, et al: Repeated diazepam dosing in cirrhotic patients: cumulation and sedation. *Clin Pharmacol Ther* 33:471–476, 1983.

37. Coffey B, Shader RI, Greenblatt DJ: Pharmacokinetics of benzodiazepines and psychostimulants in children. *J Clin Psychopharmacol* 3:217–225, 1983.

38. Boston Collaborative Drug Surveillance Program: Clinical depression of the central nervous system due to diazepam and chlordiazepoxide in relation to cigarette smoking and age. *N Engl J Med* 288:277–280, 1973.

39. Reidenberg MM, Levy M, Warner H, et al: Relationship between diazepam dose, plasma level, age, and central nervous system depression. *Clin Pharmacol Ther* 23:371–374, 1978.

40. Elia J, Katz IR, Simpson GM: Teratogenicity of psychotherapeutic medications. *Psychopharmacol Bull* 23:531–586, 1987.

41. Cree JE, Meyer J, Hailey DM: Diazepam in labour: its metabolism and effect on the clinical condition and thermogenesis of the newborn. *Br Med J* 4:251–253, 1973.

42. Cole AP, Hailey DM: Diazepam and active metabolite in breast milk and their transfer to the neonate. *Arch Dis Child* 50:741–742, 1975.

▬ B ▬

Buspirone Database

FORMULATIONS

Buspirone tablets: 5 mg, 10 mg
Brand names: BuSpar (Mead-Johnson)

BASIC PHARMACOLOGY

Buspirone is a member of the azaspirodecanedione class of drugs (Fig. 4B.1). It is the first nonbenzodiazepine antianxiety drug to be introduced in decades. Buspirone is chemically unrelated to the benzodiazepines, barbiturates, β-adrenergic blockers, and other drugs that have been used as antianxiety agents. In contrast to the benzodiazepines, it lacks anticonvulsant and muscle-relaxant properties (1). In addition, it is less sedating than the benzodiazepines and no more than placebo. This is a useful clinical advantage as, theoretically, sedation and antianxiety effects are separate properties.

Buspirone has complex neurochemical effects, which raises important issues for pharmacologists. Since the discovery of high affinity receptors for benzodiazepines in the CNS and their linkage to GABA receptors (see Chapter 1B), it has been assumed that effective antianxiety drugs interact with these structures in vivo. In contrast to the benzodiazepine actions on GABA neurotransmission, buspirone only indirectly affects the GABA-benzodiazepine receptor complex (2). It has no effect on the in vitro binding of radiolabeled flunitrazepam or diazepam in rat brain tissue. However, pretreatment of rodents with buspirone in some experiments resulted in moderate increases in benzodiazepine receptor binding (3). Although the mechanism of buspirone's antianxiety effects cannot be ascribed to direct occupation of brain benzodiazepine receptors, buspirone may alter the apparent affinity and/or number of benzodiazepine and associated GABA receptors by an indirect mechanism. It seems to influence neurotransmission in a complex manner, involving serotoninergic, noradrenergic, and dopaminergic activity in the brain (see Chapter 1B). The drug has affinity for dopamine receptors, but its antianxiety effects more likely involve interactions with serotonin (5-HT)-1A receptors (2). Buspirone lacks direct effects on α_1, α_2, and β-adrenergic receptors in vitro and does not block the reuptake of catecholamines. Buspirone does not seem to alter monoamine oxidase activity. These actions imply that a complex process is involved in producing antianxiety effects. Elucidation of buspirone's mechanism of action should add substantially to our understanding of the physiological basis of anxiety.

Buspirone's actions on dopamine neurotransmission are thought to be responsible for increasing prolactin and growth hormone secretion (4). In normal daily doses, buspirone has little effect on physiological monitoring parameters. Its effects on sleep parameters are slight, but it may decrease total rapid eye movement (REM) time and increase REM onset time (5). Buspirone's

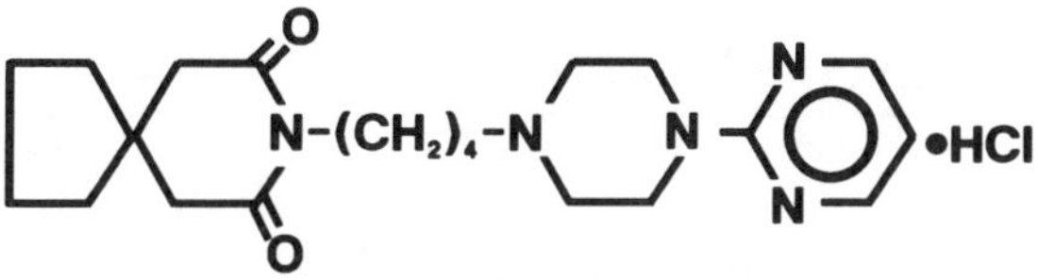

Figure 4B.1.   Structure of buspirone.

Table 4B.1.
Expected Physiological Effects from Buspirone Therapy for Monitoring[a]

Parameter	Drug Effect
Cardiovascular status	
Heart rate	Slight or no increase
ECG	No effects
Blood pressure	No effects
Renal function	
Serum creatinine and clearance, BUN	Normal values should not change in most adults.
Hepatic function	
AST (SGOT), ALT (SGPT), alkaline phosphatase	Normal values should not change. Infrequent increases in AST and ALT have occurred, usually in combination with trazodone.
Hematology status	
CBC	Normal values should not change. Rarely, eosinophilia, leukopenia, and thrombocytopenia have occurred.
Neuroendocrine status	
Cortisol	No effect expected
Growth hormone	Slight or no elevation
Prolactin	Dose-dependent elevations during therapy

[a]For abbreviations, see Table 4A.1.

expected effects on various physiological parameters and laboratory tests are outlined in Table 4B.1.

PHARMACOKINETIC PROPERTIES

Plasma concentrations of buspirone are low after oral administration. Single doses of 10 to 20 mg result in peak concentrations of less than 10 ng/ml. Thus, defining its kinetic profile has been difficult and only possible with sensitive analytical methods (6). The absorption of buspirone seems to be rapid, with peak concentrations usually occurring in 1 hour or less. During absorption, the drug seems to undergo an extensive presystemic elimination. The major metabolites are 5-hydroxybuspirone and 1-(2-pyrimidinyl)piperazine (1-PP). When taken with a meal, buspirone's plasma concentration is higher than when the drug is administered in a fasting state. This effect probably results from a decrease in first-pass metabolism mediated by the coadministration of food.

The 1-PP metabolite seems to be pharmacologically active (7). In animal studies, it exists in higher concentrations in plasma and brain than does buspirone (8). This observation suggests some contribution by 1-PP to the overall actions of buspirone. As discussed in Chapter 1D, defining the contribution of active

Table 4B.2.
Pharmacokinetic Parameters of Buspirone

Parameter	Range
Bioavailability	Well absorbed
Time of peak concentration after single dose	1 hour
Plasma protein binding	95%
Volume of distribution	5.3 ± 2.6 liters/kg
Total plasma clearance	1.7 ± 0.6 liters/hr/kg
Renal clearance	Negligible
Elimination half-life	2.4 ± 1 hr
Active metabolites	Pyrimidinylpiperazine (1-PP)
Steady-state metabolite to parent concentration ratio	Greater than 1.0
Therapeutic range for antianxiety effect	Not yet determined

metabolites to the actions of psychoactive drugs continues to be a major challenge to researchers in clinical psychopharmacology.

Buspirone is highly plasma protein-bound, approximately 95%, with binding to both albumin and α_1-acid glycoprotein (9). Thus, displacement interactions with coadministered drugs could be clinically important, although this issue has not received much research attention. The distribution of buspirone within animal tissues is extensive. Concentrations have been found to be higher in several organs of the rat compared to plasma. Buspirone's volume of distribution in healthy adults, averaging 5.3 liters/kg, suggests a broad distribution in humans outside of the systemic circulation.

Buspirone's elimination half-life averages 2 to 4 hours. Linearity can be assumed within the usual daily dose range, but half-life is likely to be prolonged in patients with either renal or hepatic impairment. The elimination half-life of 1-PP can be expected to be longer than that of buspirone and averages about 6 hours. A summary of buspirone's pharmacokinetic parameters is given in Table 4B.2.

INDICATIONS

Buspirone has been approved for the treatment of generalized anxiety disorder. Premarketing clinical trials demonstrated that buspirone was superior to placebo and as efficacious as standard benzodiazepines (diazepam or alprazolam) in the treatment of mild-to-moderate anxiety (10–12). Subtle differences between the benzodiazepines and buspirone in clinical trials suggest a basis for discrimination in drug selection for specific patients.

Compared to the benzodiazepines, buspirone may be more effective for anger and hostility associated with anxiety. Buspirone would be preferred in some patients with a history of aggression or loss of impulse control as disinhibition sometimes occurs with benzodiazepine use.

As buspirone has only a minimal effect in producing sedation, patients with psychomotor agitation may be better treated with a benzodiazepine. Also, for patients with a high degree of somatic anxiety and muscle tension, a benzodiazepine may be beneficial because of its sedative and muscle relaxant qualities.

For some patients who have never received an antianxiety drug, buspirone may be preferred because of its lack of sedation. Patients with a history of benzodiazepine use often have specific expectations from antianxiety therapy. These patients may become disappointed with buspirone's slow onset of therapeutic activity.

Buspirone has been shown in double-blind studies to be effective for relief of anxiety in the presence of depression (13); however, other data suggest that buspirone has equivocal effects as an antidepressant. At present, depression does not constitute an indication for buspirone. In anxious patients who do not respond adequately to buspirone therapy in several weeks, underlying depression should be suspected and treated specifically if found to exist.

Buspirone's dopaminergic activity would suggest possible beneficial effects for Parkinson's disease and schizophrenia (14, 15), disorders with a recognized pathophysiological basis involving dopamine. In limited studies, buspirone did not seem to have promising activity for either of these indications. Buspirone was tried in high doses, from 600 to 2400 mg/day, in 10 schizophrenic patients without success (15).

DOSAGE REGIMEN DESIGN

The recommended starting dose of buspirone is 15 mg daily divided into three dosage intervals. At intervals of 2 to 3 days, dosage may be increased at a rate of 5 mg/day up to a maximum of 60 mg/day. The most common dosage is 20 to 30 mg/day.

Compared to the benzodiazepines, buspirone has a slower onset of action. Optimal benefits may not accrue for 4 weeks or longer. However, demonstration of long-term benefits from buspirone therapy through controlled clinical trials is lacking. Although this situation also exists with the benzodiazepines, many anxious patients report benefit for longer than 4 months. Nevertheless, a reassessment of continued benefits should be made at regular intervals. Patients should be encouraged to develop coping strategies to deal with stress and to minimize the use of antianxiety agents.

The combination of psychological and pharmacological therapy for anxiety is more likely to benefit patients than either treatment alone. Buspirone therapy should be accompanied by supportive care, including education about the causes of anxiety and reassurance about the future.

THERAPEUTIC DRUG MONITORING

There have been no reports of plasma buspirone concentrations correlating with clinical effects. This situation is caused partly by a lack of suitable analytical methods that can be widely utilized in clinical practice. Traditionally, plasma monitoring of antianxiety drug concentrations has been of little value. The benzodiazepines have such a safe dose-response curve that plasma concentrations have been of limited utility in avoiding toxicity.

Monitoring buspirone therapy is by means of target symptoms of anxiety. Consideration should be given to duration, frequency, and intensity of symptoms. In the 1st week, some patients have noted an increased ability to concentrate and reduced worrying, irritability, and agitation. Rating scales such as the Hopkins Symptom Check List, which covers both psychological and somatic symptoms, may be of value. Effective monitoring of buspirone can be performed by careful clinical observation.

CONTRAINDICATIONS—WARNINGS—PRECAUTIONS

Most sedatives interact adversely with alcohol and other CNS depressants. Buspirone is an exception. Buspirone can cause drowsiness and fatigue, but these effects are usually minimal and caused no impairment of driving-related skills (16, 17). In addition, buspirone was found to lack euphoriant effects or addictive potential (18). Some patients may experience dizziness if single doses as high as 40 mg are taken. Buspirone may be preferred for patients who are likely to combine antianxiety therapy with depressants like alcohol.

For patients receiving benzodiazepines who are switched to buspirone, tapering of the benzodiazepine must be initiated as buspirone does not block benzodiazepine withdrawal symptoms. It is recommended that the same benzodiazepine dose be kept until buspirone has been titrated up to an acceptable daily dose, around 30 mg/day. At this time, the benzodiazepine dose can be slowly decreased. Similarly, when buspirone must be discontinued, tapering should also be instituted, although a specific withdrawal syndrome has not yet been described.

DRUG INTERACTIONS

The most important sedative-anxiolytic drug interactions are with alcohol. Buspirone does not seem to potentiate alcohol blood concentrations nor to enhance alcohol's cognitive and psychomotor impairment (17). Patients should still be advised not to combine CNS depressants with antianxiety therapy. This would include over-the-counter sedatives, antihistamines, and cough suppressants.

Buspirone has been reported to result in blood pressure elevations when combined with monoamine oxidase inhibitor therapy (phenelzine or tranylcypromine). Until this potential interaction is further investigated, it is prudent to avoid this drug combination (T Donosky, Mead-Johnson Pharmaceutical Company, personal communication, April 27, 1987).

Buspirone has been studied in combination with cimetidine (T Donosky, personal communication). This histamine receptor (H2) antagonist interferes with the hepatic metabolism of several psychoactive drugs, including imipramine and amitriptyline (19). Only a minimal effect by cimetidine on buspirone disposition has been noted. Generally, ranitidine is involved in far fewer drug interactions than cimetidine when an H2 antagonist must be combined with psychoactive drug therapy.

In a pharmacokinetic study of combined haloperidol and buspirone, serum haloperidol concentrations were significantly increased when the two drugs were administered concomitantly (T Donosky, personal communication). This interaction may be due to competitive inhibition of haloperidol dealkylation by buspirone. Addition of buspirone to the dosage regimen of patients receiving haloperidol should be performed cautiously with due consideration of the possibility of exaggerated antipsychotic drug effects. No reports of buspirone interactions with other antipsychotics have been published.

Depressed patients frequently demonstrate accompanying anxiety. Buspirone did not change either amitriptyline or nortriptyline steady-state plasma concentrations when combined with these antidepressants (T Donosky, personal communication). These drug combinations can apparently be used without concern of a pharmacokinetic interaction.

Table 4B.3.
Drug Interactions with Buspirone

Interacting Drug	Effect
Haloperidol	Buspirone may inhibit metabolism and raise haloperidol plasma concentrations.
Trazodone	The combination has resulted in elevation of hepatic enzymes, but no definite pharmacodynamic interaction has been noted. Attempts to replicate this interaction have not been successful.
Amitriptyline, nortriptyline	No kinetic or dynamic interaction reported
Monoamine oxidase inhibitors (phenelzine or tranylcypromine)	Elevations in blood pressure

Table 4B.4.
Expected Side Effects from Buspirone Therapy

Effect	Rare	Less Common	More Common
Gastrointestinal complaints			X
Nausea			X
Drowsiness		X	
Dizziness			X
Headache			X
Nervousness			X
Skin rash	X		
Sweating/clamminess		X	
Galactorrhea	X		

Overall, the significance of drug interactions with buspirone seems to be slight. A summary of current findings is given in Table 4B.3.

ADVERSE REACTIONS—OCCURRENCE AND MANAGEMENT

The side-effect profile of buspirone indicates a low incidence of side effects when compared to placebo or to benzodiazepines (20). The most frequent side effects are dizziness, headache, nausea, and (to a lesser degree) nervousness. Drowsiness is generally less than in patients receiving diazepam, lorazepam, or alprazolam. Table 4B.4 summarizes the expected side effects.

MANAGEMENT OF OVERDOSE

Overdosage with buspirone seems to be relatively safe, not dissimilar to the situation with the benzodiazepines. Due to buspirone's dopaminergic actions, overdoses could potentially produce extrapyramidal reactions. Supportive care should be given as no specific antidote is available.

USE IN RENAL AND/OR HEPATIC DISEASE

Liver disease has been shown to impair the metabolism of buspirone (21). In cirrhotic patients, the half-life was 6.1 hours compared to 3.2 hours in healthy controls. This effect was probably due to decreased hepatic clearance of buspirone and was reflected in an area under the curve after a single dose greater than 10-fold higher in cirrhotic men than in healthy volunteers. These data suggest that patients with significant liver disease should be dosed cautiously with buspirone, initially with reduced dosage.

Buspirone has also been reported to have a prolonged half-life in renal impairment, although this effect is unexpected because of its low degree of urinary excretion (22). Nevertheless, reduced dosage is recommended for these patients beginning buspirone therapy.

USE IN CHILDREN AND ADOLESCENTS

Studies using buspirone in children have not been reported, and this drug is not recommended for use in this population. Potential uses include aggression and agitation associated with pervasive developmental disorder, especially as buspirone does not cause ataxia. However, no reports have yet appeared of buspirone use in children.

USE IN ELDERLY

Buspirone's disposition has not been shown to be altered in the elderly as occurs with other psychoactive drugs. However, in tradition with geriatric prescribing, dosage should be started low, as much as a third of the usual adult dosage. As elderly patients have reduced renal and hepatic function, which accompanies ageing, there exists a physiological basis for recommending low starting doses. Maximal daily doses should not exceed 60 mg. Overall clinical experience suggests that many geriatric patients will experience no greater degree of side effects from buspirone therapy than do younger patients.

USE IN PREGNANCY

Buspirone has not produced evidence of teratogenesis in common animal studies utilitizing rats and rabbits. It is listed under the FDA pregnancy category B. For patients who plan to become pregnant during therapy, counseling should be performed about the uncertain risk of receiving any drug during gestation.

PATIENT INFORMATION

Patients should be told of the common side effects and warned about standing too quickly if dizziness becomes apparent during therapy. Realistic expectations from therapy should be discussed with patients and emphasis placed on avoiding a reliance upon drugs to offset normal stress. Patients should be instructed not to take more than the prescribed dosage and not to discontinue the drug abruptly without medical advice.

REFERENCES

1. Riblet LA, Taylor DP, Eison MS, et al: Pharmacology and neurochemistry of buspirone. *J Clin Psychiatry* 43:11–15, 1982.
2. Skolnick P, Paul SM, Weissman BA: Preclinical pharmacology of buspirone hydrochloride. *Pharmacotherapy* 4:308–314, 1984.
3. Goeders NE, Ritz MC, Kuhar MJ: Buspirone enhances benzodiazepine receptor binding in vivo. *Neuropharmacology* 27:275–280, 1988.
4. Meltzer HY, Flemming R, Robertson A: The effect of buspirone on prolactin and growth hormone secretion in man. *Arch Gen Psychiatry* 40:1099–1102, 1983.
5. Seidel WJ, Cohen SA, Bliwise NG, et al: Buspirone: an anxiolytic without sedative effect. *Psychopharmacology* 87:371–373, 1985.

6. Gammans RE, Mayol RJ, Labudde JA, et al: Metabolic fate of 14C/15N-buspirone in man. *Fed Proc* 41:1335, 1982.
7. Bianchi G, Garattini S: Blockade of alpha-2-adrenoceptors by 1-(2-pyrimidinyl)-piperazine in vivo and its relation to the activity of buspirone. *Eur J Pharmacol* 147:343–350, 1988.
8. Caccia S, Conti I, Vigano G, et al: 1(2-Pyrimidinyl)-piperazine, an active metabolite of buspirone in man and rat. *Pharmacology* 33:46–51, 1986.
9. Bullen WW, Bivens DL, Gammans RE, et al: The binding of buspirone to human plasma proteins. *Fed Proc* 44:1123, 1985.
10. Rickels K, Weisman K, Norstad N, et al: Buspirone and diazepam in anxiety: a controlled study. *J Clin Psychiatry* 43:81–86, 1982.
11. Feighner JP, Merideth CH, Hendrickson GA: A double-blind comparison of buspirone and diazepam in outpatients with generalized anxiety disorder. *J Clin Psychiatry* 43:103–107, 1982.
12. Goldberg GL, Finnerty RJ: The comparative efficacy of buspirone and diazepam in the treatment of anxiety. *Am J Psychiatry* 136:1184–1187, 1979.
13. Riblet LA, Eison AS, Eison MS, Newton RE, Taylor DP, Temple DL Jr: Buspirone: an anxioselective alternative for the management of anxiety disorders. *Prog Neuropsychopharmacol Biol Psychiatry* 7:663–668, 1983.
14. Ludwig CL, Weinberger DR, Bruno G, et al: Buspirone, Parkinson's disease and the locus coeruleus. *Clin Neuropharmacol* 9:373–378, 1986.
15. Sathananthan GL, Sanbghvi I, Phillips N, et al: NJM 9022: correlation between neuroleptic potential and stereotypy. *Curr Ther Res* 18:701–705, 1975.
16. Mattila MJ, Aranko K, Seppala T: Acute effects of buspirone and alcohol on psychomotor skills. *J Clin Psychiatry* 43:56–60, 1982.
17. Moskowitz H, Smiley A: Effects of chronically administered buspirone and diazepam on driving related skills performance. *J Clin Psychiatry* 43:45–55, 1982.
18. Cole JO, Orzack MH, Beake B, et al: Assessment of the abuse liability of buspirone in recreational sedative users. *J Clin Psychiatry* 43:69–74, 1982.
19. Curry SH, DeVane CL, Wolfe MM: Cimetidine interactions with amitriptyline. *Eur J Clin Pharmacol* 29:429–433, 1985.
20. Newton RE, Marunycz JD, Alderdice MT, Napoliello MJ: Review of the side-effect profile of buspirone. *Am J Med* 80(suppl 3B):17–21, 1986.
21. Dalhoff K, Poulsen HE, Garred P, Placchi M, Gammans RE, Mayol RF, Pfeffer M: Buspirone pharmacokinetics in patients with cirrhosis. *Br J Clin Pharmacol* 24:547–550, 1987.
22. Gammans RE, Mayol RF, Labudde JA: Metabolism and disposition of buspirone. *Am J Med* 80:41–51, 1986.

C

Intraclass Comparisons of Anxiolytics

Numerous clinical trials have demonstrated the benzodiazepines' efficacy in reducing excessive anxiety. These drugs have consistently been found to be superior to placebo. On the basis of their comparative efficacy, it is difficult to choose one benzodiazepine as best for all patients. They have more similarities than differences. The choice of a particular benzodiazepine is based on the patient's therapeutic needs, pharmacokinetic considerations, and other factors,

Table 4C.1.
Pharmacological Comparison of Benzodiazepines

Basis of Comparison	Clinical Implication
Intrinsic potency	Partly determines differences in daily milligram dose administered to achieve equivalent antianxiety effects (see Chapter 1C)
Absorption rate	Rate-limiting step for entry of drug into the brain; affects onset of acute clinical effects. The greater the lipid solubility, the faster the rate and onset of action.
Plasma protein binding	The smaller the fraction bound in plasma, the greater the amount of drug available to diffuse into the brain.
Volume of distribution	Along with clearance, one of the two major determinants of half-life; a reflection of the extent of drug distribution beyond the systemic circulation (see Chapter 1D).
Hepatic clearance	Determines the extent of drug accumulation at steady state; along with volume of distribution, determines the half-life and therefore the time to achieve steady state and time for drug to wash out of the body after stopping therapy; relates to duration of action (see Chapter 1D)
Predominant metabolism by oxidative pathways (phase I)	Production of active metabolites; predicts prolonged half-lives in elderly, greater likelihood of some drug interactions and influence on disposition from liver disease
Predominant metabolism by conjugation pathways (phase II)	Less influence from ageing, smoking, liver disease, enzyme inhibitors on elimination rate

which include availability of dosage forms, assessment of patient compliance, and medication cost.

The benzodiazepines have major differences in their physiochemical and pharmacokinetic properties. Table 4C.1 summarizes these properties. The factors listed are largely interdependent and are discussed below as they relate to selection of rational drug therapy. The benzodiazepines marketed as anxiolytics in the United States are listed in Table 4C.2. Some additional drugs used as anxiolytics from other pharmacological classes are discussed below.

INTRINSIC POTENCY

This concept is described in Chapter 1C. The potency of various benzodiazepines is determined primarily by their inherent ability to interact with receptors. The various benzodiazepines seem to bind at the same sites in the brain but with different affinities. Differences in potency are reflected in the average daily doses required to produce antianxiety effects (Table 4C.2).

Benzodiazepine potency is a relatively unimportant characteristic because it makes little difference whether 2 or 20 mg of a drug is administered to achieve the same pharmacological effect. This is especially true when side effect profiles

Table 4C.2.
Benzodiazepine Anxiolytics and Their Usual Daily Oral Doses

Medication	Brand Names	Daily Dose Range (mg)
Alprazolam	Xanax	1–4
Clorazepate	Tranxene	15–60
Chlordiazepoxide	Librium, other generics	15–60
Diazepam	Valium, other generics	4–40
Halazepam	Paxipam	60–160
Lorazepam	Ativan	1–6
Oxazepam	Serax, other generics	10–120
Prazepam	Centrax	20–60

of different drugs in the same class are similar, as is the case with most of the drugs in this class. Within other psychoactive drug classes, particularly the antipsychotics, side effect profiles differ substantially and potency becomes an important basis for drug selection.

Regardless of potency differences, pharmacokinetic determinants of the amount of a drug that is available at receptor sites and the duration of its availability can strongly affect efficacy. Thus, kinetic differences are a primary basis for drug selection. For example, benzodiazepines have frequently been considered as either "long"- or "short"-acting compounds. However, when given in an appropriate dosage regimen to minimize kinetic differences, the benzodiazepines do not consistently differ from each other in the ability to reduce the symptoms of anxiety globally (1).

ABSORPTION RATE

Lipid solubility is one of the major determinants of benzodiazepine absorption rate (2). As discussed in Chapter 1D, most drugs are absorbed from the proximal small intestine by passive diffusion. All of the anxiolytic benzodiazepines possess enough lipid solubility to be nearly totally absorbed after oral administration, even though the various drugs possess different rates of absorption.

The onset of antianxiety effects after single doses correlates with benzodiazepine absorption rate. The time that peak concentration occurs in the blood varies with different drugs between 30 minutes and 4 hours. Relative absorption rates and other pharmacokinetic parameters are listed in Table 4C.3. The most rapidly absorbed drugs are diazepam and clorazepate. Drugs that have an intermediate absorption rate include lorazepam and chlordiazepoxide, and the most slowly absorbed are prazepam, oxazepam, and halazepam.

As expected, diazepam produces subjective effects soon after administration, usually within 30 minutes. This can be a clinical advantage when immediate effects are sought from an oral dosage form. This allows diazepam to be an effective "prn" drug, administered as needed, despite its long half-life. When rapid onset of effects is unimportant relative to how long antianxiety effects last after each dose, elimination rate becomes a greater consideration in choosing among the various drugs.

Nearly all drugs are best absorbed on an empty stomach. The presence of food or antacid in the gastrointestinal tract can moderate drug absorption. The effects of coadministered antacid can be considered with the example of clorazepate (3). This prodrug, which is inactive in its administered dosage form, is converted to desmethyldiazepam in the stomach before absorption. This pro-

Table 4C.3.
Pharmacokinetic Parameters of Various Benzodiazepines

Drug	Absorption Rate	Half-life (hours)	Active Metabolites in Plasma	Metabolite Half-life (hours)
Drugs Undergoing Phase I Metabolism				
Clorazepate	Rapid	—[a]	Desmethyldiazepam	36–96
Diazepam	Rapid	20–70	Desmethyldiazepam	36–96
Alprazolam	Intermediate	6–16		
Chlordiazepoxide	Intermediate	5–30	Desmethylchlordiazepoxide	10–30
			Demoxazepam	30–80
			Desmethyldiazepam	36–96
Halazepam	Intermediate to slow	14–35	Desmethyldiazepam	36–96
Prazepam	Slow	—[a]	Desmethyldiazepam	36–96
Drugs Undergoing Phase II Metabolism				
Lorazepam	Intermediate	10–20		
Oxazepam	Intermediate to slow	5–15		
Temazepam	Slow	8–20		

[a]Prodrug not present in plasma.

cess occurs by hydrolysis, that is, splitting of the administered prodrug into fragments by the addition of water. Clorazepate's hydrolysis is dependent upon gastrointestinal pH. The lower the pH, the faster the hydrolysis. Therefore, an increased pH beyond normal could decrease the liberation of desmethyldiazepam. In a comparison of the kinetics of clorazepate administered with and without magnesium-aluminum hydroxide antacid, the presence of antacid reduced the rate and extent of appearance in blood of desmethyldiazepam, the active form of clorazepate. Thus, in patients taking antacids along with clorazepate, attenuated clinical effects could be expected. Antacids taken with other benzodiazepines may decrease the rate but not necessarily the extent of their absorption (4, 5).

The presence of food in the stomach has been shown to decrease the rate of diazepam absorption into the circulation (4). The time for peak diazepam plasma concentration to occur was delayed when the drug was taken with a meal, and the maximal plasma concentration was decreased. However, no reduction was observed in the area under the plasma concentration-time curve during the study period. This finding implies that the extent of absorption was unchanged (see Chapter 1D).

The clinical implication of absorption rate is that, when a benzodiazepine is needed for antianxiety effects in an acutely stressful situation, a rapidly absorbed drug may be of clinical advantage (Table 4C.3). The presence of food or antacid may blunt drug effectiveness by decreasing absorption rate. However, if the extent of drug absorption is not decreased, coadministration of food should have little impact on clinical effects during long-term therapy.

VOLUME OF DISTRIBUTION

The benzodiazepines are widely distributed in the body. The extent of distribution is another characteristic influenced by lipid solubility (6). Diazepam is the most lipid-soluble of these drugs. The practical result of this property after oral absorption is for diazepam to be quickly distributed to the brain. The onset of clinical effects occurs more rapidly after a single diazepam dose than, for example, with lorazepam, which is less lipid-soluble (7). However, rapid distribution of diazepam also occurs from the CNS to peripheral tissues. This redistribution results in an earlier termination of action after a single diazepam dose than for less lipid-soluble benzodiazepines like oxazepam and lorazepam (2).

In summary, rapid drug absorption and distribution to the CNS may cause clinical effects such as drowsiness, dizziness, or feelings of well-being to be felt quickly after single doses of highly lipid-soluble benzodiazepines like diazepam or clorazepate; however, their plasma concentrations fall rapidly because of extensive tissue distribution, which diminishes clinical effects. Less rapidly distributed drugs like alprazolam or lorazepam may result in clinical effects persisting for a longer time after single doses. Upon chronic dosing, however, clinical effects are largely a function of elimination rate. The slower the clearance and the longer the half-life, the greater the accumulation and persistence of clinical effects, even after discontinuing therapy. The drugs listed in Table 4C.3 that produce desmethyldiazepam as a metabolite should all have sustained anxiolytic effects throughout the day during chronic therapy and for several days after therapy is discontinued.

PLASMA PROTEIN BINDING

Knowledge of the extent of plasma protein binding is of limited value in choosing a benzodiazepine even though a broad variability, over a 30% difference, exists in the free fraction in plasma. The degree of protein binding seems to be independent of drug concentration (2). This means that increasing the dose of any of these medicines will not result in an increase in the free fraction of drug in plasma. Therefore, increases in dose produce a proportional increase in free drug in plasma and in the amount of drug available at receptor sites. Protein binding considerations can generally be ignored in choosing a benzodiazepine for therapy.

HEPATIC CLEARANCE

The benzodiazepines are eliminated from the body almost entirely by hepatic metabolism. Renal clearance of these drugs in their unchanged form is minimal. As discussed in Chapter 1D, the clearance of a drug determines its extent of accumulation at steady state. Although this knowledge alone is not useful in selecting a particular benzodiazepine, it is useful to know for which drugs clearance is altered by the presence of disease states, advanced age, drug interactions, or environmental factors.

Generally, liver disease and ageing are associated with decreases in the clearance of most drugs. Some benzodiazepines are affected more than others. Those metabolized by phase I reactions, explained below, can be expected to show the most pronounced changes. Those drugs metabolized by phase II reactions show the least influence from ageing and hepatic impairment. A change in clearance, without a change in volume of distribution, will result in a proportional change in drug half-life in the opposite direction (see equation 17, Chapter 1D). The half-life of a benzodiazepine is relevant in determining how soon anxiety recurs or withdrawal symptoms appear after drug therapy is discontinued.

PREDOMINANT METABOLIC PATHWAYS

Drug metabolism can be divided into two stages called phase I and phase II. *Phase I metabolism* refers to biotransformations that are mostly oxidations or reductions, that is, functional groups on drug molecules are altered in some fashion. Some examples include N-dealkylations, hydroxylation of carbon atoms, deaminations, or hydrolysis of esters or ethers. *Phase II metabolism* refers to processes that are synthetic in nature, that is, functional groups are added to the drug molecule. Examples include methylation reactions, acetylations, and formation of conjugates. Conjugation reactions occur mostly by the combining of drug molecules with either sulfate or glucuronic acid. These reactions occur mostly in the liver.

Many drug metabolites, having been first formed by phase I reactions, undergo phase II reactions and are then excreted into the bile or are renally cleared. One of the major functions of drug metabolism is to make molecules more water-soluble (less lipid-soluble), which facilitates renal excretion either by glomerular filtration, renal tubular secretion, or both of these mechanisms.

The majority of drugs are first oxidized by phase I reactions. For four of the major benzodiazepines (diazepam, clorazepate, chlordiazepoxide, and halazepam), this biotransformation step results in the generation of an active metabolite, N-desmethyldiazepam. The significance of this metabolite is that it has a far longer half-life (ranging from 36 to 96 hours) than has its precursor (8, 9). Thus, clinical effects after dosing with these drugs persist longer than would be expected on the basis of the parent drug's half-life.

Three of the benzodiazepines (lorazepam, oxazepam, and temazepam) undergo phase II reactions only, first being conjugated with glucuronic acid and then excreted in the urine. Active metabolites are not produced because glucuronide conjugation is believed to be an inactivating process. Therefore, phase II metabolites in plasma do not complicate the assessment of drugs' clinical effects. Compared to the other benzodiazepines that produce phase I metabolites, lorazepam, oxazepam, and temazepam participate in fewer drug interactions and are less subject to the enzyme-inducing effects from smoking and the decreased metabolic ability that accompanies advanced age or liver disease. Each of these factors is further considered below.

ADDITIONAL FACTORS INFLUENCING DRUG SELECTION AND DOSAGE REGIMEN DESIGN

Tobacco smoke contains over 3000 chemicals. Smoking allows nicotine and various aromatic hydrocarbon byproducts to be absorbed into the systemic circulation. These compounds then cause hepatic microsomal enzyme induction, thereby enhancing the ability of the liver to metabolize many drugs (10). Thus, some drugs will demonstrate shorter half-lives in smokers compared to nonsmokers. In the Boston Collaborative Drug Surveillance Program, smokers treated with diazepam experienced less drowsiness than nonsmokers receiving the drug (11). These data suggest that a faster disposition of diazepam in smokers was accompanied by reduced clinical effects.

In general, the effect of smoking on drug disposition is greater for drugs that undergo primarily phase I metabolism than for drugs undergoing only conjugation (phase II) reactions (Table 4C.3). Accordingly, the disposition of oxazepam, lorazepam, and temazepam should be less affected by smoking than that of other benzodiazepines.

Table 4C.4.
Effects of Ageing on Half-life of Some Benzodiazepines

	Half-life (hours)	
Drug	Healthy Adults	Elderly
Alprazolam	6–16	12–27
Diazepam	20–70	30–200
Desmethyldiazepam	36–96	45–200
Flurazepam (desalkylflurazepam)	35–150	70–290
Oxazepam	5–15	5–20

Advanced age is widely appreciated to be accompanied by a general decrease in the ability to metabolize and eliminate many drugs. This applies to the benzodiazepines (12). The impact of ageing is more pronounced for the benzodiazepines metabolized by phase I reactions than those metabolized by phase II processes. Both the half-life of diazepam and that of desmethyldiazepam, its principle active metabolite, are prolonged in elderly patients (13, 14). Age has a minimal effect on elimination half-life of oxazepam or temazepam (14, 15). Advanced age implies that diazepam, flurazepam, and other highly metabolized benzodiazepines should be given to the elderly in initially smaller doses to avoid enhanced CNS depression. Examples of the effect of ageing on benzodiazepine kinetics are given in Table 4C.4.

Several drugs interact with benzodiazepines to alter their elimination from the body. One of the most thoroughly studied interactions occurs with histamine-2 (H2) receptor blockers. Cimetidine, the prototype drug in this class, acts as a hepatic enzyme inhibitor to prolong the elimination and effects of drugs metabolized by phase I reactions. Cimetidine's inhibitory effects on phase II processes are far less prominent. Combining cimetidine and oxazepam, for example, would be less likely to result in altered pharmacokinetics or prolonged clinical effects from usual doses of oxazepam than the combination of cimetidine with diazepam (16). Even though the kinetics of benzodiazepines may be substantially altered by cimetidine, the large therapeutic index of these drugs suggests that, in usual doses, the cimetidine-benzodiazepine interaction would have minimal clinical importance (17). In the elderly or in patients on relatively high doses, monitoring for prolonged clinical effects may be useful in determining the need for a downward adjustment of dosage when these drugs are combined. Ranitidine, another H2 antagonist, is less likely to interfere with the disposition of any of the benzodiazepines compared to cimetidine (18).

Disulfiram interferes with the metabolism of benzodiazepines. This interaction is discussed in Chapter 6A. Such a drug combination may occasionally be used in the treatment of chronic alcohol abuse. Diazepam, chlordiazepoxide, and probably other benzodiazepines eliminated through phase I reactions seem to be especially affected; their elimination rate is prolonged (19). Less effect can be expected from disulfiram combined with oxazepam. Thus, the depressant effects of benzodiazepines on the CNS might be further enhanced by combination therapy with disulfiram and any of the drugs metabolized by phase I reactions.

Liver disease is a factor with differential effects on benzodiazepine kinetics. Phase I processes seem to be more susceptible to compromise in alcoholic liver disease than conjugation reactions. Patients with cirrhosis of the liver can be expected to show more pronounced clinical sedation when treated with diazepam (20). Oxazepam kinetics have been shown to be less affected by liver disease (21). When using a benzodiazepine in a patient with chronic liver disease, the initial dose should be reduced, especially if using one of the drugs with oxidatively formed active metabolites (Table 4C.3).

Recognition of the psychological and physical dependence properties of the benzodiazepines is well established (22). Predisposing factors include length of therapy and high dosage. Seizures secondary to benzodiazepine withdrawal are generally associated with long-term, high dose usage. However, even in relatively low therapeutic dosage, withdrawal symptoms may appear after abrupt discontinuation. A mild abstinence syndrome may occur, consisting of subjective symptoms of anxiety and flu-like symptoms. The shorter the drug's half-life, the earlier this discontinuation syndrome is seen (23). Thus, the rate of fall of plasma concentrations of administered drug and active metabolites after therapy is stopped relates to the time of onset of a withdrawal syndrome. A tapering of one-eight to one-fourth of the daily dose every 1 to 2 weeks is recommended for patients who have received daily therapy with a benzodiazepine for more than 2 months. Normal-dose dependency can and does occur. The shorter the drug's half-life, the more care should be taken in discontinuing therapy.

INDIVIDUAL AGENTS

Alprazolam

Among the benzodiazepines, alprazolam has the most proven effectiveness for treatment of panic disorder (24). Clonazepam ranks second, and only limited data exist for the efficacy of diazepam. The usual effective oral daily dose range of alprazolam for anxiety is 1 to 4 mg/day but, for effective treatment of panic disorder, the daily dosage may range up to 6 mg/day. Pharmacokinetic studies suggest that alprazolam should be effective when administered sublingually as the completeness of absorption has been shown to be similar to that with the oral route. This may be useful information for an occasional patient.

Alprazolam is also distinguished by having shown effectiveness for depression and anxiety associated with depression (25). Several multicenter trials found it to be equivalent in many standard measures to cyclic antidepressants. However, the dosage at which antidepressant effects occur, in the range of 4 to 8 mg/day, is generally higher than doses needed for anxiolytic effects.

Alprazolam has been the most thoroughly studied benzodiazepine for antidepressant effects. The possibility exists that other benzodiazepines may also be useful for depression. Adinazolam, another triazolobenzodiazepine, is currently in clinical trials for this indication.

The moderate half-life of alprazolam, in the range of 6 to 16 hours, means that plasma concentrations will fall substantially during a twice daily dosage schedule. This has led to the reemergence of panic symptoms in some patients. Thus, a more frequent dosage schedule may be necessary to maintain the duration of action. Monitoring of daily symptoms (Chapter 1F) will help determine this need.

Like the other benzodiazepines, alprazolam has been implicated as causing withdrawal symptoms when therapy is stopped. There is controversy as to whether alprazolam may be worse than other benzodiazepines in this characteristic (26). The drug should be tapered when discontinued to minimize these effects. Some patients could benefit from overlap with another, long-acting benzodiazepine when discontinuing alprazolam. Diazepam, in a dosage of 10 mg/day for each 1 mg of alprazolam per day, has been recommended with a tapering schedule of 10 mg weekly. Clonazepam (half-life of 45 hours) has proven successful for this situation. Any of the benzodiazepines with long half-lives should help in discontinuing alprazolam. A preferred approach is to use a slow tapering schedule, decreasing the daily dose by only 0.5 mg/week. This usually avoids withdrawal problems in most patients. However, anxiety disorders such as panic disorder are chronic in their clinical course, and reemergence of symptoms may occur during the attempt to discontinue drug therapy. Buspirone will not suppress benzodiazepine withdrawal symptoms and cannot be used for this purpose.

Buspirone

Buspirone is discussed in detail in Chapter 4B. It is the first drug to be marketed from the class of azaspirodecanediones. It may have a slower onset of anxiolytic activity than the benzodiazepines, but it has clinical advantages by participating in fewer drug interactions and possessing minimal dependence potential and low sedating effects when compared to the benzodiazepines.

Clonidine

Clonidine is an α_2-agonist marketed as an antihypertensive drug. It has been useful in clinical psychopharmacology for moderating the withdrawal from opiate addiction (27). It has been proposed as a treatment for various mental disorders, including schizophrenia, Korsakoff's psychosis, tardive dyskinesia, obsessive-compulsive disorder, and Gilles de la Tourette syndrome, and for reduction of the craving for alcohol, nicotine, and cocaine (28). Most studies have found limited effectiveness for these indications. Studies of clonidine in panic anxiety have suggested only a moderate effect (29). A tolerance to its benefits has also been noted with a decrease in efficacy over time.

There are theoretical reasons for manipulating the noradrenergic system in anxiety disorders (30), and clonidine is likely to continue to be investigated as a psychopharmacological agent. Its physiological effects for monitoring are summarized in Table 4C.5.

The use of clonidine is complicated by side effects. Most prominent are those affecting the cardiovascular system. Mean arterial blood pressure will decrease during therapy. Frequent side effects include sedation, dry mouth, and constipation. Less frequent effects are changes in sleep patterns, nightmares, headaches, and disturbances in sexual function. Of concern is the rebound in blood pressure that may occur upon abrupt discontinuation of clonidine. Within 12 to 24 hours after stopping the drug, restlessness, irritability, and tremor may occur. Behavioral symptoms such as anxiety and nervousness have been noted. Rapid withdrawal should be avoided by tapering the drug when stopping therapy.

Clorazepate

As a prodrug for desmethyldiazepam, clorazepate would not seem to have any distinct advantage over diazepam. An occasional patient who may be sensitive to the early subjective effects of diazepam may be suitably treated with clorazepate. Because of its long half-life, its use in elderly patients should be accompanied by smaller initial doses and less frequent dosage adjustments (9).

Table 4C.5.
Expected Physiological Effects from Clonidine Therapy for Monitoring[a]

Parameter	Drug Effect
Cardiovascular status	
Heart rate	Decrease within 30 minutes after oral dose, peak at 2 hours, lasting 24 to 36 hours
Blood pressure	Decrease in systolic and diastolic
	Rebound hypertension if drug is abruptly stopped
ECG	Rare A-V block; digitalis may predispose patients to this effect.
Renal function	
Serum creatinine and clearance, BUN	Normal values should not change.
Hepatic function	
AST (SGOT), ALT (SGPT), alkaline phosphatase	Transient increases during therapy
Hematology status	
CBC	No changes expected
Neuroendocrine status	
Cortisol	No changes expected
Other observations	Acute and sustained decreases in plasma epinephrine and norepinephrine

[a]For abbreviations, see Table 4A.1. A-V, atrioventricular.

Chlordiazepoxide

This drug has been widely promoted for use in alcohol withdrawal. Its availability in a parenteral dosage form has been useful but, based on pharmacodynamic and pharmacokinetic considerations, there exists no particular reason why chlordiazepoxide should have any superior effects in moderating drug withdrawal symptoms over other moderate to long-acting benzodiazepines. Oral halazepam has also been found to be effective. When given by intramuscular injection, the absorption of chlordiazepoxide can be slow and erratic (31). Its moderate half-life with a range of 5 to 30 hours in healthy young adults is extended in liver disease to greater than 60 hours (32).

Diazepam

Diazepam is the prototype benzodiazepine and is discussed in Chapter 4A. It is an extremely useful drug available in a variety of dosage forms. Because it has been discussed so much in the lay press, patients may have developed distinct opinions of it and even fear its dependence-producing potential. These patients should be reassured about the goals and expectations of pharmacotherapy.

Halazepam

This drug is slowly absorbed, with peak concentrations occurring in about 2 hours (33). Thus, its acute effects may be delayed compared to other, more rapidly absorbed drugs in its class. Halazepam may have a lower abuse potential compared to diazepam because its peak intensity and onset of effects are slower. Halazepam is similar in structure to diazepam and produces the same metabolite, desmethyldiazepam. It has been suggested to cause minimal, paradoxical reactions of hostility compared to other benzodiazepines (34). The evidence for this advantage is minimal and without supportive data from controlled clinical trials.

Hydroxyzine

Hydroxyzine is an antihistamine that is sometimes used in place of a benzodiazepine as a sedative in alcohol-dependent patients. Many clinicians wisely avoid the use of any drug with dependence-producing properties in alcoholics and patients with a history of substance abuse. Hydroxyzine and another commonly used antihistamine, diphenhydramine, do not have dependence-producing properties, although clinical experience suggests that some patients abuse diphenhydramine to produce an anticholinergic delirium. These drugs may have only slight anxiolytic effects, far less than the benzodiazepines, and at doses causing relatively high sedation.

Lorazepam

An advantage of lorazepam is that it is conjugated and excreted in the urine as its major pathway of elimination (7). Thus, its disposition is minimally affected by ageing, drug interactions, or liver disease. It is the only benzodiazepine that is principally metabolized by phase II processes available for parenteral and intravenous administration. Lorazepam, like clonazepam, is becoming favored as a benzodiazepine alternative to neuroleptics in the treatment of manic agitation. It may also be occasionally useful to treat neuroleptic-induced akathisia.

Lorazepam may cause similar or more severe anterograde amnesia than that caused by other benzodiazepines. This effect on memory can be an advantage when a benzodiazepine is used as a premedication before surgery or endoscopic procedures. There seems to be no adverse effect on recall of material previously learned. Lorazepam causes impairment in a variety of laboratory-administered performance tests, effects that are counteracted by caffeine. Memory problems can occur with other benzodiazepines (for example, diazepam), and they seem to be more frequent with parenteral administration and rare with oral dosing. Overall, lorazepam is a suitable benzodiazepine for many anxious patients.

Midazolam

This is a short-acting benzodiazepine (half-life, 1 to 4 hours), available only for intravenous use as a preanesthetic.

Oxazepam

Oxazepam seems to be especially useful in patients with liver disease or when other factors are present that would alter phase I metabolism (12). Unfortunately, oxazepam is not available in a parenteral dosage form. Oxazepam seems to have some advantages over diazepam in the management of anxiety in the elderly because of its lack of accumulation (14).

Prazepam

Prazepam and clorazepate are prodrugs for desmethyldiazepam (8, 9). Prazepam is converted to desmethyldiazepam by dealkylation in the liver, a process that results in slower appearance of desmethyldiazepam in the blood than gastrointestinal hydrolysis of clorazepate. This difference provides a basis for a choice between these drugs. Both drugs would be expected to provide a long duration of action, but initially perceived clinical effects will vary.

Propranolol

β-Adrenergic blockers are sometimes used in anxiety disorders with the belief that blocking the peripheral manifestations of anxiety, such as tachycardia and tremor, will alleviate the subjective impression of anxiety. Propranolol has been the most widely used β-blocker in this regard. Social phobias such as stage fright or fear of public speaking may show good response, but, overall, β-adrenergic blockers have only minimal anxiolytic effects compared to the benzodiazepines.

Frequent side effects include sedation, feelings of lethargy and fatigue, and impaired concentration. Less common side effects are sleep disturbances, nightmares, and depressed mood. Less lipid-soluble β-blockers such as metoprolol or atenolol are sometimes substituted for propranolol. This would presumably minimize CNS side effects. However, the various β-blockers can all enter the CNS, although at different rates according to their lipid solubility.

REFERENCES

1. Greenblatt DD, Shader RI: *Benzodiazepines in Clinical Practice*, Raven Press, New York, 1974.
2. Greenblatt DJ, Shader RI: Pharmacokinetics of antianxiety agents. In: *Psychopharmacology: The Third Generation of Progress*, Meltzer HY (ed), Raven Press, New York, 1987, pp 1377–1386.
3. Shader RI, Georgotas A, Greenblatt DJ, et al: Impaired absorption of desmethyldiazepam from clorazepate by magnesium aluminum hydroxide. *Clin Pharmacol Ther* 24:308–315, 1978.
4. Greenblatt DJ, Allen MD, MacLaughlin DS, et al: Diazepam absorption: effect of antacids and food. *Clin Pharmacol Ther* 24:600–609, 1978.
5. Greenblatt DF, Shader RI, Harmatz BA, Franke K, Koch-Weser J: Influence of magnesium and aluminum hydroxide mixture on chlordiazepoxide absorption. *Clin Pharmacol Ther* 19:234–239, 1976.
6. Arendt RM, Greenblatt DJ, Divoll M, et al: Predicting in vivo benzodiazepine distribution based on in vitro lipophilicity. *Clin Pharmacol Ther* 31:200–201, 1982.
7. Ameer B, Greenblatt DJ: Lorazepam: a review of its clinical pharmacological properties and therapeutic uses. *Drugs* 21:161–200, 1981.
8. Allen ME, Greenblatt DJ, Harmatz JS, Shader RI: Desmethyldiazepam kinetics in the elderly after oral prazepam. *Clin Pharmacol Ther* 28:196–202, 1980.
9. Shader RI, Greenblatt DJ, Ciraulo DA, Divoll M, Harmatz JS, Georgotas A: Effect of age and sex on disposition of desmethyldiazepam formed from its precursor clorazepate. *Psychopharmacology* 75:193–197, 1981.
10. Jusko WJ: Influence of cigarette smoking on drug metabolism in man. *Drug Metab Rev* 9:221–236, 1979.
11. Boston Collaborative Drug Surveillance Program: Clinical depression of the central nervous system due to diazepam and chlordiazepoxide in relation to cigarette smoking and age. *N Engl J Med* 288:277–280, 1973.
12. Wilkinson GR: Effects of aging on the disposition of benzodiazepines in human beings: binding and distribution considerations. In: *Age and the Pharmacology of Psychoactive Drugs*, Raskin A, Robinson DS, Levine J (eds), Elsevier, New York, 1981, pp 3–15.
13. Greenblatt DJ, Allen MD, Harmatz JS, Shader RI: Diazepam disposition determinants. *Clin Pharmacol Ther* 27:301–312, 1980.
14. Salzman C, Shader RI, Greenblatt DJ, Harmatz JS: Long v. short half-life benzodiazepines in the elderly: kinetics and clinical effects of diazepam and oxazepam in the elderly. *Arch Gen Psychiatry* 40:293–297, 1983.

15. Divoll M, Greenblatt DJ, Harmatz JS, et al: Effect of age and gender on disposition of temazepam. *J Pharm Sci* 70:1104–1107, 1981.
16. Klotz U, Reimann I: Influence of cimetidine on the pharmacokinetics of desmethyldiazepam and oxazepam. *Eur J Clin Pharmacol* 18:517–520, 1980.
17. Greenblatt DJ, Abernethy DR, Morse DS, Harmatz JS, Shader RI: Clinical importance of the interaction of diazepam and cimetidine. *N Engl J Med* 310:1639–1643, 1984.
18. Abernethy DR, Greenblatt DJ, Eshelman FN, Shader RI: Ranitidine does not impair oxidative or conjugative metabolism: noninteraction with antipyrine, diazepam, and lorazepam. *Clin Pharmacol Ther* 35:188–192, 1984.
19. MacLeod SM, Sellers EM, Giles HG, Billings BJ, Martin PR, Greenblatt DJ, Marshman JA: Interaction of disulfiram with benzodiazepines. *Clin Pharmacol Ther* 24:583–589, 1978.
20. Ochs HR, Greenblatt DJ, Eckardt B, Harmatz JS, Shader RI: Repeated diazepam dosing in cirrhotic patients: cumulation and sedation. *Clin Pharmacol Ther* 33:471–476, 1983.
21. Sellers EM, Greenblatt DJ, Giles HG, Naranjo CA, Kaplan H, MacLeod SM: Chlordiazepoxide and oxazepam disposition in cirrhosis. *Clin Pharmacol Ther* 26:240–246, 1979.
22. Greenblatt DJ, Shader RI: Dependence, tolerance and addiction to benzodiazepines: clinical and pharmacokinetic considerations. *Drug Metab Rev* 8:13–28, 1978.
23. Tyrer P, Rutherford D, Huggett T: Benzodiazepine withdrawal symptoms and propranolol. *Lancet* 1:520–522, 1981.
24. Ballenger JC, Burrows GD, DuPont RL Jr, Lesser IM, Noyes R Jr, Pecknold JC, Rifkin A, Swinson RP: Alprazolam in panic disorder and agoraphobia: results from a multicenter trial. I: Efficacy in short-term treatment. *Arch Gen Psychiatry* 45:413–422, 1988.
25. Dawson GW, Jue SG, Brogden RN: Alprazolam: a review of its pharmacodynamic properties and efficacy in the treatment of anxiety and depression. *Drugs* 27:132–147, 1984.
26. Brown JL, Hauge KJ: A review of alprazolam withdrawal. *Drug Intell Clin Pharm* 20:837–841, 1986.
27. Gold MS, Pottash ALC, Sweeney DR, Kleber HD: Efficacy of clonidine in opiate withdrawal: a study of thirty patients. *Drug Alcohol Depend* 6:201–208, 1980.
28. Bond WS: Psychiatric indications for clonidine: the neuropharmacologic and clinical basis. *J Clin Psychopharmacol* 6:81–87, 1986.
29. Hoehn-Saric R, Merchant AF, Keyser ML, Smith VK: Effects of clonidine on anxiety disorders. *Arch Gen Psychiatry* 38:1278–1282, 1981.
30. Gorman JM, Liebowitz MR, Fyer AJ, Stein J: A neuroanatomical hypothesis for panic disorder. *Am J Psychiatry* 146:148–161, 1989.
31. Greenblatt DJ, Shader RI, Koch-Weser J, Franke K: Slow absorption of intramuscular chlordiazepoxide. *N Engl J Med* 291:1116–1118, 1974.
32. Greenblatt DJ, Shader RI, MacLeod SM, Sellers EM: Clinical pharmacokinetics of chlordiazepoxide. *Clin Pharmacokinet* 3:381–394, 1978.
33. Chung M, Hilbert JM, Gural RP, Radwanski E, Symchowicz N, Zampaglione N: Multiple-dose halazepam kinetics. *Clin Pharmacol Ther* 35:838–842, 1984.
34. Zisook S, Rogers PJ, Faschingbauer TR, Devaul RA: Absence of hostility in outpatients after administration of halazepam—a new benzodiazepine. *J Clin Psychiatry* 39:683–686, 1978.

Flurazepam Database

FORMULATIONS

Flurazepam capsules: 15 mg, 30 mg
Brand names: Dalmane (Roche); various generic brands

BASIC PHARMACOLOGY

Flurazepam is a member of the 1,4-benzodiazepine class of drugs (Fig. 4D.1). Since its introduction in 1970, its major use has been as a sedative-hypnotic because of its ability to decrease sleep latency, reduce the number of nighttime awakenings, and prolong total sleep. Its efficacy has been proven in controlled clinical trials for up to 4 weeks of continuous therapy (1, 2). In contrast to other classes of psychoactive drugs, including the barbiturates, tricyclic antidepressants, and monoamine oxidase inhibitors, flurazepam has only a minor effect on decreasing rapid eye movement (REM) sleep (2). A slight REM rebound occurs when the drug is stopped.

The benzodiazepines seem to potentiate inhibition of neurotransmission via γ-aminobutyric acid (GABA) at the limbic, thalamic, and hypothalamic levels of the CNS. Furthermore, the benzodiazepines apparently enhance GABA effects without themselves becoming GABA-mimetic compounds, probably by binding to endogenous, saturable, benzodiazepine-specific regulatory sites adjacent to the GABA receptor (3). Flurazepam is less potent than diazepam as a muscle relaxant and anticonvulsant. It produces only mild, transient cardiovascular and respiratory effects. The expected effects on physiological status and various laboratory tests are outlined in Table 4D.1.

PHARMACOKINETIC PROPERTIES

Flurazepam is rapidly absorbed from the gastrointestinal tract. After a single oral dose, peak plasma concentration occurs at 30 to 60 minutes. A rapid decrease in concentration follows the peak, and flurazepam becomes barely detectable during continuous dosing. The major metabolite, desalkyl-flurazepam, reaches a steady-state concentration after 7 to 10 days of dosing (4, 5).

Flurazepam has a high volume of distribution as expected from a high degree of lipophilicity, and it widely distributes in body tissues. It crosses the placenta and is secreted into breast milk. The plasma protein binding is extensive, estimated at greater than 90%.

Approximately 70% of flurazepam is rapidly oxidized to metabolites during its first pass through the liver by the microsomal enzyme systems. There are at least six nonconjugated metabolites of flurazepam, some of which have various degrees of pharmacological activity (5). The parent compound disappears rapidly from the blood, and less than 0.2% of flurazepam is recovered in the urine in

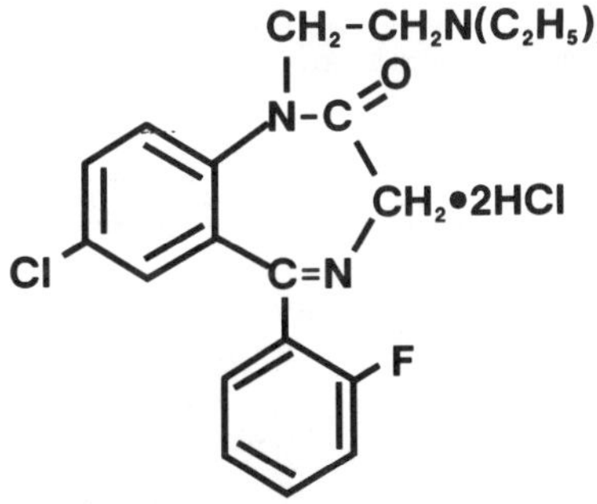

$$CH_2-CH_2N(C_2H_5)_2$$

Figure 4D.1.   Structure of flurazepam.

Table 4D.1.
Expected Physiological Effects from Flurazepam Therapy for Monitoring[a]

Parameter	Drug Effect
Cardiovascular status	
Heart rate	No effects are expected unless a slight slowing.
ECG	No expected effects
Blood pressure	Mild and clinically unimportant decrease
Renal function	
Serum creatinine and clearance, BUN	Normal values should not change in most adults.
Hepatic function	
AST (SGOT), ALT (SGPT), alkaline phosphatase	Normal values should not change in most adults.
Hematology status	
CBC	Normal values should not change in most adults. Rare case of leukopenia is reported.
Neuroendocrine status	
Cortisol	Normal values should not change in most adults.

[a]For abbreviations, see Table 4A.1.

an unchanged form. There is some evidence that the benzodiazepines undergo enterohepatic recirculation that can result in delayed secondary plasma concentration peaks. The apparent half-life of flurazepam is less than 2 hours. Desalkylflurazepam is pharmacologically active, with a half-life ranging from 36 to 100 hours (5).

The hypnotic profile of flurazepam is a reflection of its pharmacokinetic properties. The rapid absorption after oral administration quickly produces an effective brain concentration because of the drug's high degree of lipophilicity (6). This results in rapid sedative effects, and, as a result, flurazepam decreases the latency to onset of sleep. The formation of the active metabolite desalkylflurazepam maintains hypnotic efficacy, minimizing sleep awakenings throughout the night. Total sleep time is prolonged. Unfortunately, the slow disappearance rate of desalkylflurazepam produces an uncomfortable daytime sedation for occasional patients. However, patients whose insomnia is accompanied by

Table 4D.2.
Pharmacokinetic Parameters of Flurazepam

Parameter	Range
Bioavailability	Nearly complete
Time of peak concentration after a single dose	30 to 60 minutes
Plasma protein binding	Greater than 90%
Renal clearance	Negligible
Elimination half-life	Flurazepam: less than 2 hours
Active metabolites	Desalkylflurazepam (half-life range of 36 to 100 hours)
	N-1-Hydroxyethylflurazepam (half-life of 2 to 4 hours)
Steady-state metabolite to parent concentration ratio	Desalkyl metabolite concentrations are 5 to 6 times greater than the 24-hour concentrations after chronic dosing
Therapeutic range for antianxiety effect	No defined concentration range exists.

daytime anxiety may benefit from this action the following day. A summary of flurazepam's pharmacokinetic properties is given in Table 4D.2.

INDICATIONS

Flurazepam is approved for the short-term (up to 4 weeks) treatment of insomnia characterized by difficulty in falling asleep, frequent nocturnal awakenings, and/or early morning awakening. Flurazepam can be used effectively in patients with recurring insomnia or poor sleeping habits. Because the long-acting metabolite accumulates during 2 weeks of continuous therapy, a "carryover" or hangover effect occurs frequently. As a result, flurazepam can be more effective on the second and third nights of administration than on the first night. The slow clearance of the metabolite and its persistence in the body after flurazepam dosing is discontinued explain why sedative effects continue for 1 to 2 nights after the drug is discontinued. This long duration of action minimizes any rebound of REM sleep. Flurazepam is superior to the older barbiturates as a sedative (7). The drug is not approved for the treatment of anxiety although, as a benzodiazepine, flurazapam could be expected to have antianxiety effects.

Although flurazepam is indicated for symptomatic relief of insomnia, the cause of sleep complaints should always be sought. Depression, anxiety, and other mental or medical disorders can result in poor sleep. Reviews of rational sedative-hypnotic prescribing are readily available (8, 9).

DOSAGE REGIMEN DESIGN

The dosage of flurazepam should be individualized for optimal effects. A prudent approach is to start with the lower dosage, especially in the elderly, of 15 mg and increase to 30 mg, if needed. The adult dosage is 15 to 30 mg before retiring. Elderly and/or debilitated patients should be started only on 15 mg and increased to 30 mg if needed. It should not be necessary to increase the dosage beyond 30 mg nightly. Flurazepam is not recommended for children or adolescents under 15 years of age.

Withdrawal symptoms have been observed upon abrupt discontinuation of anxiolytic benzodiazepines taken continuously for several months, generally at higher than therapeutic doses (10, 11). Severe symptoms of withdrawal include extreme agitation, confusion, and seizures. Although these have not been reported specifically for flurazepam, gradual tapering of doses after prolonged usage is recommended; abrupt discontinuance should be avoided. As with any hypnotic, caution should be exercised in administering flurazepam to any individuals known to be dependence-prone or those whose history may suggest that they might increase dosage on their own initiative.

A hazard of withdrawing sedative-hypnotic use is rebound insomnia and anxiety (12, 13). This syndrome is characterized by worsening of sleep parameters above baseline levels. Drugs with short half-lives, whether administered for a few nights or chronically, are more likely to cause this effect than is flurazepam.

THERAPEUTIC DRUG MONITORING

There is little justification for plasma concentration monitoring of flurazepam. For therapeutic effects, improvement in sleep onset and duration and quality of sleep should be monitored. For toxic effects, signs of excessive CNS-related drowsiness (i.e., morning hangover) should be observable. The long half-life of desalkylflurazepam provides an explanation of why some patients experience daytime sedation. If daytime drowsiness becomes a problem, then a reduction in dosage or the use of an alternative benzodiazepine with a shorter half-life might be a useful alternative.

CONTRAINDICATIONS—WARNINGS—PRECAUTIONS

Contraindications include known hypersensitivity to flurazepam and use in pregnancy (see below). Physical and psychological dependence are rare in patients taking flurazepam; however, prolonged therapy with doses greater than those recommended increases the risks.

Benzodiazepines are subject to abuse and dependence. Withdrawal symptoms may occur after the abrupt discontinuance of dosing; however, this problem may be less with flurazepam than other sedative-hypnotics because of the slow elimination of desalkylflurazepam.

Flurazepam may impair physical and/or mental abilities required for operating a motor vehicle or other hazardous machinery. Ambulatory patients should be cautioned accordingly about engaging in such activities while taking this drug.

Flurazepam has the potential for additive effects with alcohol and other CNS depressants. The potential for this interaction continues for several days after discontinuation of the drug, until substantial amounts of active metabolites have been eliminated.

It is recommended that the dose of flurazepam be limited to 15 mg for elderly and debilitated patients because the risk of oversedation, dizziness, confusion, or ataxia is substantially increased with larger doses in such patients (5, 14). Flurazepam should be used with caution in patients with impaired renal or hepatic function and chronic pulmonary insufficiency.

DRUG INTERACTIONS

Additive depressant effects may occur when flurazepam is used concurrently with alcohol, CNS depressants, antianxiety agents, antihistamines, or any other agent with CNS depressant or hypnotic effects. This additive effect may still occur if alcohol is consumed the day after the use of flurazepam for nighttime sedation. This potential persists for several days after the discontinuance of flurazepam.

Antacids or the presence of food in the stomach may decrease the rate of benzodiazepine absorption (13). The extent of absorption is usually unaffected. It is recommended to take flurazepam on an empty stomach.

Concurrent therapy with other drugs that are metabolic inhibitors or inducers may intensify or decrease the effects of flurazepam, although these interactions have not been specifically studied. Cimetidine and disulfiram decrease the clearance of benzodiazepines by approximately 25 to 50%. Isoniazid impairs the metabolism of benzodiazepines (increases their half-lives), whereas rifampin induces benzodiazepine metabolism (decreasing their half-lives). Flurazepam is not an inducer of hepatic microsomal enzymes and may be safely administered to patients receiving oral anticoagulants. Table 4A.4 gives a more complete list of benzodiazepine drug interactions.

ADVERSE REACTIONS—OCCURRENCE AND MANAGEMENT

Adverse effects related to depressed CNS function include dizziness, drowsiness, ataxia, falling (especially in elderly or debilitated patients), and disorientation. The most common are drowsiness and hangover (14). Rarely, paradoxical excitement (including nervousness, talkativeness, irritability, and apprehension) has been observed.

Gastrointestinal side effects include nausea, vomiting, and diarrhea. Occasionally, constipation or gastrointestinal pain have been reported. Miscellaneous side effects include weakness, palpitations, chest pains, and other somatic complaints. Very rarely leukopenia, granulocytopenia, diaphoresis, blurred vision, hypotension, shortness of breath, and anorexia have occurred. A summary of flurazepam's adverse reactions is given in Table 4D.3.

MANAGEMENT OF OVERDOSE

The benzodiazepine toxicity profile is relatively nonspecific. Because of its mild symptoms, diagnosis should be based on history and/or physical findings. Somnolence and confusion occur in most cases. Occasionally, coma has resulted from benzodiazepine overdose. The vast majority of overdose fatalities suggest benzodiazepines only as a factor in multiple drug ingestions (15). Fewer than a dozen poorly documented deaths possibly resulting from oral benzodiazepines have been reported in the literature. Overall, the benzodiazepines are extremely safe. Early case reports of patients ingesting as much as 360 mg demonstrated the good prognosis of patients overdosed with flurazepam (16).

General treatment includes monitoring of vital signs (respiration, pulse, blood pressure) and maintenance of an adequate airway as needed, including an artificial airway if necessary. Preventing absorption is mandatory. Depending on the level of consciousness of the patient, the stomach may be emptied of flurazepam by either initiating emesis with syrup of ipecac or, if the patient is comatose, convulsing, or uncooperative, using gastric lavage. Activated charcoal may be administered in an adult dose of 60 to 100 gm or 30 to 60 gm for a child. Saline cathartics (e.g., magnesium sulfate) may also be useful.

Table 4D.3.
Expected Side Effects from Flurazepam Therapy

Effect	Rare	Less Common	More Common
Dry mouth		X	
Blurred vision		X	
Nausea		X	
Vomiting		X	
Diarrhea			
Drowsiness			X
Dizziness			X
Ataxia			X
Mental confusion			X
Disorientation			X
Headache		X	
Restlessness or paradoxical stimulation	X		
Difficult urination	X		
Constipation		X	
Hypotension		X	
Tachycardia	X		
Jaundice	X		

Generally, the above is the only treatment required. In the rare event of respiratory or circulatory compromise associated with benzodiazepine overdose (particularly with multiple drug ingestions), urgent attention to the airway, ventilation, and circulatory support are essential.

USE IN RENAL AND/OR HEPATIC DISEASE

Because flurazepam is extensively metabolized in the liver, no dosage adjustment is recommended for patients with renal disease. Furthermore, because of its high degree of protein binding, no adjustment in dosage is required for patients undergoing hemodialysis.

Because flurazepam is extensively metabolized, its clearance is markedly decreased in patients with liver disease. This drug should be used with caution in such patients and on the basis of careful monitoring of clinical signs. Quantitative recommendations for decreasing the dosage of flurazepam cannot be made because the degree of impaired drug clearance cannot be directly related to any of the standard liver function tests.

USE IN CHILDREN AND ADOLESCENTS

Because of the lack of clinical investigation into the use of flurazepam in children, the drug is not recommended for use in children under 15 years of age.

USE IN ELDERLY

Some elderly patients seem inherently more sensitive to the effects of flurazepam (as well as other sedative-hypnotics) and require smaller doses than do younger patients. One reason may be lower plasma protein binding of the drug in the elderly (allowing a greater percentage of the drug to enter the CNS). Due to the decrease in hepatic function associated with ageing, the half-life of the drug is prolonged and its clearance is considerably decreased, resulting in higher than usual plasma concentrations (5, 13). Consequently, flurazepam should be used with caution in elderly patients and dosage adjustments should be made on the basis of careful clinical monitoring.

USE IN PREGNANCY

Benzodiazepines cross the placenta. Human teratogenicity studies are not conclusive, but there are indications of an increased risk of congenital malformations (especially oral clefts) when diazepam and chlordiazepoxide have been used during the first trimester. Furthermore, symptoms of neonatal depression have been observed in an infant whose mother received 30 mg of flurazepam nightly for 10 days before delivery. Flurazepam should be avoided in pregnant patients.

Benzodiazepines are excreted in breast milk in clinically significant amounts. Lethargy, poor feeding, and weight loss have been reported in breast-fed infants. Infants under 2 weeks of age metabolize benzodiazepines poorly and, as a result, the drug and its active metabolites may accumulate in excessive amounts. For these reasons, flurazepam is not recommended when patients are mothers nursing their infants.

PATIENT INFORMATION

Patients should be told to avoid simultaneous ingestion of alcohol or other CNS depressants (antihistamines, nonprescription sleep aids, etc.) as additive sedative effects may occur. The prescribed dosage should not be exceeded, and the medication should not be abruptly discontinued after prolonged therapy. Additionally, patients should be told of the possibility of daytime drowsiness. They should exercise caution while driving a car or operating machinery.

REFERENCES

1. Greenblatt DJ, Shader RI, Koch-Weser J: Flurazepam hydrochloride. Clin Pharmacol Ther 17:1–14, 1975.
2. Kales A, Kales JD, Scharf MB, Tan T-L: All-night EEG studies of chloral hydrate, flurazepam and methaqualone. Arch Gen Psychiatry 23:219–225, 1970.
3. Paul SM, Marangos PJ, Goodwin FK, Skolnick P: Brain-specific benzodiazepine receptors and putative endogenous benzodiazepine-like compounds. Biol Psychiatry 15:407–428, 1980.
4. Kaplan SA, deSilva JAF, Jack ML, et al: Blood level profile in man following oral administration of flurazepam hydrochloride. J Pharm Sci 62:1932–1935, 1973.
5. Greenblatt DJ, Divoll M, Harmatz JS, et al: Kinetics and clinical effects of flurazepam in young and elderly noninsomniacs. Clin Pharmacol Ther 30:475–486, 1981.
6. Chiueh CC, Ohata M, Jonas LA, et al: Brain uptake of flurazepam and of N-1-desalkyl flurazepam after administration of flurazepam to the cat. Drug Metab Dispos 13:1–4, 1985.
7. Kales A, Kales JD, Bixler EO, Scharf MB: Effectiveness of hypnotics drugs with prolonged use: flurazepam and pentobarbital. Clin Pharmacol Ther 18:356–363, 1975.
8. Dement WC: Rational basis for the use of sleeping pill. Pharmacology 27(suppl 2):3–38, 1983.
9. Sleep Disorders Classification Committee, Association of Sleep Disorders Centers: Diagnostic classification of sleep and arousal disorders. Sleep 2:1–137, 1979.
10. Greenblatt DJ, Shader RI: Dependence, tolerance and addiction to benzodiazepines: clinical and pharmacokinetic considerations. Drug Metab Rev 8:13–28, 1978.
11. Hallstrom C, Lader MH: Benzodiazepine withdrawal phenomena. Int Pharmacopsychiatry 16:235–244, 1981.
12. Kales A, Bixler EO, Tan T-L, Scharf M, Kales JD: Chronic hypnotic-drug use: ineffectiveness, drug-withdrawal insomnia, and dependence. JAMA 227:513–517, 1974.

13. Kales A, Scharf MB, Kales JD: Rebound insomnia: a new clinical syndrome. *Science* 201:1039–1041, 1978.
14. Greenblatt DJ, Allen MD, Shader RI: Toxicity of high-dose flurazepam in the elderly. *Clin Pharmacol Ther* 21:355–361, 1977.
15. Greenblatt DJ, Allen MD, Noel BJ, Shader RI: Acute overdosage with benzodiazepine derivatives. *Clin Pharmacol Ther* 21:497–514, 1977.
16. O'Neil JT, Pogge RC: Relative safety of self-inflicted overdose with relatively newer medications. *Ariz Med* 30:484–485, 1973.

▬E

Intraclass Comparisons of Sedative-Hypnotics

A comparison of pharmacological factors favors the choice of benzodiazepines as sedative-hypnotics over the barbiturates and older nonbarbiturate sedatives (1, 2) (Table 4E.1). Addiction and habituation occur to a lesser degree relative to the other drugs that have traditionally been used as sedatives. True addiction (i.e., physiological dependence) occurs, but the hazards associated with benzodiazepine use have probably been exaggerated. The benzodiazepines have a remarkably low order of toxicity (3). The consequences of overdosage are far less severe than from ethchlorvynol, glutethimide, meprobamate, and methaqualone. Clinically significant enzyme induction in humans receiving therapeutic doses of benzodiazepines is unlikely. This contrasts with the effects of glutethimide, meprobamate, and methaprylon.

Although several benzodiazepines could be effectively used as sedative-hypnotics (4), only three are specifically marketed for this purpose in the United States. Clinical trials have proven flurazepam, temazepam, and triazolam effective for promoting sleep and improving the quality of sleep (5, 6). Differences between these drugs become apparent by considering their effects on sleep architecture and their pharmacokinetic properties (7).

NORMAL SLEEP ARCHITECTURE

Electrophysiological studies in sleep laboratories have defined characteristic patterns of brain activity and physiological status that are referred to as sleep stages (8). There are four stages collectively known as nonrapid eye movement (NREM) sleep. This designation is used to distinguish these sleep stages from REM sleep. These sleep states are determined in the laboratory by analysis of recorded electroencephalograms (EEGs) of brain activity, electrooculograms (EOGs) of eye movement, and electromyograms (EMGs) of muscle tension. The physiological significance of the various sleep stages is still being defined.

The onset of sleep is preceded by a latency period, the time it takes to fall asleep, usually ranging from 10 to 20 minutes. When normal sleep begins, EEG activity changes from low voltage with fast activity to a pattern of slower activity. This signals the onset of stage 1 sleep. About 5% of total sleep time in adults is spent in this sleep stage. The percentage increases with age. In stage 2, the

Table 4E.1.
Pharmacological Comparison of Sedative-Hypnotics in Short-Term Therapy

Drug	Lethality in Overdose	Enzyme Induction	Physiological Dependence	Sleep Rebound	Sleep Efficacy
Chloral hydrate	+	+	+	0, +	+
Benzodiazepines	0	0	+	variable	+ +
Barbiturates (pentobarbital, secobarbital)	+ +	+ +	+ +	+ +	+ +
Glutethimide	+ +	+	+	+ +	+
Methyprylon	+ +	+	+	+ +	+
Ethchlorvynol	+ +	0, +	+	+ +	+

EEG activity remains slow and contains recognizable waveforms called "K-complexes" and "spindles." In stages 3 and 4, known as deep sleep, the EEG shows high amplitude, slow activity waves. Normal adults spend 19 to 23% of total sleep time in the deep stages of NREM sleep.

The onset of REM sleep occurs with episodic bursts of rapid eye movements (9). The EEG is characterized by low voltage with mixed frequency accompanied by low EMG activity. Dreaming occurs during this sleep stage. A normal sleeper proceeds through stages 1, 2, 3, and 4, then typically returns briefly to stages 3 and 2, before entering the first REM period, which occurs after about 90 minutes of NREM sleep. Several of these cycles usually occur each night. A summary of the characteristics of sleep stages is given in Table 4E.2.

INSOMNIA COMPLAINTS

Insomnia is defined as a relative lack of sleep that is accompanied by a complaint. For many patients, this will be difficulty in falling asleep or maintaining sleep, reduced total sleep time, or early morning awakening. Disturbed sleep may be characterized by several parameters measurable in the sleep laboratory. In patients with insomnia, REM may be more fragmented and occurs earlier in the night. Insomnia patients are also more restless with more leg movements during the night. There is no single predominant pattern that characterizes insomnia, but sleep laboratory studies are continuing to define the meaning of normal and disturbed sleep and the changes in sleep that occur with ageing.

Latency to onset represents the time lapse from preparing to sleep until the onset of stage 1. An increased latency is probably the most common sleep complaint. Excessive wakefulness during the night is also common. Most normal sleepers awaken several times during the night but fall asleep again within a few minutes. Many insomnia patients have prolonged periods of wakefulness with difficulty returning to sleep. Total sleep time decreases with age, from an average of 16 hours at birth to 8 hours in adulthood. The elderly sleep even less.

There are numerous causes of insomnia. Foremost are secondary medical or psychiatric disorders. A thorough medical and psychiatric history is necessary to rule out secondary causes. For example, depression and anxiety are commonly associated with a complaint of insomnia. These disorders should be suspected and treated appropriately if found to be present. The complaint of insomnia will often disappear when secondary causes are treated. A partial list of disorders commonly associated with a complaint of insomnia is presented in Table 4E.3.

Table 4E.2.
Physiological Characteristics of Sleep Stages

Sleep Stage	EEG	EOG	EMG	Comment
Stage 1	Low amplitude, mixed frequency	Slow, rolling eye movements	Decreased tone compared to wakefulness	May be perceived as drowsiness or sleep
Stage 2	Similar to stage 1 with spindles and K-complexes	Absent eye movements	Further decrease from stage 1	General decrease in many body functions
Stage 3	High amplitude, slow frequency	Absent eye movements	Lower tone compared to wakefulness	Stages 3 and 4 are known as slowwave or delta sleep
Stage 4	High amplitude, slow frequency	Absent eye movements	Lower tone compared to wakefulness	
REM sleep	Low amplitude, mixed frequency similar to stage 1; EEG is activated	Episodic bursts of rapid eye movements	Lowest muscle tone during sleep	Dreaming often occurs

When patients complain of excessive daytime sleepiness, sleep attacks, or unusual snorting or gasping sounds during sleep, sleep apnea should be suspected (10). This is an indication for evaluation by a sleep laboratory. Bed partners should be asked to corroborate the patient's complaints. Sedative-hypnotics are not indicated for this disorder as a risk exists of further decreasing the ventilatory drive. Current experimental treatments include medroxyprogesterone and protriptyline, a tricyclic antidepressant.

The DSM-III-R classifies sleep disorders that are chronic (more than 1 month's duration) into dyssomnias and parasomnias. The former category relates to disturbances in the amount, quality, or timing of sleep, and the later group of disorders includes as an essential feature an abnormal event that occurs during sleep or at the threshold between wakefulness and sleep. Examples of parasomnias include sleep terrors and sleepwalking. Sedative-hypnotics are not necessarily indicated in these conditions. A comprehensive discussion of the various sleep disorders can be found in recent reviews (11, 12).

For evaluating the majority of complaints of insomnia, sleep laboratory studies are not necessary. Sleep disturbances can be usefully divided into transient insomnia, short-term insomnia, and long-term insomnia (13). Transient or situational insomnia frequently occurs in healthy individuals in response to a stressful event; for example, the need to sleep away from home during brief hospitalization or travel. Observing good sleep hygiene is useful in these patients, but some patients may benefit from brief pharmacotherapy lasting less than 1 week.

Table 4E.3.
Partial List of Medical and Psychiatric Conditions Commonly Associated with a Complaint of Insomnia

Psychiatric	Medical
Affective disorders	Painful states (cancer, migraine headache)
Anxiety disorders	Cardiovascular disease (angina, congestive heart failure)
Substance use disorders	
Somatoform disorders	
Adjustment disorder (with depressed mood, anxious mood, or mixed features)	Duodenal ulcer
	Chronic renal disease
	Asthma, other pulmonary disease
	Hypothyroidism
	Parkinson's disease

Short-term insomnia, amenable to drug therapy with benzodiazepines, may last up to 3 weeks. Long-term insomnia, persisting beyond 1 month, should be evaluated carefully for the presence of underlying psychiatric or medical conditions or the presence of a specific sleep disorder. Substance abuse disorders commonly produce complaints of sleeplessness and should be ruled out. The long-term use of benzodiazepines in these patients is controversial. This point is emphasized as efficacy beyond 1 month has been difficult to demonstrate and the risk of dependence increases with length of therapy.

When evaluating insomnia, the specific source of the complaint related to the common sleep parameters should be sought. Is there an increased sleep latency, a decrease in the duration of sleep, or the presence of increased nocturnal awakenings? The clinical course of the complaint should be determined from the time it first became apparent to the patient. Treatment is directed at minimizing or correcting the major complaint. The sleep history indicates the target symptoms to be monitored during pharmacotherapy.

EFFECTS OF DRUGS ON SLEEP

Although all sedative-hypnotics are CNS depressants, their effects on the architecture of sleep differ. Ethchlorvynol and antihistamines decrease REM sleep, and the barbiturates and glutethimide decrease both REM and stage 4 sleep. The benzodiazepines cause the least alteration in normal sleep during use and after withdrawal (14). Although benzodiazepines cause little or no change in REM sleep, they suppress stage 4 sleep. This has therapeutic advantages in the treatment of somnambulism and pavor nocturnus (night terror). Benzodiazepines retain their effectiveness in inducing and maintaining sleep for longer periods of continuous use than do other hypnotics. Flurazepam has the longest demonstrated efficacy, lasting for at least a month of continuous use (15).

The phenomenon of rebound insomnia may occur after discontinuance of sedative therapy (16). The shorter the half-life of the chosen drug, the more likely this condition will occur. It consists of an increase in wake time during sleep compared to the baseline state before beginning therapy.

BENZODIAZEPINE PHARMACOKINETICS

Choosing the most appropriate benzodiazepine from among the three currently marketed specifically for insomnia requires knowledge of their pharmacokinetic properties (7). A large individual variability exists in pharmacological

Table 4E.4.
Pharmacokinetic Parameters of Sedative-Hypnotic Benzodiazepines

	Time of Maximal Concentration (min)	Elimination Half-life (hr)	Active Metabolites Present in Plasma (Half-life) (hr)
Flurazepam	30–60	<2	Hydroxyethylflurazepam, 2–4
			Desalkylflurazepam, 36–120
Triazolam	60–70	1.5–5	None
Temazepam	45–120	8–20	None
Quazepam	45–120	15–35	Oxoquazepam, 25–35
			Desalkylflurazepam, 36–120

response to sedative-hypnotic benzodiazepines. Thus, the choice of drug and dosage must be individualized. Currently, no single benzodiazepine hypnotic seems best for all patients. Considerations for pharmacotherapy include rate of absorption, the elimination half-life, presence or absence of active metabolites, and side effect profile. The more rapid the absorption, generally the greater the benefits for reducing sleep latency. The presence of active metabolites correlates with sleep maintenance during the night and reduction of early morning awakening but may produce daytime drowsiness. A further benefit of long-acting metabolites is the self-tapering effect and minimal rebound insomnia occurring upon discontinuance of the drug. The pharmacokinetic properties of the benzodiazepine sedative-hypnotics are compared in Table 4E.4.

INDIVIDUAL AGENTS

Chloral Hydrate

Chloral hydrate has been used as a sedative for decades. It obtained a somewhat tainted reputation as the principal ingredient in the "Mickey Finn" cocktail when combined with alcohol. It is regarded as a weak enzyme inducer. It has proven effective for inducing and maintaining sleep with initial and short-term use, but its benefits decrease with continued therapy (14). Patients who take chloral hydrate for months or years are probably deriving little benefit from this practice. Chloral hydrate should be reserved for treatment of transient insomnia. Doses range between 500 and 1500 mg/night.

A metabolite of chloral hydrate, trichloroacetic acid, is highly plasma protein-bound and can displace warfarin from binding sites on albumin. This can result in an increase in the hypoprothrombinemic effect of warfarin (17). This drug interaction was thoroughly studied in the 1970s with conflicting results. Given the safety of the benzodiazepines when combined with warfarin, chloral hydrate should be avoided during anticoagulant therapy.

Flurazepam

Flurazepam is discussed in detail in Chapter 4D. The majority of patients with a complaint of insomnia who have difficulty falling asleep will benefit from treatment with flurazepam. Therapy can be initiated with 15 mg in patients of all ages, particularly sedative-naive patients. This dose should always be used before the 30-mg dose in the elderly.

The half-life of intact flurazepam is short, less than 2 hours, and very sensitive analytical techniques are needed to measure its concentration in blood. However, it generally produces sedative effects lasting the entire night after a single dose. For some individuals, sedative effects are felt the following day.

This is partly due to the presence of N-desalkylflurazepam in plasma, an active metabolite with a long elimination half-life (Table 4E.4). Flurazepam apparently produces sedative effects immediately because of its rapid absorption and maintains efficacy because of the slow formation and elimination of desalkyl-flurazepam. In the elderly, the half-life of this metabolite can be extended beyond 10 days.

The elderly should be given reduced dosages of flurazepam and monitored closely for the presence of excessive daytime sedation. Driving ability may be impaired, and some patients may feel compromised in performing other skilled and dangerous tasks. The intake of caffeine-containing beverages may not be sufficient to reverse the hypnotic-induced depressant effects of flurazepam. The risk of hip fractures is increased in the elderly with the use of benzodiazepines with long elimination half-lives (18).

Temazepam

Temazepam should cause less daytime sedation than flurazepam because its metabolic profile is free of slowly accumulating active metabolites (19). The major metabolite is temazepam glucuronide, which is inactive and is excreted in the urine. The average half-life of temazepam, 8 to 20 hours, suggests that it should be nearly ideal to maintain sleep without excessive daytime sedation; however, temazepam is relatively slowly absorbed, reaching peak concentrations as late as 2 hours after a single dose. Therefore, it does not consistently reduce sleep latency. Pharmaceutical formulation factors seem to influence this aspect of temazepam's pharmacokinetics. A dosage form with a more rapid dissolution rate could become available in the future. Until this time, it may be beneficial to administer temazepam an hour or more before bedtime.

As temazepam's major route of elimination is by conjugation, it is less subject to the effects of ageing on its disposition compared to flurazepam (see Chapter 4C). This is a potential advantage of temazepam in the elderly, although this effect has not been clearly established with published research.

Triazolam

Triazolam has useful sedative properties: it produces a rapid onset of effects, reduces nocturnal awakenings, causes minimal daytime sedation, and has a pharmacokinetic profile that precludes accumulation, even in the elderly, upon chronic dosing (20). A disadvantage is that psychomotor impairment after its use may be worse than that from the other benzodiazepines (21). Another disadvantage is its propensity to cause a rebound insomnia. One or two nights of disturbed sleep may occur when the drug is discontinued. A brief tapering period over 4 days has reduced the symptoms of rebound insomnia (22). Triazolam's very rapid onset of action may possibly produce euphoria in occasional patients. The usual nightly dose is 0.25 mg. For elderly patients, the dose should not exceed 0.125 mg.

L-Tryptophan

The amino acid L-tryptophan is a precursor of serotonin. In doses of 1 to 5 gm at bedtime, it has some efficacy as a sedative; however, its failure rate may be higher than that of other sedatives. It can be expected to be most effective in reducing sleep latency, with lesser effects of maintaining sleep throughout the night. L-tryptophan is available as an over-the-counter product from health food stores and pharmacies as a dietary supplement.

Table 4E.5.
Pharmacodynamic Comparison of Sedative-Hypnotic Benzodiazepines

Parameter	Flurazepam	Triazolam	Temazepam	Quazepam
Reducing sleep latency	+ +	+ +	0, +	+
Prolonging total sleep time	+ +	+	+ +	+ +
Preventing early morning awakening	+ +	+	+ +	+ +
Daytime drowsiness	+ +	0	+	+ +
Rebound insomnia	0, +	+ +	+	0, +

Quazepam

Quazepam is expected to be the fourth benzodiazepine available in the United States for use as a sedative-hypnotic (23). It undergoes oxidative metabolism, ultimately producing desalkylflurazepam, the long-acting metabolite (half-life of 36 to 100 hours) of flurazepam. Thus, it can be expected to reduce wake time during the night and for 1 or 2 days after drug therapy is stopped. It is more slowly absorbed than flurazepam and may have less pronounced effects on decreasing sleep latency, at least during the first 2 to 4 nights of therapy. In sleep laboratory reports, it seems to be an effective sedative.

SUMMARY

The benzodiazepines offer clear advantages over previously available drugs for use as sedative-hypnotics (Table 4E.1). Differences in their pharmacokinetic and dynamic properties allow a rational choice of drug directed toward a patient's specific sleep complaints. These differences are summarized in Tables 4E.4 and 4E.5.

When a specific complaint of sleep onset difficulties is present, flurazepam or triazolam may be a good choice. When a rapid onset of action is needed, triazolam is equal to flurazepam and may be better. Both drugs will outperform temazepam in improving this sleep parameter.

When only short-term therapy is needed, i.e., for less than five nights, triazolam is an appropriate choice, especially if daytime alertness is a priority and if the patient would not need to perform complicated psychomotor activities should nocturnal awakening occur. For occasional or for short-term use, rebound insomnia should not be a problem with triazolam. However, for long-term use, the available efficacy data favor the selection of flurazepam.

Some data suggest that hypnotic efficacy is less in middle age (40 to 50 years) than would be suggested from studies in young adults. This observation relates to the greater disturbance of sleep during this time of life when drug disposition ability is not yet impaired due to advanced age.

The elderly are well known to have a predisposition to the sedating effects of benzodiazepines. Decreased body clearance of flurazepam has been documented with pharmacokinetic studies. Although the short half-life of triazolam would seem to be an advantage in this population, the negative effects on cognitive performance outweigh the pharmacokinetic advantages, and one should be hesitant to initiate triazolam therapy in these patients. Flurazepam's rapid onset of effects exceeds that of temazepam and will be preferred for some patients.

Generally, all sleep medication is overprescribed, especially the use of the higher milligram dosage forms. Sedative-hypnotics should be used only on an as needed basis, rather than routinely, and for the shortest time possible. Persistent complaints of insomnia should prompt the search for a secondary cause and an accurate diagnosis.

REFERENCES

1. Lader MH, Bond AJ, James DC: Clinical comparison of anxiolytic drug therapy. *Psychol Med* 4:381–387, 1974.
2. Greenblatt DJ, Shader RI: The clinical choice of sedative-hypnotics. *Ann Intern Med* 77:91–100, 1972.
3. Greenblatt DJ, Allen MD, Noel BJ, Shader RI: Acute overdosage with benzodiazepine derivatives. *Clin Pharmacol Ther* 21:497–514, 1977.
4. Kales A, Soldatos CR, Bixler EO, Kales JD, Vela-Bueno A: Diazepam: effects on sleep and withdrawal phenomena. *J Clin Psychopharmacol* 8:340–346, 1988.
5. Kales A, Bixler EO, Schard MB, Kales JD: Sleep laboratory studies of flurazepam: a model for evaluating hypnotic drugs. *Clin Pharmacol Ther* 19:576–583, 1975.
6. Wincor MZ: Insomnia and the new benzodiazepines. *Clin Pharm* 1:425–432, 1982.
7. Greenblatt DJ, Divoll M, Abernethy DR, Shader RI: Benzodiazepine hypnotics: kinetic and therapeutic options. *Sleep* 5:S18–S27, 1982.
8. Kales A, Allen C, Scharf MD, Kales JD: Hypnotic drugs and their effectiveness: all-night EEG studies of insomniac patients. *Arch Gen Psychiatry* 23:226–232, 1970.
9. Dement WC, Kleitman N: The relation of eye movements during sleep to dream activity: an objective method for the study of dreaming. *J Exp Psychol* 53:339–346, 1957.
10. Bixler EO, Kales A, Soldatos CR, Vela-Bueno A, Jacoby JA, Scarone S: Sleep apneic activity in a normal population. *Res Commun Chem Pathol Pharmacol* 36:141–152, 1982.
11. Kales A, Kales JD, Soldatos CR: Insomnia and other sleep disorders. *Med Clin North Am* 66:971–991, 1982.
12. Williams RL, Karacan I: *Sleep Disorders: Diagnosis and Treatment*, John Wiley & Sons, New York, 1978.
13. Drugs and insomnia. *JAMA* 251:2410–2414, 1984.
14. Kales A, Bixler EO, Kales JD, Scharf MB: Comparative effectiveness of nine hypnotic drugs: sleep laboratory studies. *J Clin Pharmacol* 17:207–213, 1977.
15. Mendelson WB, Weingartner H, Greenblatt DJ, Garnett D, Gillin JC: A clinical study of flurazepam. *Sleep* 5:350–360, 1982.
16. Kales A, Soldatos CR, Bixler EO, Kales JD: Rebound insomnia and rebound anxiety: a review. *Pharmacology* 26:121–137, 1983.
17. Sellers EM, Koch-Weser J: Potentiation of warfarin-induced hypoprothrombinemia by chloral hydrate. *N Engl J Med* 283:827–831, 1970.
18. Ray WA, Griffin MR, Schaffner W, Baugh DK, Melton LJ III: Psychotropic drug use and the risk of hip fracture. *N Engl J Med* 316:363–406, 1987.
19. Mitler MM: Evaluation of temazepam as a hypnotic. *Pharmacotherapy* 1:3–13, 1981.
20. Eberts FS Jr, Philopoulos Y, Reineke LM, Vliek RW: Triazolam disposition. *Clin Pharmacol Ther* 29:81–93, 1981.
21. Roth T, Roehrs TA, Zorick FJ: Pharmacology and hypnotic efficacy of triazolam. *Pharmacotherapy* 3:137–148, 1983.
22. Greenblatt DJ, Harmatz JS, Zinny MA, Shader RI: A brief tapering period over four days has reduced the symptoms of rebound insomnia. *N Engl J Med* 317:722–728, 1987.
23. Kales A, Scharf MB, Bixler EO, Schweitzer PK, Jacoby JA, Soldatos CR: Dose-response studies of quazepam. *Clin Pharmacol Ther* 30:194–200, 1981.

–5
Drug Therapy for Childhood Mental Disorders

The most pervasive childhood mental disorders are attention deficit hyperactivity disorder (ADHD), childhood schizophrenia, major depression and bipolar mood disorder, and enuresis. Developmental disorders and behavioral problems related to impulsiveness and aggressivity are other common disorders of interest in childhood psychopharmacology. Table 5.1 lists the problems in children and adolescents for which drug therapy has been used. The use of the prototype agent of each major psychoactive drug class is discussed in previous databases.

Methylphenidate is the most extensively used drug in childhood psychopharmacology. It is discussed in detail in Chapter 5A. Methylphenidate supplanted amphetamine as a stimulant for use in ADHD because of lower abuse potential and a better side effect profile.

There is a paucity of data from clinical trials using benzodiazepines in children for uses other than as anticonvulsants. Caution is called for in using benzodiazepines in children with schizophrenia or impulsive-aggressive behavior because symptoms may become worse with the use of these drugs.

Indications for antipsychotics include infantile autism, pervasive developmental disorder, schizophrenic disorders of childhood and adolescence, and Gilles de la Tourette's syndrome. Adverse effects of antipsychotics in children are similar to the side effect profile in adults. Drowsiness, extrapyramidal reactions, and tardive dyskinesia may occur. Female patients seem to be at higher risk for antipsychotic-related problems than are male patients, but total dose and duration of treatment correlate with the frequency of problems. The clinical profile of antipsychotics seems to be similar in adults and children. In a clinical comparison of thiothixene with thioridazine in schizophrenic adolescents, clinical efficacy was similar, but the high potency drug, thiothixene, predictably produced less sedation.

The antipsychotics are extensively used to control severe behavioral symptoms in mental retardation and pervasive developmental disorders. Antipsychotics are not a specific treatment for mental retardation. They are useful only for controlling behavior that would otherwise make it impossible to provide educational training for these patients because of excessive environmental aggressiveness. The use of antipsychotics is predicated on the belief that behavioral control will enable other useful therapeutic interventions.

Childhood manic-depressive disorder seems to be rare before the age of 10; however, many adults with bipolar disorder had their first manic episode before the age of 20. The response and adverse effects of adolescents to lithium seem to be similar to those of adults. Serum concentrations must be monitored,

239

Table 5.1.
Potential Indications for Psychoactive Drugs in Children and Adolescents

Drug Group	Potential Indications
Stimulents	Attention deficit hyperactivity disorder
Benzodiazepines	Seizure disorders
Lithium	Bipolar mood disorder, conduct disorder
Antipsychotics	Infantile autism, disruptive behavioral problems in developmental disorders, Gilles de la Tourette's syndrome
Cyclic antidepressants	Major depression, enuresis, encopresis, attention deficit hyperactivity disorder, school phobia (separation anxiety disorder), bulimia

but required doses may seem higher given the higher renal function compared to adults. Saliva lithium measurements have been proposed as a noninvasive method to monitor lithium concentrations, and the results have been promising but nonconfirmatory.

Lithium has been reported to be more effective than placebo and to result in fewer, less severe side effects than haloperidol in the treatment of chronic aggressiveness in children and adolescents. The major side effects of lithium are stomachache, headache, and tremor of the hands. Haloperidol causes excessive sedation, acute dystonic reactions, and drooling. Both drugs are significantly better than placebo, whereas lithium seems to have the most specific benefit. Both drugs should have only mild effects on cognition. Children with ADHD have not been reported to respond well to lithium.

Amantadine has been reported in a preliminary study to decrease the wetting frequency in enuretic children. Its use is based on the hypothesis that enuresis results from an imbalance in dopamine and norepinephrine. Tricyclic antidepressants influence both of these neurotransmitters, but imipramine, the most widely used and only approved tricyclic for enuresis, exerts more of an effect on norepinephrine. If proven useful, amantadine would have theoretical advantages in some patients who cannot be easily treated with imipramine because of anticholinergic and other side effects.

A

Methylphenidate Database

FORMULATIONS

Methylphenidate tablets: 5 mg; 10 mg; 20 mg; 20 mg in a sustained release formulation
Brand names: Ritalin (Ciba); various others

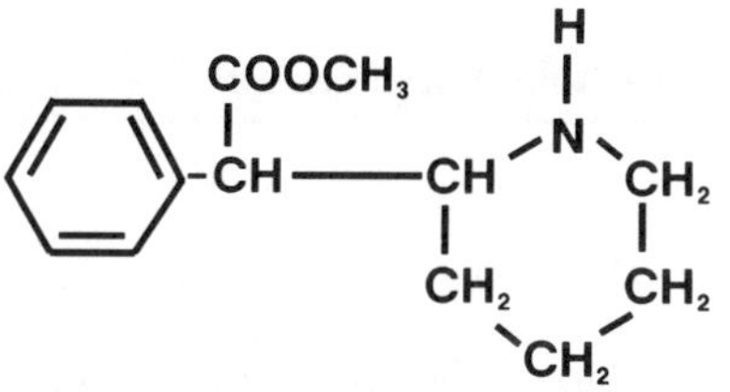

Figure 5A.1.   Structure of methylphenidate.

BASIC PHARMACOLOGY

Methylphenidate is a central nervous system (CNS) stimulant with indirect sympathomimetic activity (Fig. 5A.1). Its effects are thought to result from release of norepinephrine and dopamine into the synaptic cleft and stimulation of postsynaptic receptors (1). Although these pharmacological actions are qualitatively similar to those of amphetamine, methylphenidate's effects are more prominent on mental rather than motor activities, an advantage over other CNS stimulants. Its characteristics differ from those of the amphetamines in having only moderate effects on the peripheral circulatory system and minor anorexic effects. In children with hyperactivity associated with ADHD, methylphenidate has a paradoxical calming effect.

Cardiovascular and endocrine status is influenced by methylphenidate. Heart rate increases in a dose-dependent fashion and a 10-beats/minute increase is common in patients taking therapeutic doses. In controlled settings, both systolic and diastolic blood pressure also increase shortly after a dose and return slowly to baseline over the course of a dosage interval (2). These effects are mild and are usually not problematic during therapy. In healthy adults, a single dose of methylphenidate had no effect on serum cortisol (3). Concern has been expressed about possible depression of growth rate in children, which may occur with methylphenidate. Growth rate is expected to increase to normal when the drug is discontinued.

There is controversy as to whether methylphenidate produces euphoria in children. In adults, a single 10- or 20-mg dose had a positive effect on subjective assessment of well-being with improvement in self-rating of vigor and elation (4). Although some children seem to be happier while taking the drug, therapeutic use of methylphenidate in ADHD is not expected to lead to a later drug dependence. The expected effects on various laboratory tests are outlined in Table 5A.1.

PHARMACOKINETIC PROPERTIES

The disposition of methylphenidate has been reported in adults and children (5, 6). After oral administration, methylphenidate is rapidly and nearly completely absorbed, usually reaching a peak plasma concentration by 2 hours. Extended-release tablets are absorbed more slowly but to a similar extent as conventional tablets.

The primary route of metabolism for methylphenidate is biotransformation to ritalinic acid, a metabolite that has poor lipid solubility and is presumed to be pharmacologically inactive (6). Other metabolic products occur from para-hydroxylation or oxidation. One metabolite, para-hydroxymethylphenidate, has measurable pharmacological activity but does not seem to accumulate appreciably in plasma.

Table 5A.1.
Expected Physiological Effects from Methylphenidate Therapy for Monitoring[a]

Parameter	Drug Effect
Cardiovascular status	
Heart rate	Can be expected to increase 10 beats/minute or more
ECG	
Blood pressure	Slight increases in systolic and diastolic pressure have been noted.
Renal function	
Serum creatinine and clearance, BUN	Normal values are not expected to change.
Hepatic function	
AST (SGOT), ALT (SGPT), alkaline phosphatase	Normal values should not change in most patients.
Hematology status	
CBC	An occasional case of eosinophilia has been noted. A hematological screen is recommended once a year.
Neuroendocrine status	
Cortisol	No effect expected

[a]Abbreviations: ECG, electrocardiogram; BUN, blood urea nitrogen; AST, aspartate aminotransferase; SGOT, serum glutamic-oxaloacetic transaminase; ALT, alanine aminotransferase; SGPT, serum glutamic-pyruvic transaminase; CBC, complete blood count.

Less than 1% of a methylphenidate dose is excreted in an unchanged form in the urine; ritalinic acid accounts for 80% of the excreted dose. The elimination half-life of methylphenidate is usually between 2 and 7 hours. The total body clearance is approximately 3.0 to 9.0 liters/kg/hour. A high clearance contributes to relatively low steady-state plasma concentrations, frequently in the range of 10 to 30 ng/ml (7). Both the inter- and intrapatient variability in steady-state serum concentrations is considerable. These properties are reflected by the need for multiple daily doses, individualized according to subjective response. A summary of methylphenidate's pharmacokinetics is given in Table 5A.2.

INDICATIONS

The major indication for methylphenidate is in the treatment of ADHD. Before the advent of DSM-III-R, patients with ADHD were frequently diagnosed as having minimal brain dysfunction or hyperkinetic child syndrome. Patients with ADHD are usually children older than 7 years of age, although symptoms will have been present before this age. These children show inappropriate degrees of inattention, impulsiveness, and hyperactivity. These behaviors often lead to difficulties in school performance and maintaining constructive relationships with family members and peers.

Methylphenidate has been proven in double-blind, placebo-controlled studies to improve behavior, concentration, and learning ability in most children with ADHD (8). It has been compared to other psychostimulants and found to be superior to caffeine and amphetamine (9). Methylphenidate has the advantage of producing fewer adverse effects than amphetamine.

Table 5A.2.
Pharmacokinetic Parameters of Methylphenidate

Parameter	Range
Bioavailability	80% or more
Time of peak concentration after a single dose	Oral: 2 to 4 hours
Plasma protein binding	15.2 ± 5.2% bound
Volume of distribution	20.13 ± 9 liters/kg
Total plasma clearance	5.5 ± 2.2 liters/kg/hr
Renal clearance	Negligible
Elimination half-life	2 to 7 hours in adults or children
Metabolites	Ritalinic acid (inactive) Para-hydroxymethylphenidate (active)
Therapeutic range for benefits in attention deficit disorder	Cannot be stated; large intra- and intersubject variability noted in plasma concentrations; frequent steady-state concentrations of 10 to 30 ng/ml

Other uses for methylphenidate include symptomatic treatment of narcolepsy and treatment of apathetic or withdrawn behavior due to a variety of causes, including depression. Its effectiveness for these uses is not completely established.

The search for drugs that facilitate memory, or cognition enhancers, is currently a major research effort for the pharmaceutical industry. CNS stimulants have long been thought to be theoretically useful. However, clinical studies in normal adults have shown that methylphenidate may actually impair learning and memory because of a disruption in attention (10). Methylphenidate does not seem to be a useful drug to enhance memory or retard memory loss. There is no evidence that it improves performance on general cognitive measures such as intelligence tests or language skills.

Provocative tests to diagnose tardive dyskinesia (TD) early during antipsychotic therapy have long been sought. Methylphenidate was shown to exaggerate the movements of patients with TD, suggesting that it may be a useful tool for diagnosis, although not for treatment (11). The effects of methylphenidate on motor activity in TD may be related to an increased catecholaminergic state or dopaminergic effects. Diagnosis of TD is not an indication for methylphenidate.

DOSAGE REGIMEN DESIGN

The dosage of methylphenidate must be carefully adjusted according to individual response. When therapy is initiated, the extended release preparation should not be used until the daily dosage is titrated to optimal response using the conventional tablets. Also, the last daily dose should be given several hours before bedtime to lessen the possibility of producing insomnia.

Methylphenidate is not approved for use in children younger than 6 years of age. For older children, initial treatment can be started with 5 mg twice daily, preferably 30 to 45 minutes before breakfast and lunch. The dose may be gradually increased by 5 or 10 mg at weekly intervals. The usually effective dosage range is 0.3 to 0.5 mg/kg/day (usually 10 to 20 mg/day). The maximal daily dosage recommended for children is 2 mg/kg or approximately 60 mg. If no improvement is observed after 1 month of treatment with a usual dose, methylphenidate should be discontinued. If the extended release form of the drug is used, it is preferably given once daily before breakfast.

For adults, the usual dose required is 10 mg two or three times a day, with a range of 10 to 60 mg. A major problem during the treatment of narcolepsy in adults is tolerance when large doses are used daily for prolonged periods. Occasional drug holidays may help to restore sensitivity and allow a reduced dosage to be used when therapy is reinstated.

Abrupt discontinuation of methylphenidate after short-term use has not been shown to cause any problems. However, after prolonged administration of large doses, abrupt withdrawal should be avoided and the dosage tapered.

THERAPEUTIC DRUG MONITORING

Studies have assessed the relationship between methylphenidate plasma concentration and behavioral effects. In one report (12), only a weak relationship was found between improvement in academic performance and serum concentration. The small number of patients studied did not allow definition of a therapeutic serum concentration range. Overall, the evidence suggesting that monitoring plasma concentrations of methylphenidate is therapeutically useful is weak.

CONTRAINDICATIONS—WARNINGS—PRECAUTIONS

Methylphenidate should not be used in a patient with a history of marked anxiety, tension, and agitation because it may aggravate these symptoms. It is also contraindicated in patients who are hypersensitive to the drug, patients with glaucoma, and patients with motor tics, a family history or diagnosis of Gilles de la Tourette's syndrome, or anorexia nervosa. In developmental disorders that resemble adult schizophrenia, methylphenidate could exacerbate psychotic symptoms and should be avoided.

Methylphenidate should not be used for severe depression or for the prevention or treatment of normal fatigue states. In patients with hypertension and patients with a prior history of seizures, methylphenidate should be used with caution, if at all.

During prolonged therapy it is advised to have periodic complete blood counts and differential and platelet counts, especially in children. The drug should be administered with caution to adults with a history of drug dependence because such patients may increase the dosage on their own initiative. Chronic excessive use may result in a marked tolerance and psychic dependence.

DRUG INTERACTIONS

The concurrent use of methylphenidate and monoamine oxidase inhibitors (MAOIs) may cause potentiation of the stimulatory effects of methylphenidate. This could adversely affect blood pressure. Therefore, methylphenidate should not be administered during or within 14 days after the administration of MAOIs.

The concurrent use of methylphenidate and guanethidine should be avoided if possible because methylphenidate will antagonize the adrenergic neuronal blockade produced by guanethidine, thereby inhibiting guanethidine's hypotensive effects. Other antihypertensive agents are available to avoid this interaction. Patients taking antihypertensives should have close monitoring of their blood pressure and cardiovascular status.

Methylphenidate seems to inhibit the metabolism of tricyclic antidepressants and may increase their blood levels appreciably. An inhibition of hydroxylation pathways seems to be a likely mechanism. Although this combination of drugs was briefly investigated as a therapeutic approach for the treatment of depression, it has been essentially abandoned for lack of documented efficacy. If this combination is used, close monitoring for tricyclic side effects is recommended.

Methylphenidate may inhibit the metabolism of coumarin anticoagulants, thereby prolonging their half-lives and pharmacological effects. Although evidence of this interaction is weak, frequent monitoring of the prothrombin time is recommended.

Methylphenidate may cause an increase in the serum levels of anticonvulsants because of inhibition of their metabolism. When using these drugs together, one should keep in mind that certain susceptible patients might manifest toxicity associated with elevated serum levels of phenytoin or other anticonvulsants.

ADVERSE REACTIONS—OCCURRENCE AND MANAGEMENT

Methylphenidate is considered to be a safe and effective drug in pediatric psychopharmacology. The common side effects include headache, insomnia, appetite reduction, and irritability. Side effects can be expected to disappear when therapy ceases. However, a few cases of movement disorders persisting after the discontinuance of therapy have been described (13, 14). Tics and, rarely, a progression to Gilles de la Tourette's syndrome have occurred. These side effects are rare but prompt the recommendation that a family history of at least two generations should be sought for movement disorders when considering methylphenidate therapy. Table 5A.3 lists the common side effects and their anticipated frequency of occurrence.

The most common adverse reactions are nervousness and insomnia. These are usually controlled by decreasing the dose and omitting the drug during the afternoon or evening. Adverse reactions that occur less commonly include dizziness, drowsiness, headache, nausea, abdominal pain, and changes in pulse rate. Side effects that occur rarely include hypersensitivity reactions, profound mood changes, leukopenia, anemia, tics resembling Gilles de la Tourette's syndrome, and seizures. Tachycardia, insomnia, anorexia, and weight loss seem to occur more frequently in children than in adults.

It is reported that long-term treatment with methylphenidate, especially in high doses, may result in some minor suppression of growth in hyperactive children. However, these effects seem transient, and overall stature is not expected to be reduced from therapy. Summer holidays from drug therapy may minimize any effect on growth rate.

MANAGEMENT OF OVERDOSE

The signs and symptoms of acute methylphenidate overdosage result principally from overstimulation of the CNS and from excessive sympathomimetic

Table 5A.3.
Expected Side Effects from Methylphenidate Therapy

Effect	Rare	Less Common	More Common
Headache		X	
Insomnia			X
Drowsiness		X	
Loss of appetite			X
Loss of weight		X	
Nausea		X	
Abdominal pain		X	
Nervousness			X
Mood changes		X	
Dry mouth		X	
Blurred vision		X	
Disorientation	X		
Tic-like movements of head, face	X		
Skin rash	X		
Blood pressure increase		X	
Tachycardia		X	
Anemia	X		

effects. Cardiovascular symptoms include flushing, palpitation, hypertension, cardiac arrhythmias, and tachycardia. Mental disturbances that may occur include confusion, delirium, euphoria, hallucinations, and delirium. Other symptoms include agitation, headache, vomiting, dryness of mucous membranes, mydriasis, hyperpyrexia, sweating, tremors, hyperreflexia, muscle twitching, and seizures.

In the treatment of overdosage, appropriate supportive measures, including maintenance of adequate circulation and respiratory exchange, should be instituted immediately. The patient should be protected against self-injury and isolated to avoid excessive external stimuli. Emesis should be initiated unless the patient is comatose, convulsing, or has lost the gag reflex. Activated charcoal could be administered (adults, 60 to 100 gm; children, 30 to 60 gm) along with a cathartic such as magnesium sulfate (adults, 30 gm; children, 250 mg/kg). The efficacy of hemodialysis or peritoneal dialysis for the treatment of methylphenidate overdosage has not been established.

USE IN RENAL AND/OR HEPATIC DISEASE

No specific data seem to be available about the use of methylphenidate during hepatic or renal disease. As the drug is extensively metabolized, little additional methylphenidate accumulation above normal would be expected in renal dysfunction. Nevertheless, changes in drug sensitivity frequently accompany renal dysfunction, and methylphenidate use should be closely monitored.

USE IN CHILDREN AND ADOLESCENTS

Methylphenidate is used primarily in children. When treating ADHD, the improvement rate can be expected to range between 60% and 90%. Enhanced attention and improved interpersonal interactions have been reported in numerous studies. The most consistent positive effect of the drug is on disruptive and socially inappropriate behavior of problem children. Lesser effects are seen on emotional symptoms. However, some shy children have been reported to show more outgoing behavior.

Before beginning methylphenidate, baseline assessment should be made to identify target behaviors of most concern to the child, parents, and teachers. Some psychometric measures of learning and academic achievement are useful. In the physical examination, weight and height should be recorded. A neurological examination is recommended to detect any predisposition to movement disorders. Counseling with the parents, the school teachers, and the child should be conducted before starting drug therapy. The child should understand the nature of the difficulties and become part of the therapeutic planning process.

There are no established guidelines for when to discontinue medication. Some patients may benefit from therapy for several years; however, an attempt should be made to give the child a drug-free trial during each school year.

Methylphenidate should not be used in children younger than 6 years of age. Safety and efficacy in this age group have not been established.

USE IN ELDERLY

Methylphenidate may cause a brief elevation in mood. This effect has been useful in patients with mild despondency. Nevertheless, there is little evidence to suggest that methylphenidate is as effective as the specific antidepressants in this age group when endogenous depression exists. The drug has been used as a general psychostimulant, but this is not an established indication.

USE IN PREGNANCY

Safe use of methylphenidate during pregnancy or lactation has not been established. It is likely to pass the placental membranes into the fetal environment given its high lipid solublity.

PATIENT INFORMATION

The following are general considerations when discussing methylphenidate use with patients: If you experience sleeping difficulties, this problem may be reduced by taking the last dose earlier in the day, i.e., no later than 3 hours before bedtime. This medication may mask symptoms of fatigue, impair physical coordination, or produce dizziness or drowsiness.

REFERENCES

1. Ferris RM, Tang FLM: Comparison of the effects of the isomers of amphetamine, methylphenidate and deoxypipradrol on the uptake of 1-H-3-norepinephrine and H-3 dopamine by synaptic vesicles from rat whole brain, striatum and hypothalamus. *J Pharmacol Exp Ther* 210:422–428, 1979.
2. Joyce PR, Nicholls MG, Donald RA: Methylphenidate increases heart rate, blood pressure and plasma epinephrine in normal subjects. *Life Sci* 34:1707–1711, 1984.
3. Brown WA, Corriveau DP, Ebert MH: Acute psychologic and neuroendocrine effects of dextroamphetamine and methylphenidate. *Psychopharmacology* 58:189–195, 1978.
4. Huey LY, Janowsky DS, Judd LL, et al: Effects of lithium carbonate on methylphenidate-induced mood, behavior, and cognitive processes. *Psychopharmacology* 73:161–164, 1981.
5. Hungund BL, Perel JM, Hurwic MJ, Sverd J, Winsberg BG: Pharmacokinetics of methylphenidate in hyperkinetic children. *Br J Clin Pharmacol* 8:571–576, 1979.

6. Faraj BA, Israili ZH, Perel JM, Jenkins ML, Holtzman SG, Cucinell SA, Dayton PG: Metabolism and disposition of methylphenidate-C-14: studies in man and animals. *J Pharmacol Exp Ther* 191:535–547, 1974.
7. Gualtieri CT, Wargin W, Kanoy R, Patrick K, Shen CD, Youngblood W, Mueller RA, Breese GR: Clinical studies of methylphenidate serum levels in children and adults. *J Am Acad Child Psychiatry* 21:19–26, 1982.
8. Barkley RA: A review of stimulant drug research with hyperactive children. *J Child Psychol Psychiatry* 18:137–165, 1977.
9. Huestis RD, Arnold LE, Smeltzer DJ: Caffeine versus methylphenidate and d-amphetamine in minimal brain dysfunction: a double-blind comparison. *Am J Psychiatry* 132:868–870, 1975.
10. Wetzel CD, Squire LR, Janowsky DS: Methylphenidate impairs learning and memory in normal adults. *Behav Neurol Biol* 31:413–424, 1981.
11. Radonjic D, Lapierre YD, Knott V: The effect of methylphenidate on tardive dyskinesia. *Prog Neuropsychopharmacol* 5:491–494, 1981.
12. Kupietz SS, Winsberg BG, Sverd J: Learning ability and methylphenidate plasma concentration in hyperactive children. *J Am Acad Child Psychiatry* 21:27–30, 1982.
13. Denckla MB, Bemporad JR, McKay MC: Tics following methylphenidate administration: a report of 20 cases. *JAMA* 235:1349–1351, 1976.
14. Bremness AB, Sverd J: Methylphenidate-induced Tourette syndrome: case report. *Am J Psychiatry* 136:1334–1335, 1979.

6

Drug Therapy for Psychoactive Substance Abuse

Substance abuse disorders occupy the largest number of listings in the DSM-III-R. This partly reflects the wide variety of abusable substances available in our culture. Unfortunately, specific treatments that cure abuse are not yet available, nor do we fully understand the pathophysiological basis for addiction. Two drugs, disulfiram (Chapter 6A) and methadone (Chapter 6B) are widely used to decrease abuse of alcohol and opiates, respectively.

A

Disulfiram Database

FORMULATIONS

Disulfiram tablets: 250 mg, 500 mg
Brand names: Antabuse (Ayerst); various generic names

BASIC PHARMACOLOGY

Disulfiram (tetraethylthiuram disulfide) (Fig. 6A.1) has been extensively used for the treatment of alcoholism for over 35 years. Approximately 200,000 people use it regularly in the United States. Its use as an alcohol deterrent is based on the fact that it produces physiological changes after ethanol consumption that are sufficently aversive to reinforce the alcoholic's motivation toward abstinence (1). These adverse effects, the disulfiram-ethanol reaction (DER), occur as a result of accumulation of acetaldehyde in the body. Ordinarily, acetaldehyde, the initial metabolite of ethanol, is converted to acetic acid through the action of the enzyme aldehyde dehydrogenase. Disulfiram inhibits this enzymatic reaction and, as a result, acetaldehyde accumulates to many times its usual concentration (2). Disulfiram does not directly influence alcohol elimination, only the conversion of acetaldehyde to acetic acid, so alcohol levels do not increase. Acetaldehyde accumulation results in nausea, vomiting, flushing, headache, tachycardia, hypotension, tachypnea, and other adverse reactions. The time course of behavioral and physical effects of the DER is outlined in Table 6A.1.

Although it is generally accepted that the primary mechanism of the DER is excessive acetaldehyde levels, studies in rodents suggest that the severity of the

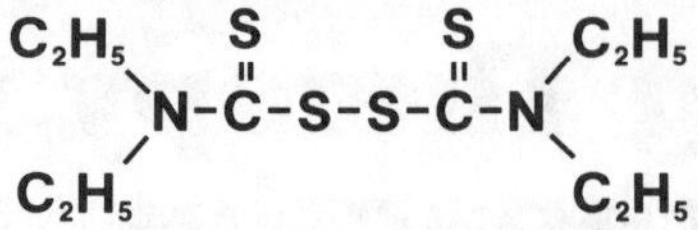

$$C_2H_5 \underset{C_2H_5}{\overset{}{\diagdown}} N - \overset{\overset{S}{\|}}{C} - S - S - \overset{\overset{S}{\|}}{C} - N \underset{C_2H_5}{\overset{C_2H_5}{\diagup}}$$

Figure 6A.1.   Structure of disulfiram.

Table 6A.1.
Characteristics of the Disulfiram-Alcohol Interaction

Time Course after Taking Ethanol	Effects
As soon as 10 minutes; peak at 20–30 minutes, lasting for 1.5 hours	Flushing, sensation of warmth in the face Vasodilation of peripheral blood vessels causing a red appearance Throbbing headache, feeling of tightness (simulating chest pain), and respiratory difficulty Weakness, vertigo, confusion
Thirty to 60 minutes, lasting for as long as 6 hours	Nausea, flushing replaced by pallor Hypotension, tachycardia, palpitations ECG changes: flattening of T-waves, depression of S-T segment, Q-T prolongation Hyperventilation Protracted vomiting Blurred vision, dizziness, ataxia Feelings of impending doom Physical exhaustion followed by sleep

DER is also related to changes in catecholamine metabolism. Inhibition of dopamine-β-hydroxylase occurs, causing increased dopamine levels and decreased norepinephrine levels in the brain (3) (see Chapter 1B). The expected effects of disulfiram on physiological status and various laboratory tests are outlined in Table 6A.2.

PHARMACOKINETIC PROPERTIES

Disulfiram is well absorbed after oral administration. Peak concentration occurs in an average of 9 hours (4). The drug is highly lipid-soluble and distributes extensively in the body. In rodents it has been found in liver, kidney, muscle, intestinal, cardiac, and other tissues.

Disulfiram is biotransformed into four major metabolites (5). It is rapidly reduced after absorption to a thiol, diethyldithiocarbamic acid (DDC). DDC is further metabolized to DDC methyl ester, diethylamine, and carbon disulfide. Studies in rodents suggest that 50% of a dose is excreted in urine as the glucuronide metabolite; however, recent studies in humans using specific analytical methods suggest that the most important pathway for elimination in humans is excretion of carbon disulfide in exhaled breath (4). This is sometimes noticeable in patient's taking disulfiram as a breath odor similar to acetone.

The biological half-life of disulfiram averages 7 hours; however, the drug causes an irreversible inhibition of hepatic enzymes, thereby producing a much longer pharmacodynamic half-life. About 12 hours is required from the initiation of therapy until disulfiram's full inhibitory effects are operative. Reactions

Table 6A.2.
Expected Physiological Effects from Disulfiram Therapy for Monitoring[a]

Parameter	Drug Effect
Cardiovascular status	
Heart rate	No effect or increase in patients with lung disease
ECG	No expected effects except in combination with alcohol (see Table 6A.1)
Blood pressure	Modest reduction in systolic pressure
Renal function	
Serum creatinine and clearance, BUN	Normal values should not change in most adults.
Hepatic function	
AST (SGOT), ALT (SGPT), alkaline phosphatase	These may become elevated during therapy, and the determination of baseline levels is recommended before starting therapy. Hepatitis and hepatotoxicity have been reported.
Cholesterol, triglycerides	Serum concentrations may rise during therapy.
Hematology status	
CBC	No effects expected
Neuroendocrine status	
Thyroid indices	These may be altered, but the patient remains euthyroid.

[a]Abbreviations: ECG, electrocardiogram; BUN, blood urea nitrogen; ALT, alanine aminotransferase; SGPT, serum glutamic-pyruvic transaminase; CBC, complete blood count.

to disulfiram have been reported to occur as long as a week after discontinuance of therapy. A summary of disulfiram's kinetic properties is given in Table 6A.3.

INDICATIONS

Disulfiram is indicated as an aid in the management of alcoholism. There are limited data from controlled clinical trials of its efficacy in maintaining long-term sobriety (6). Patients do best who are highly motivated and who feel the need for an external aid in an abstinence program.

The effectiveness of disulfiram depends on the patient's willingness to initiate and comply with treatment. In one study (7), patients who accepted disulfiram tended to be younger and were more likely to be acceptors of most other types of treatment recommendations for problem drinking. A large number of alcoholics refuse to take the drug. Psychological testing has suggested that patients who accept the drug have a strong belief that disulfiram will generally help them to remain sober and will help them to resist the urge to drink (7, 8). It may be beneficial to try to convince skeptical patients that the drug can be helpful. Sources of doubt about the drug's effects and value should be identified, and misconceptions about side effects should be clarified.

DOSAGE REGIMEN DESIGN

The recommended initial dose is 250 or 500 mg daily. It is not necessary to give a loading dose of disulfiram. Maintenance therapy can be given at 250 mg daily; some patients may be maintained on smaller doses. A dosage of 500 mg

Table 6A.3.
Pharmacokinetic Parameters of Disulfiram

Parameter	Range
Bioavailability	Oral: nearly complete
Time of peak concentration after single dose	9.2 ± 0.3 (SD) hours
Renal clearance	Negligible; glucuronide metabolites are excreted.
Elimination half-life	Average of 7 hours
Active metabolites (half-life)	Diethyldithiocarbamate (15 hr)
	Diethyldithiocarbamate-methyl ester (22 hr)
	Diethylamine (14 hr)
	Carbon disulfide (9 hr)

daily should not be exceeded. Patients are commonly continued on therapy for months or even years until they are fully recovered socially.

A disulfiram challenge test has been used in some treatment programs but is no longer considered necessary or even desirable. This test consisted of taking enough alcohol in combination with disulfiram to produce the DER. Deaths have resulted from this type of aversive therapy, and this procedure is discouraged. Patients can be fully informed about the DER to achieve the same purpose.

Because drowsiness is the most common side effect of disulfiram, it may be useful to take the drug at bedtime. Drowsiness usually does not persist into the following day. When sedation continues to be a problem, the dose should be reduced.

Before beginning the drug, the patient should be completely free of alcohol. At least 12 to 24 hours should elapse between the last drink and the initiation of disulfiram therapy. When the recent history of alcohol consumption is in doubt, 24 hours or more should elapse before initiating disulfiram therapy.

THERAPEUTIC DRUG MONITORING

Plasma concentration monitoring capability for disulfiram is not generally available. As the drug is an irreversible enzyme inhibitor, it is expected that plasma drug concentrations would have little relationship to enzyme inhibition.

Measurements of erythrocyte acetaldehyde oxidizing capacity (AOC) are probably better than measurements of plasma concentrations of disulfiram for identifying patients who are undertreated. AOC is maximally suppressed after 6 days of treatment (9). When patients report that they are able to drink with impunity while taking disulfiram, noncompliance should be suspected. For the promotion of abstinence, regular follow-up sessions with an understanding primary clinician are essential.

CONTRAINDICATIONS—WARNINGS—PRECAUTIONS

There are several relative contraindications to the use of disulfiram. These include a history of an unusually severe reaction, a history of severe cardiovascular disease, diabetes mellitus, cirrhosis of the liver, hypothyroidism, or a psychiatric history of major affective disorder, schizophrenia, or dementia. A patient with a history of rubber contact dermatitis may be at high risk for an allergic reaction to disulfiram. Pregnancy should be considered a contraindication.

In patients with cardiovascular disease, excessive accumulation of acetaldehyde may cause shock and myocardial infarction. Deaths due to the DER have been reported. Patients with ischemic heart disease should not be treated with disulfiram.

DRUG INTERACTIONS

Disulfiram increases the half-life of antipyrine by inhibition of hepatic microsomal mixed function oxidases (10). Antipyrine is a model compound widely used as an index of hepatic mixed function oxidase activity in vivo. It is a low extraction drug and therefore its clearance is minimally influenced by hepatic blood flow (see Chapter 1D). The effects of disulfiram on its clearance suggest that disulfiram would inhibit the clearance of many highly metabolized drugs.

Not surprisingly, disulfiram enhanced the effects of warfarin, another low extraction drug, by inhibiting its hydroxylation (11). Phenytoin toxicity has occurred when disulfiram was combined in an anticonvulsant regimen. The exaggerated sedative effect of diazepam when combined with disulfiram is discussed in Chapter 4A.

The clearance of antipsychotics and antidepressants is predictably decreased by disulfiram. When single doses of imipramine and desipramine were administered to two alcoholics before and during disulfiram treatment, decreased tricyclic clearance was noted along with increased elimination half-life (12). Thus, dosage adjustments may be necessary to prevent toxicity if these combinations are used; however, some clinicians avoid disulfiram altogether in patients who require therapy with these drugs.

Disulfiram decreased the clearance of caffeine in both normal subjects and recovering alcoholics by 24 to 30% (13). This observation suggests an increased risk of side effects from higher concentrations of caffeine, a situation that might complicate withdrawal from alcohol, as coffee consumption is high among recovering alcoholics. A summary of drug interactions is given in Table 6A.4.

ADVERSE REACTIONS—OCCURRENCE AND MANAGEMENT

Disulfiram can produce unwanted effects that are not due to interference with acetaldehyde metabolism. The most common side effect is drowsiness. Fatigability, headache, and restlessness are also usual complaints. More serious reactions include peripheral neuropathy and effects on vision from optic or retrobulbar neuritis (14). Occasionally, a skin rash occurs, which can be managed by antihistamine administration or a reduction in the daily dose. A metallic or garlic-like taste frequently occurs during the first 2 weeks of therapy. A summary of expected disulfiram side effects is given in Table 6A.5.

In a review of the medical literature, 52 reports of psychoses after the use of disulfiram were collected (15). A plausible mechanism for this adverse effect is the inhibition of dopamine β-hydroxylase (see Chapter 1B), which would increase stimulation of postsynaptic dopamine receptors. Recently, cases of manic psychoses have been reported in patients with family histories of affective disorder (16, 17). It is suggested that disulfiram be used cautiously in patients with either a personal or a family history of bipolar disorder or schizophrenia.

Table 6A.4.
Drug Interactions with Disulfiram

Interacting Drug	Effect
Coffee	Decreased clearance; possible increased stimulation
Ethanol-containing beverages, foods, products	Disulfiram-ethanol reaction (Table 6A.1)
Isoniazid	Decreased clearance; exaggerated effects
Benzodiazepines	Decreased clearance; increased sedation
Warfarin	Decreased clearance; enhanced hypoprothrombinemic effects possible
Phenytoin	Decreased clearance; possible toxicity
Cyclic antidepressants	Decreased clearance; increased side effect risk
Metronidazole	Possible precipitation of acute toxic reaction
Marijuana	Synergistic central nervous stimulation?

Table 6A.5.
Expected Side Effects from Disulfiram Therapy

Effect	Rare	Less Common	More Common
Dry mouth		X	
Blurred vision		X	
Nausea		X	
Vomiting		X	
Drowsiness			X
Dizziness			X
Ataxia		X	
Headache			X
Restlessness			X
Excitement			X
Skin rash		X	
Blood pressure decrease		X	
Tachycardia		X	
Jaundice	X		
Hepatitis	X		
Peripheral neuritis	X		

As hepatitis has been reported, baseline liver function tests are recommended before starting therapy (18–20). The onset of hepatitis has occurred in as little as 10 days after initiation of therapy. Most cases have occurred within 3 months. Prodromal symptoms include nausea, fatigue, and fever proceeding to jaundice. Liver function tests (bilirubin and alkaline phosphatase) can be expected to be abnormally elevated. After withdrawal of disulfiram, improvement should occur usually within 2 weeks. In alcoholic liver disease, the aspartate aminotransferase (AST) (serum glutamic-oxaloacetic transaminase (SGOT)) is usually less than 300 units; however, in difulfiram-induced hepatotoxicity, it can be expected to be much higher, usually in excess of 800 units.

Peripheral neuropathies have been reported during disulfiram therapy but can be expected to improve upon stopping the drug. The usual time course for a sensorimotor neuropathy to develop is between 10 days and 18 months after initiation of treatment (14). However, one case is reported in which neurological deficits developed after disulfiram was taken for over 30 years (21). A period of months may be required for substantial improvement to occur after discontinuing the drug.

An encephalopathy may also occur, arising days to months after the medicine is begun (22). A mild, diffuse slowing of the electroencephalogram may be apparent (23). Alcoholics are prone to seizures, and they may be more susceptible during disulfiram therapy (24).

MANAGEMENT OF OVERDOSE

Acute overdose of disulfiram is rare. A recent case report described a 31-year-old man who was presumed to have taken as much as 7.5 gm in an overdosage (25). He demonstrated delirium, somnolence, and catatonic behavior over 2 days. He recovered without neurological deficits after conservative treatment with haloperidol for delirium. No seizures occurred. Treatment of disulfiram overdosage is aimed toward specific symptoms with observance of general principles of poison treatment. No specific antidote is available. Treatment for shock may be necessary.

USE IN RENAL AND/OR HEPATIC DISEASE

Disulfiram has been implicated in causing hepatotoxicity resembling viral or alcoholic hepatitis (19). If jaundice occurs during therapy, the drug should be discontinued as soon as this symptom is noted. Patients have died from complications of liver damage. Unfortunately, daily dosage does not predict problems with liver damage.

In a large Veterans Administration trial of alcoholic subjects who were randomly assigned to either disulfiram or placebo for up to 12 months (18), there was no relationship between liver function tests and disulfiram treatment. However, increases in transaminase and bilirubin levels identified patients on disulfiram who were still drinking. Liver function test abnormalities were frequent. The DER in subjects with severe liver disease can persist for an long as 96 hours after disulfiram withdrawal compared to 24 hours in subjects with normal liver function (26). Patients with severe liver or renal disease should not be candidates for disulfiram therapy.

USE IN CHILDREN AND ADOLESCENTS

Disulfiram should not be used in children or adolescents. There is essentially no experience in this area of pharmacotherapeutics. Alcohol problems in adolescents should be managed through intensive behavioral treatment programs.

USE IN ELDERLY

The severity of the DER shows considerable variability. Clinical experience suggests that the decrease in blood pressure during the DER is more pronounced for patients older than 40 years. Cardiovascular tolerance may decrease with ageing, making the risk of a severe DER greater in older patients (9).

USE IN PREGNANCY

Pregnancy is a contraindication to the use of disulfiram. Reports exist of maldevelopment of limbs of infants born to women taking disulfiram (27).

PATIENT INFORMATION

Patients must be fully informed of the purpose of disulfiram treatment, the mechanism of the reaction, and the expected consequences of drinking alcohol. It should be presumed that many patients will experience the reaction, and they should be told of what to do in this situation.

Patients should understand that the DER may not occur immediately after imbibing alcohol. A delay in the reaction may be as long as 24 hours. It is best to present the patient with a written description of these symptoms, express them verbally, and include a signed consent form in the patient's records.

Patients should be informed that alcohol is an ingredient in many foods, medicines, and preparations that are applied to the skin, in addition to alcoholic beverages. Complete lists, which should be given to the patient, are available from the manufacturer of Antabuse (Ayerst).

REFERENCES

1. Lundwall L, Baekeland F: Disulfiram treatment of alcoholism: a review. *J Nerv Ment Dis* 153:381–394, 1971.
2. Haley TJ: Disulfiram (tetraethylthioperoxydicarbonic diamide): a reappraisal of its toxicity and therapeutic application. *Drug Metab Rev* 9:319–335, 1979.
3. Goldstein M, Nakajima K: The effect of disulfiram on catecholamine levels in the brain. *J Pharmacol Exp Ther* 157:96–102, 1967.
4. Faiman MD, Jensen JC, Lacoursiere RB: Elimination kinetics of disulfiram in alcoholics after single and repeated doses. *Clin Pharmacol Ther* 36:520–526, 1984.
5. Eneanya DI, Bianchine JR, Duran DO, Andresen BD: The actions and metabolic fate of disulfiram. *Ann Rev Pharmcol Toxicol* 21:575–596, 1981.
6. Fuller RK, Branchey L, Brightwell DR, et al: Disulfiram treatment of alcoholism: a Veterans Administration co-operative study. *JAMA* 256:1449–1455, 1986.
7. Rush BR, Malla A: A comparison of disulfiram acceptors and refusers on selected demographics and clinical characteristics. *Drug Alcohol Depend* 14:75–85, 1984.
8. Brubaker RG, Prue DM, Rychtarik RG: Determinants of disulfiram acceptance among alcoholic patients: a test of the theory of reasoned action. *Addict Behav* 12:43–51, 1987.
9. Beyeler C, Fisch H-U, Preisig R: The disulfiram-alcohol reaction: factors determining and potential tests predicting severity. *Alcoholism* 9:118–124, 1985.
10. Vessel ES, Passananti GT, Cynthia H: Impairment of drug metabolism by disulfiram in man. *Clin Pharmacol Ther* 12:785–792, 1971.
11. O'Reilly R: Interaction of sodium warfarin and disulfiram (Antabuse) in man. *Ann Intern Med* 78:73–76, 1973.
12. Ciraulo DA, Barnhill J, Boxenbaum H: Pharmacokinetic interaction of disulfiram and antidepressants. *Am J Psychiatry* 142:1373–1374, 1985.
13. Beach CA, Mays DC, Guiler RC, Jacober CH, Gerber N: Inhibition of elimination of caffeine by disulfiram in normal subjects and recovering alcoholics. *Clin Pharmacol Ther* 39:265–270, 1986.
14. Ansbacher LE, Borch EP, Cancilla PA: Disulfiram neuropathy: a neurofilamentous distal axonopathy. *Neurology* 32:424–428, 1982.
15. Liddon SC, Satran R: Disulfiram (Antabuse) psychosis. *Am J Psychiatry* 123:1284–1289, 1967.
16. Nunes E, Quitkin F: Disulfiram and bipolar affective disorder. *J Clin Psychopharmacol* 7:284, 1987 (letter).
17. Bakish D, Lapierre YD: Disulfiram and bipolar affective disorder: a case report. *J Clin Psychopharmacol* 6:178–180, 1986.
18. Iber FL, Lee K, Lacoursiere R, Fuller R: Liver toxicity encountered in the Veterans Administration trial of disulfiram in alcoholics. *Alcoholism* 11:301–304, 1987.

19. Black JL, Richardson JW: Disulfiram hepatotoxicity: case report. *J Clin Psychiatry* 46:67–68, 1985.
20. Keeffe EB, Smith FW: Disulfiram hypersensitivity. *JAMA* 230:435–436, 1974.
21. Borrett D, Ashby P, Bilbao J, Carlen P: Reversible, late-onset disulfiram-induced neuropathy and encephalopathy. *Ann Neurol* 17:396–399, 1985.
22. Knee ST, Razani J: Acute organic brain syndrome: a complication of disulfiram therapy. *Am J Psychiatry* 131:1281–1282, 1974.
23. Busse E, Barnes RH, Ebaugh FG: Effect of Antabuse on the electroencephalogram. *Am J Med Sci* 223:126–130, 1952.
24. Price T, Silberfarb P: Convulsions following disulfiram treatment. *Am J Psychiatry* 133:235, 1976 (letter).
25. Kirubakaran V, Liskow B, Mayfield D, Faiman MD: Case-report of acute disulfiram overdose. *Am J Psychiatry* 140:1513–1514, 1983.
26. Iber FL, Chowdhury B: The persistance of the alcohol-disulfiram reaction after discontinuation of drug in patients with and without liver disease. *Alcoholism* 1:365–370, 1977.
27. Nora AH, Nora JJ, Blue J: Limb-reduction anomalies in infants born to disulfiram-treated alcoholic mothers. *Lancet* 2:664, 1977 (letter).

B

Methadone Database

FORMULATIONS

Methadone hydrochloride tablets: 5 mg, 10 mg
Methadone hydrochloride dispersible tablets: 40 mg
Methadone hydrochloride oral solution: 5 mg or 10 mg/5 ml
Methadone hydrochloride for injection: 10 mg/ml
Brand names: Dolophine HCl (Lilly); Methadone HCl (Roxane)

BASIC PHARMACOLOGY

Methadone is a synthetic opiate receptor agonist with pharmacological properties similar to those of morphine (1) (Fig. 6B.1). It acts as an agonist at μ-receptors, one of the subtypes of opiate receptors. Methadone produces effective analgesic activity and prominent antitussive actions. Miosis, respiratory depression, and decreased gastrointestinal motility are other significant effects produced by methadone. Its pharmacological effects are long-lasting after single doses. Although analgesic effects may last for less than 6 to 8 hours, the respiratory and miotic effects from acute methadone administration last for more than 48 hours (2).

Methadone can induce significant insomnia. In sleep laboratory studies, using nondependent volunteers, it increased total wakefulness by increasing the number of awake episodes during the night, the latency to rapid eye movement (REM) sleep, and muscle tension and by decreasing total REM sleep (3). During long-term therapy, blood pressure, heart rate, and respiratory rate may slightly decrease. The expected effects of methadone on physiological status and various laboratory tests are outlined in Table 6B.1.

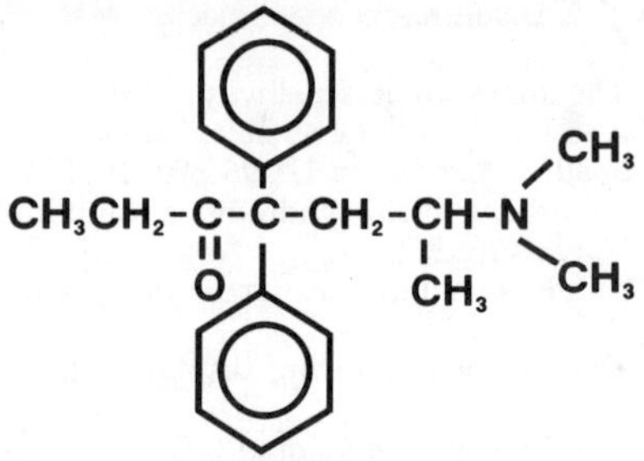

Figure 6B.1.   Structure of methadone.

Table 6B.1.
Expected Physiological Effects from Methadone Therapy for Monitoring[a]

Parameter	Drug Effect
Cardiovascular status	
Heart rate	No effect or slight decrease
ECG	
Blood pressure	Modest or no reduction in systolic pressure
Renal function	
Serum creatinine and clearance, BUN	Normal values should not change in most adults
Hepatic function	
AST (SGOT), ALT (SGPT), alkaline phosphatase	No changes expected due to methadone, but many patients will have concurrent hepatitis or alcoholic liver disease
Hematology status	
CBC	No changes expected
Neuroendocrine status	
Cortisol	No change or decrease in plasma cortisol; potential interference with dexamethasone suppression test
Other signs/symptoms	
Pupillary response	Miosis
Respiration	Frequency decreased; little effect on tidal volume
Body temperature	No expected effect or slight increase

[a]For abbreviations, see footnote *a* to Table 6A.2.

Methadone was discovered in the 1940s to have addictive liability similar to morphine, but its use as an analgesic seemed to produce a low incidence of abuse. Methadone has become a standard of pharmacotherapy for narcotic dependence since the 1960s. It provides cross-tolerance to opiate drugs and presumably reduces the euphoric effects of illicit drugs. However, since the 1970s, increasing concern has arisen over the drug's abuse potential and its diversion from methadone maintenance clinics.

Heroin, methadone, and morphine are equally euphorigenic when given intravenously (4). The extent of oral methadone's reinforcing effects has been questioned (5). This has led to controversy as to whether acceptance of methadone therapy is a result of avoidance of withdrawal symptoms or the inherent reinforcing properties of oral methadone. It is likely that methadone functions as a reinforcer for some clients when it is made available for treatment of opiate addiction. Thus, the potential for methadone abuse is a pertinent issue when evaluating candidates for maintenance therapy.

PHARMACOKINETIC PROPERTIES

Methadone is well absorbed after oral administration, producing peak plasma concentrations within 4 hours. Methadone is extensively bound to plasma proteins. Binding is more avid to α_1-acid glycoprotein (AGP) in plasma than to albumin (6). The average binding in healthy subjects is nearly 90%, although there is considerable individual variability. The degree of binding has correlated directly with the concentration of AGP. Therefore, in some disease states, increases can be anticipated in the extent of methadone's plasma protein binding. In inflammatory states, a shorter half-life of methadone could result from increased binding. However, changes in protein binding may not necessarily result in changes in pharmacological effects, especially for high clearance drugs with nonrestrictive binding. More avid binding may result in an increase in total plasma drug concentration with no change in free drug concentration, the pharmacologically active species. Nevertheless, the large variability in the degree of plasma protein binding of methadone contributes to difficulties in relating its plasma concentration to clinical effects (7).

Methadone is metabolized to inactive N-demethylated products. Urinary excretion of methadone and its major metabolites accounts for 10 to 43% of a given dose. In one pharmacokinetic study, the daily methadone dose was increased from 10 to 80 mg over a 5- to 6-week period. Over this time interval, an increase was noted in the urinary excretion of the metabolite compared to methadone. This observation suggests an enhancement in metabolism during chronic therapy (8), but autoinduction is not a recognized property of methadone.

The renal clearance of methadone is influenced by urinary pH. At acidic pH, clearance is increased, probably due to an increased ionization resulting in less renal tubular reabsorption (9). This is clinically unimportant as renal clearance is usually low, less than 10 to 25% of total body clearance.

The average elimination half-life of methadone is approximately 24 hours. This accounts for its long analgesic activity relative to morphine (Table 6B.2). A long half-life also allows methadone to be dosed once daily in addiction treatment programs.

In comparison to the pharmacokinetics of other opiate agonists, heroin and morphine (Table 6B.2), methadone has a much slower clearance and longer half-life. Heroin is essentially a prodrug, being rapidly converted by extensive presystemic elimination to its active metabolites, 6-acetylmorphine and morphine.

INDICATIONS

Methadone is an opiate analgesic indicated for relief of severe pain. It is also used for detoxification and temporary maintenance treatment of narcotic addiction. The difference between these concepts relates to duration of therapy. When detoxification continues for longer than 3 weeks, maintenance therapy is considered to be occurring and must be undertaken in a methadone program approved by the Food and Drug Administration. When used as an analgesic, methadone may be dispensed by any licensed pharmacy.

Table 6B.2.
Pharmacokinetic Parameters of Opiates

Parameter	Methadone	Morphine	Heroin
Onset of effects after oral dosing, minutes	30 to 60	15 to 60	15 to 60
Oral bioavailability, percentage	High, but reduced from presystemic elimination	100; reduced to 15 to 64 from presystemic elimination	100; reduced to 79 from presystemic elimination
Time of peak concentration after single dose, hr	0.5 to 4	0.5 to 1	
Plasma protein binding, percentage	89 ± 0.9	12 to 38	
Volume of distribution, liters/kg	3.6	1 to 6	
Total plasma clearance, ml/min/kg	2.5 to 5	5 to 20	30
Renal clearance, ml/min	1 to 20	100 to 170	
Elimination half-life	7 to 48 hr	1 to 8 hr	2 to 6 min
Major metabolites	N-Desmethyl	Morphine glucuronide	6-Acetylmorphine, morphine

The quality of pain relief with methadone was found to be similar to that of morphine in postoperative patients in a double-blind parallel group comparison (10); however, the duration of pain relief with methadone was considerably longer than with morphine. This longer duration of action probably results from methadone's slower clearance compared to that of morphine (Table 6B.2).

Methadone's major use is for treatment of narcotic addiction. Many addicts continue their illicit drug use to avoid the narcotic abstinence syndrome. This syndrome is similar whether the abused substance is a natural or synthetic opiate, although the time course for appearance and resolution of symptoms differs. For morphine and heroin, withdrawal symptoms appear at a time when the next dose would ordinarily be taken, increase in intensity to a maximum within 36 to 72 hours, and then gradually subside over 5 to 10 days. With methadone, the onset of withdrawal is slower and the period for resolution of symptoms is more prolonged, up to a period of weeks. The typical symptoms of opiate withdrawal are outlined in Table 6B.3. The more prolonged and less severe withdrawal from methadone has allowed it to be used in detoxification and treatment, although not without controversy.

Methadone is available as short-term (methadone detoxification) and long-term (methadone maintenance) treatment. For detoxification, patients are first

Table 6B.3.
Narcotic Abstinence Syndrome after Last Dose

Occurring within Several Hours	Occurring within 8 to 16 Hours	Occurring within 24 Hours
Anxiety	Uncontrollable yawning	Tremor
Insomnia	Sweating	Goose flesh
Restlessness	Rhinorrhea	Chills
Irritability	Lacrimation	Anorexia
Feeling sick	Nasal congestion	Muscle cramps
Poor appetite	Sneezing	Diarrhea
Drug craving	Eyes sensitive to light	Nausea, vomiting
	Feeling of a change in temperature	Cardiovascular instability
	Stomach pain	Seizures (rarely)

stabilized over a few days on a moderate dose of methadone. The dose is then gradually reduced with the objective of having the patient opiate-free at the end of 3 weeks. For methadone maintenance, patients are maintained on a relatively higher but stable dose for an extended period, sometimes for years. The argument in favor of this therapy is that cross-tolerance produced by methadone to other opiates will diminish the intake of illicit drugs.

A similar logic is operative in increasing methadone maintenance doses given to addicts who repeatedly present with opiate-positive urines. Using a contingent-method dosing schedule may have an advantage in this situation. As methadone is known to be reinforcing, making methadone dose supplements contingent on opiate-free use has reduced the percentage of illicit opiate use compared to patients in a control group (11).

Alternatives to methadone have been tried for detoxification and maintenance treatment of narcotic addicts. Some positive results have been observed with propoxyphene but have not been substantiated (12). Methadone patients stayed in treatment longer than those treated with propoxyphene and were less likely to abuse heroin. A recently investigated alternative to methadone for opiate detoxification is clonidine, the α_2-receptor agonist (see Chapter 1B). It has been useful in drug detoxification in patients receiving methadone maintenance as well as other opiates (13). Clonidine has been favorably compared to methadone in the rapid detoxification of patients dependent on heroin (14). Both therapies were highly effective, although cardiovascular side effects were prominent with clonidine (see Chapter 4C).

DOSAGE REGIMEN DESIGN

When used as an analgesic for severe pain, the parenteral dose, either intramuscularly or subcutaneously, is 2.5 to 10 mg every 3 or 4 hours, as needed. A parenteral dose of 8 to 10 mg of methadone is considered equianalgesic to 10 mg of morphine. Subcutaneous use, which may result in local irritation, should be avoided when the need for multiple doses is anticipated. Oral administration is approximately one-half as potent as parenteral use. Recently, it has been noted that sublingual absorption of methadone is an effective route of administration (15). For patients with cancer who are unable to tolerate oral administration, this route of administration may be beneficial.

For narcotic detoxification with methadone, oral administration is preferred. A dose of 15 to 20 mg will usually suppress the narcotic withdrawal syndrome

(Table 6B.3). Patients who are physically dependent may require 40 mg. For heavy heroin users, 20 or 40 mg of methadone is given 4 to 8 hours after heroin is stopped. When there is doubt about the degree of addiction, a smaller dose should be administered. After a stabilization period of 2 to 3 days, the starting dose is decreased. Further decreases may be attempted on a daily or less frequent basis to maintain withdrawal symptoms at a tolerable level. This detoxification procedure should be completed within 21 days. An increased risk of relapse may occur if the time to complete detoxification is considerably less than 21 days.

For maintenance therapy, the dose must be individualized. Protocols vary widely among different treatment programs. A frequently used regimen is as follows. The initial dose should be large enough to suppress abstinence symptoms but not cause obvious respiratory depression. The daily dose is adjusted as necessary, up to a maximum of 120 mg/day, to avoid withdrawal symptoms. The goal is the same as in the detoxification procedure, to achieve eventual total withdrawal from opiates.

Unfortunately, a poor relationship has been found between the oral dose of methadone needed on admission to a drug dependence unit and the self-reported use of heroin (16). Part of this difference arises because of the inaccuracy of patient-reported opiate use plus the wide variability in the purity of available street drugs.

THERAPEUTIC DRUG MONITORING

Therapeutic drug monitoring of methadone is desirable to detect the extent of illicit drug use, the presence of physical dependence, the presence of withdrawal, and the degree of opiate tolerance. Unfortunately, these objectives have been difficult to achieve. Studies have indicated a large variability in plasma concentrations among patients who are maintained at a given dose. Despite stable dosage, large week-to-week variability in plasma concentrations has been noted (7). Compounding this problem is the fact that addicts often exaggerate the severity of their illicit drug use when seeking admission to maintenance programs. A challenge with naloxone, a narcotic antagonist, has been useful to assess the presence and severity of opiate dependence, but this procedure is objectionable as it may precipitate unpleasant withdrawal symptoms. Other approaches to therapeutic drug monitoring have been suggested, but all suffer from a lack of replication studies.

Pupillary response has been proposed as a practical method of therapeutic drug monitoring (17). Pupillary constriction was negatively correlated to the generally reported highest amount of illicit heroin use 2 hours after a 20-mg dose of methadone. This approach might be useful as a screening procedure for entry into methadone programs, but it needs to be replicated because of the degree of variability present in the results.

Evidence has been presented for a dispositional tolerance to methadone (18). In two groups of addicts, maintained on either 30 or 60 mg daily, the higher-dose group had a better therapeutic outcome. Those with plasma methadone concentrations greater than 200 ng/ml had fewer illicit drugs in their urine. This approach has been proposed as a method for increasing the therapeutic effectiveness of methadone maintenance therapy. Patients with lower plasma concentrations might be more likely to consume other opiates to avoid the abstinence syndrome. This work requires further research to define its utility.

The development of tolerance to opiates may be related to changes in adenylate cyclase activity (19). In former heroin addicts who had been stabilized with methadone, withdrawal of methadone was associated with a significant increase in prostaglandin E_1-sensitive platelet adenylate cyclase activity. This increase paralleled withdrawal symptoms from methadone. This monitoring approach holds promise, like the ones described above, but needs further testing and evidence of validity.

CONTRAINDICATIONS—WARNINGS—PRECAUTIONS

When methadone is withdrawn over 21 days, withdrawal symptoms are at a moderate level at the outset of treatment and remain this way for 2 weeks during the methadone dose reduction period. Symptoms may then rise to a peak at day 20 when methadone is discontinued before beginning a slow but steady decline. Withdrawal symptoms may persist for an additional 3 weeks after addicts have become drug-free. It is generally agreed that the withdrawal syndrome from methadone is more prolonged, but less severe, than with other opiates (20). This period after detoxification, when residual symptoms are present, may be an especially vulnerable period for the addict and requires continual psychological support to prevent relapse.

All narcotic analgesics share abuse potential and can lead to psychological and physical dependence if used repeatedly for long periods. Signs include tolerance to the analgesic effects and excessive demands to obtain additional drug doses.

DRUG INTERACTIONS

The experience of methadone maintenance patients suggests that oral diazepam enhances the subjective effects of methadone. However, there is no apparent peripheral pharmacokinetic basis for this interaction (Table 6B.4). Blood concentrations of methadone were unaffected by coadministration of diazepam in five male addicts on methadone maintenance (21). Neither urinary excretion nor plasma protein binding of methadone has been observed to be altered by diazepam (22). Nevertheless, a central mechanism may be operative in altering pharmacodynamic effects of methadone. Based on the available evidence, however, the treatment of methadone maintenance patients with moderate doses of diazepam should not alter the metabolism of methadone.

No changes were noted in methadone kinetics when administered with or without naloxone (23). Patients receiving methadone could experience withdrawal symptoms if treated with pentazocine because of this drug's weak antagonist properties.

Coadministered enzyme inducers would be expected to increase the clearance of methadone and, therefore, the risk of precipitating opiate withdrawal. Rifampin, a recognized enzyme inducer (see Chapter 1D, Table 1D.5), significantly lowers plasma levels of methodone, an effect that has been paralleled by the appearance of withdrawal symptoms (24). Phenytoin can also precipitate methadone abstinence symptoms in previously stable patients (25). The drug-drug interactions of methadone are summarized in Table 6B.4.

Table 6B.4.
Drug Interactions with Methadone

Interacting Drug	Effect
Magnesium-aluminum antacids	Delays rate of absorption and possibly extent
Rifampin	Increases clearance, at times enough to precipitate narcotic withdrawal
Isoniazid	Decreases clearance and prolongs elimination half-life
Disulfram	Inhibits clearance
Cimetidine	Inhibits clearance
Naloxone	No kinetic interaction; however, pharmacodynamic interaction of narcotic withdrawal has occurred
Pentazocine	Withdrawal symptoms possible from antagonist effects
Phenytoin	Pharmacodynamic withdrawal presumably from increased methadone clearance has occurred

ADVERSE REACTIONS—OCCURRENCE AND MANAGEMENT

The major hazard of methadone use is central nervous depression, including depression of the respiratory and cardiovascular systems. Common side effects are sedation, nausea, vomiting, and sweating. The frequency of methadone's adverse drug reactions are outlined in Table 6B.5.

MANAGEMENT OF OVERDOSE

Severe overdose is characterized by respiratory depression, extreme somno-lence progressing to coma, constricted pupils, cold and clammy skin, brady-

Table 6B.5.
Expected Side Effects from Methadone Therapy

Effect	Rare	Less Common	More Common
Dry mouth		X	
Blurred vision		X	
Sweating			X
Constipation			X
Nausea			X
Vomiting			X
Drowsiness			X
Dizziness			X
Ataxia		X	
Disorientation		X	
Headache		X	
Skin rash		X	
Blood pressure decrease			X
Bradycardia		X	
Jaundice	X		
Urinary retention		X	

cardia, and hypotension. Respiratory depression can be counteracted by the administration of a narcotic antagonist. If naloxone is given for overdose, caution should be observed. The duration of action of naloxone is shorter than that of methadone, and symptoms of toxicity, including respiratory depression, can return after the cessation of naloxone's effects. Oxygen, intravenous fluids, and other supportive treatment should be used appropriately in severe overdose situations.

USE IN RENAL AND/OR HEPATIC DISEASE

Some patients in methadone maintenance therapy drink heavily. Alcoholic liver disease is frequent is this population. Liver disease has equivocal effects on the disposition of narcotic drugs. It has been shown to impair the elimination of meperidine but not morphine. In a study of methadone maintenance patients with alcoholic liver disease, there were minimal kinetic differences in methadone compared to a control group with no evidence of liver disease (26). Thus, based on pharmacokinetic data, the usual methadone maintenance dose may be continued in patients despite the presence of advanced alcoholic liver disease.

When used as an analgesic in nontolerant patients with terminal illnesses and concomitant liver disease, usual doses should be used cautiously (27).

In doses of 80 to 120 mg/day in patients taking methodone for 3 years or longer, no changes were noted in liver function. Liver function test changes in addicts probably occur secondary to other drug use or disease-induced changes in liver function.

USE IN CHILDREN AND ADOLESCENTS

Methadone does not have an established dosage range in children and is not recommended for pediatric use.

USE IN ELDERLY

The elderly can be unusually sensitive to the central nervous system depressant effects of drugs, including methadone. Elderly and debilitated patients should be considered at special risk for respiratory depression and other side effects from methadone.

USE IN PREGNANCY

Safe use has not been established in pregnancy. Oral methadone maintenance is sometimes used in pregnant women to keep them from continued intravenous heroin use. The effects of methadone could reduce oxygenation to the fetus. The ventilatory response to carbon dioxide of infants after chronic prenatal methadone exposure is decreased (28). Methadone should be avoided during pregnancy unless the potential benefits outweigh the risks.

PATIENT INFORMATION

Patients should be informed of the expected side effects (Table 6B.5). They should be warned to avoid alcohol use or other central nervous system depressants, which could produce additive drowsiness. Methadone can be taken with food if gastrointestinal upset occurs. As methadone can produce impairment in mental acuity, patients should be warned of increased hazards in performing complicated psychomotor tasks such as driving an automobile.

REFERENCES

1. Jaffe JH, Martin WR: Opioid analgesics and antagonists. In: *Goodman and Gilman's The Pharmacological Basis of Therapeutics*, ed 7, Gilman AG, Goodman LS, Rall TW, Murad F (eds), Macmillan, New York, 1985, pp 491–531.
2. Olsen GD, Wilson JE, Robertson GE: Respiratory and ventilatory effects of methadone in healthy women. *Clin Pharmacol Ther* 29:373–380, 1981.
3. Pickworth WB, Neidert GL, Kay DC: Morphinelike arousal by methadone during sleep. *Clin Pharmacol Ther* 30:796–804, 1981.
4. Jasinski DR, Preston KL: Comparison of intravenously administered methadone, morphine and heroin. *Drug Alcohol Depend* 17:301–310, 1987.
5. Stitzer ML, McCaul ME, Biegelow GE, Liebson I: Oral methadone self-administration: effects of dose and alternative reinforcers. *Clin Pharmacol Ther* 34:29–35, 1983.
6. Romach MK, Piafsky KM, Abel JG, Khouw V, Sellers EM: Methadone binding to orosomucoid: determinant of free fraction in plasma. *Clin Pharmacol Ther* 29:211–217, 1981.
7. Horns WH, Goldstein A: Plasma levels and symptom complaints in patients maintained on daily dosage of methadone hydrochloride. *Clin Pharmacol Ther* 17:636–649, 1975.
8. Verebely K, Volavka J, Mule S, Resnick R: Methadone in man: pharmacokinetic and excretion studies in acute and chronic treatment. *Clin Pharmacol Ther* 18:180–190, 1975.
9. Bellward GD, Warren PM, Howald W, Axelson JE, Abbott FS: Methadone maintenance: effect of urinary pH on renal clearance in chronic high and low doses. *Clin Pharmacol Ther* 22:92–99, 1977.
10. Gourley GK, Willis RJ, Lamberty J: A double-blind comparison of the efficacy of methadone and morphine is postoperative pain control. *Anesthesiology* 64:322–327, 1986.
11. Higgins ST, Stitzer ML, Bigelow GE, Liebson IA: Contingent methadone delivery: effect on illicit opiate use. *Drug Alcohol Depend* 17:311–322, 1986.
12. Woody GE, Mintz J, Tennant F, O'Brien CP, McLellan AT, Marcovici M: Propoxyphene for maintenance treatment of narcotic addiction. *Arch Gen Psychiatry* 38:898–900, 1981.
13. Gold MS, Redmond DE, Kleber HD: Clonidine in opiate withdrawal. *Lancet* 1:929–930, 1978.
14. Cami J, de Torres S, San L, Sole A, Guerra D, Ugena B: Efficacy of clonidine and of methadone in the rapid detoxification of patients dependent on heroin. *Clin Pharmacol Ther* 38:336–341, 1985.
15. Weinberg DS, Ingurrisi CE, Reidenberg B, et al: Sublingual absorption of selected opioid analgesics. *Clin Pharmacol Ther* 44:335–342, 1988.
16. Johns AR, Gossop M: Prescribing methadone for the opiate addict: a problem of dosage conversion. *Drug Alcohol Depend* 16:61–66, 1985.
17. Higgins ST, Stitzer ML, McCaul ME, Bigelow GE, Liebson IA: Pupillary response to methadone challenge in heroin users. *Clin Pharmacol Ther* 37:460–463, 1985.
18. Holmstrand J, Anggard E, Gunne L-M: Methadone maintenance: plasma levels and therapeutic outcome. *Clin Pharmacol Ther* 23:175–180, 1978.
19. Pandey GN, DeLeon-Jones FA, Inwang EE, Davis JM: Effect of acute methadone withdrawal on prostaglandin E-stimulated 3-H-cyclic adenosine monophosphate accumulation in human platelets. *Clin Pharmacol Ther* 27:607–611, 1980.
20. Gossop M, Bradley B, Phillips GT: An investigation of withdrawal symptoms shown by opiate addicts during and subsequent to a 21-day in-patient methadone detoxification procedure. *Addict Behav* 12:1–6, 1987.
21. Preston KL, Griffiths RR, Cone EF, Darwin WD, Gorodetzky CW: Diazepam and methadone blood levels following concurrent administration of diazepam and methadone. *Drug Alcohol Depend* 18:195–202, 1986.
22. Pond SM, Tong TG, Benowitz NL, Jacob P III, Rigod J: Lack of effect of diazepam on methadone metabolism in methadone-maintained addicts. *Clin Pharmacol Ther* 31:139–143, 1982.
23. Kreek MJ, Gutjahr CL, Garfield JW, Bowen DV, Field FH: Drug interactions with methadone. *Ann NY Acad Sci* 281:350–376, 1976.

24. Kreek MJ, Garfield JW, Gutjahr CL, Giusti LM: Rifampin-induced methadone withdrawal. *N Engl J Med* 294:1104–1106, 1976.
25. Tong TG, Pond SM, Kreek MJ, Jaffery NJ, Benowitz NB: Phenytoin-induced methadone withdrawal. *Ann Intern Med* 94:349–351, 1981.
26. Novick DM, Kreek MJ, Arns PA, Lau LL, Yancovitz SR, Gelb AM: Effect of severe alcoholic liver disease on the disposition of methadone in maintenance patients. *Alcoholism* 9:349–354, 1985.
27. Saive J, Hansen J, Ginnan C, Hartvig P, Jakobsson PA, Nilsson M-I, Rane A, Anggard E: Patient-controlled dose regimen of methadone for chronic cancer pain. *Br Med J* 282:771–773, 1981.
28. Olsen GD, Lees MH: Ventilatory response to carbon dioxide of infants following chronic prenatal methadone exposure. *J Pediatr* 96:983–989, 1980.

Index

Page numbers in *italics* denote figures; those followed by "t" denote tables.